CRITICAL REVIEWS IN
TROPICAL MEDICINE
Volume 2

Editorial Advisory Board

A Continuation Order Plan is available for this series. A continuation order will bring delivery of each new volume immediately upon publication. Volumes are billed only upon actual shipment. For further information please contact the publisher.

CRITICAL REVIEWS IN
TROPICAL MEDICINE
Volume 2

Edited by
R. K. Chandra

Memorial University of Newfoundland
St. John's, Newfoundland, Canada

PLENUM PRESS · NEW YORK AND LONDON

The Library of Congress cataloged the first volume of this title as follows:

Main entry under title:

Critical reviews in tropical medicine.

Includes bibliographical references and index.
1. Tropical medicine. I. Chandra, Ranjit Kumar. [DNLM: 1. Tropical medicine—
Periodical. W1 CR216Y]
RC961.5.C74   1982   616′.00913   82-15129
ISBN-13: 978-1-4612-9689-8   e-ISBN-13: 978-1-4613-2723-3
DOI: 10.1007/978-1-4613-2723-3

Contributors

J. Azocar, Center for Microbiology and Cellular Biology, Venezuelan Institute for Scientific Research, Caracas 1010A, Venezuela

Reza Behin, World Health Organization, Immunology Research and Training Center, Biochemistry Institute, University of Lausanne, 1066 Epalinges, Switzerland

R. K. Chandra, Department of Pediatrics, Janeway Child Health Centre, Memorial University of Newfoundland, St. John's, Newfoundland, Canada A1A 1R8

G. C. Cook, Department of Clinical Tropical Medicine, London School of Hygiene and Tropical Medicine, London WC1H 7HT, England

Tim Dyson, Department of Population Studies, London School of Economics, London WC2A 2AE, England

Jacques Louis, World Health Organization, Immunology Research and Training Center, Biochemistry Institute, University of Lausanne, 1066 Epalinges, Switzerland

Dilip Mahalanabis, Kothari Centre of Gastroenterology, The Calcutta Medical Research Institute, Calcutta-700027, India

J. A. O'Daly, Center for Microbiology and Cellular Biology, Venezuelan Institute for Scientific Research, Caracas 1010A, Venezuela

David S. Rowe, Special Programme for Research and Training in Tropical Diseases, World Health Organization, 1211 Geneva 27, Switzerland

G. P. Talwar, National Institute of Immunology and Department of Biochemistry, All India Institute of Medical Sciences, New Delhi 1100029, India

Devhuti Vyas, Health Sciences Centre, Memorial University of Newfoundland, St. John's, Newfoundland, Canada A1B 3V6

Derek Wakelin, Department of Zoology, University of Nottingham, Nottingham NG7 2RD, England

Preface

At the present time there are renewed global efforts to control the major tropical infections and to stem the tide of malnutrition, the two serious, often intertwined, problems that contribute to much of the morbidity and mortality in under-privileged populations. Many international organizations have joined hands with national governments and with the private sector to search for new approaches to problems that beset much of the developing world, including countries in the tropical region. This volume continues the tradition of the previous publication in the Series. A variety of fare is offered to readers: explanations of the activities and achievements of the UNDP/World Bank/WHO Special Programme for Research and Training in Tropical Diseases; and studies of infant mortality, schistosomiasis, trypanosomiasis, helminths, lactase deficiency, oral rehydration therapy, functional consequences of iron deficiency, and fertility control. Authoritative state-of-the-art reviews provide a critical analysis of recent data. I hope the Series will continue to prove useful to all those working in the tropics and to those in the industrialized countries whose awareness of physical health problems of the Third World is relatively limited.

R. K. Chandra

St. John's, Newfoundland

Contents

Chapter 3. Oral Rehydration Therapy...................... 77

DILIP MAHALANABIS

Chapter 4. Functional Consequences of Iron Deficiency:
            Nonerythroid Effects........................ 93

R. K. CHANDRA AND DEVHUTI VYAS

Chapter 6.   Immune Response to *Leishmania*   141

REZA BEHIN AND JACQUES LOUIS

The Special Programme for Research and Training in Tropical Diseases

David S. Rowe

1. ORIGINS, OBJECTIVES, AND DISEASES

In May 1974 the World Health Assembly of the World Health Organization (WHO) passed Resolution WHA27.52, which included the following:

> Recognizing that tropical parasitic diseases are one of the main obstacles to improving the level of health and socio-economic development in countries of the tropical and sub-tropical zones;
>
> Bearing in mind the need to develop research on matters connected with the most important tropical parasitic diseases;
>
> Realizing that national, regional or global programmes of tropical parasitic disease control can be implemented only if scientifically based methods and effective means for their control are available,
>
> [the World Health Assembly of the WHO] Requests the Director-General:
>
> to intensify WHO activities in the field of research on the major tropical parasitic diseases (malaria, onchocerciasis, schistosomiasis, the trypanosomiases, etc.) taking into consideration that such activities be carried out in endemic areas whenever possible and feasible;
>
> to define the priorities in research on the problem of tropical parasitic diseases in the various regions of the world, bearing in mind the primary needs of the developing countries;
>
> and to extend cooperation with national institutions and other governmental and non-governmental organizations in regard to the coordination of research in this field.

David S. Rowe • Special Programme for Research and Training in Tropical Diseases, World Health Organization, 1211 Geneva 27, Switzerland.

Behind the formal language of this resolution lay recognition of the importance of research as an integral part of efforts to improve control of major tropical diseases and concern over the inadequacy of the then current research activities. There was also the concept that an important part of such research should be internationally based. This resolution forms the mandate and broad terms of reference for the Special Programme for Research and Training in Tropical Diseases. The first step was to develop this resolution into a Programme of well-defined scope and mode of working. This was completed and the Programme formally established in February 1978, although many activities began before that date. Recognizing that the objectives and activities of the Programme relate to the potential for economic development of tropical disease-endemic countries, the United Nations Development Programme (UNDP) and the World Bank have joined the WHO as cosponsors of the Programme, with WHO as the executing agency. From its beginning, the Programme was seen as likely to continue for 20 years or more. This account describes the Programme's objectives and *modus operandi* and reviews major activities and achievements to the end of 1982.

The Special Programme has two formal objectives:

1. To develop new preventive, diagnostic, therapeutic, and vector-control methods specifically suited to prevent, treat, and control selected tropical diseases in the countries most affected by them. The new methods must be susceptible to implementation at a cost that can be borne by developing countries, requiring minimal skills or specialized supervision, and in a manner that allows their integration into the health services—especially the primary health care systems—of developing countries.
2. To strengthen research capability in countries most affected by tropical diseases through training in biomedical sciences and through various forms of institutional support. Biomedical research capability in tropical countries must be strengthened to enable these countries to undertake research relevant to the control of indigenous diseases. Specifically, research on the specification, development, and testing of new tools must take place in countries where the diseases are endemic, so as to ensure that the tools are appropriate and effective in the circumstances in which the diseases occur.

The diseases selected for inclusion were malaria, schistosomiasis, filariasis (including onchocerciasis), both African and South American trypanosomiases, leprosy, and the leishmaniases.

The following main criteria were used for their selection:

1. Their impact as a public health problem

2. The absence of satisfactory methods for control under circumstances prevailing in tropical countries
3. The existence of research leads towards improved control methods

2. THE *MODUS OPERANDI* OF THE PROGRAMME

As regards research and development, knowledge and understanding of the varied epidemiological circumstances of the diseases is the baseline; from this the requirements and characteristics of new or improved tools and methods for control are specified. Tools under development include drugs, vaccines, agents for the biological control of vectors, and improved diagnostic tests. The social and economic circumstances of the diseases are also studied, so as to ensure that control measures are socially acceptable and economically feasible.

As regards strengthening of research capability, the policy is to assist national authorities and institutions according to the research needs they identify for the improvement of disease control. Assistance is provided for the development of institutional facilities, for scientific exchange, and for the training of scientists and technical staff.

The main groups that have been established to operate the Programme, as well as their relationships, are shown in Figure 1.

2.1. Scientific Working Groups

Research and development under the Programme is conducted by scientific working groups (SWGs), which are established for different components as needed (e.g., the Scientific Working Group on Schistosomiasis). Sometimes, for operational reasons, more than one SWG is established for a component (e.g., the SWG on Immunology of Leprosy and the SWG on Therapy of Leprosy). SWGs have also been established to deal with research that cuts across disease lines (e.g., the SWG on Epidemiology).

SWGs plan, implement, and evaluate research under the Programme related to their component. Plans are based on needs and opportunities for research to improve control, assessment of research in progress outside the Programme, and the resources available to the Programme for this research. Clearly the Programme cannot pursue all desirable lines of research; therefore SWGs establish specific goals and priorities and analyze the different tasks needed to achieve them. Thus drug development, according to the current state of knowledge, may require research according to the following sequence: fundamental studies of parasite biology, synthesis and screening of compounds, testing in animal models, and safety testing followed by clinical and field trials.

David S. Rowe

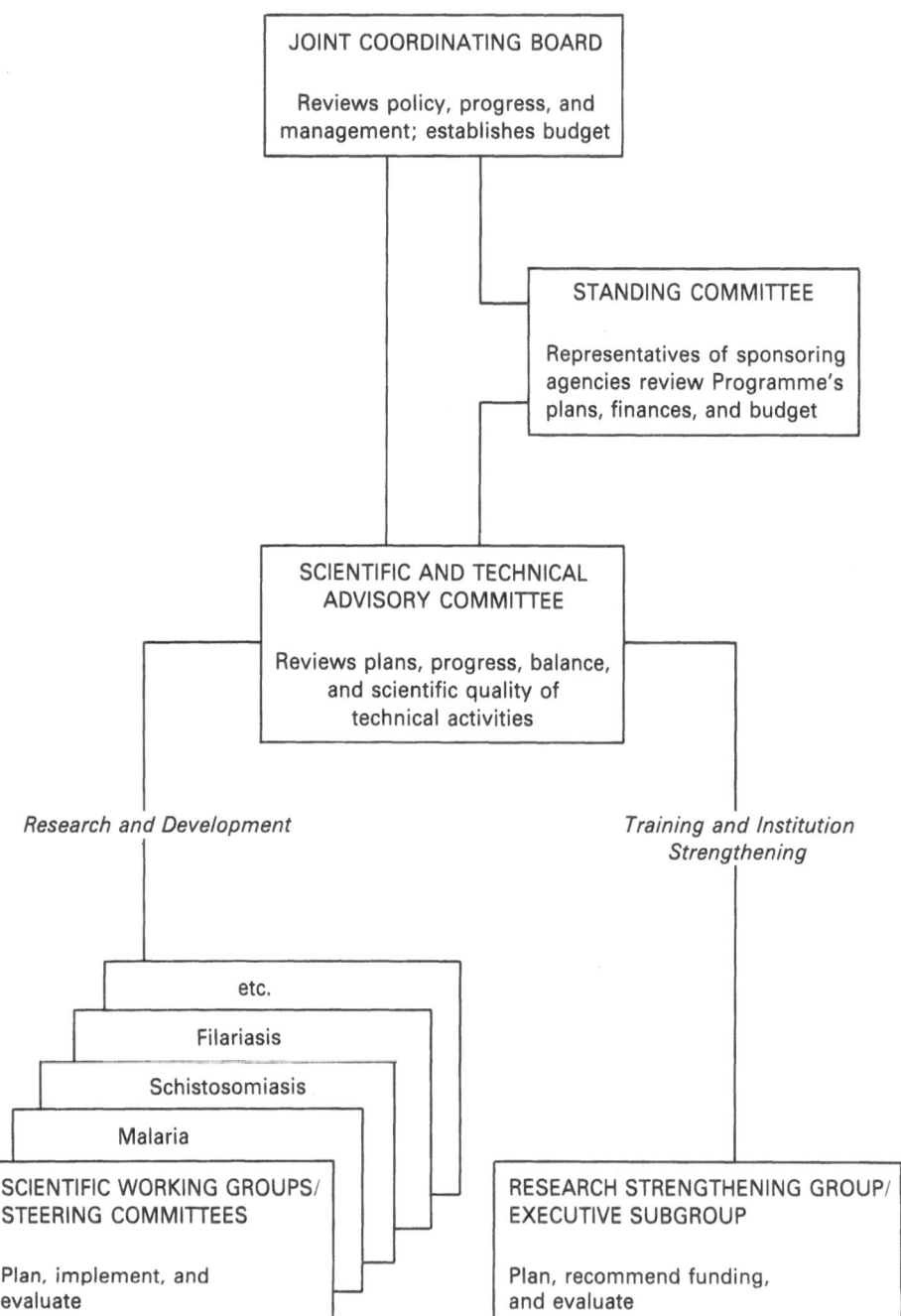

Figure 1.   Scheme of management of the Programme with WHO as executing agency.

Membership of SWGs includes all those scientists who are involved in any aspect of the SWGs' work; thus SWGs comprise all scientists who are funded to undertake projects and all who attend meetings of various types. There is no fixed membership, and scientists with different expertise are involved in different ways according to the tasks in hand.

The SWGs' research plans and activities are managed by SWG steering committees (SCs). Each SWG has one and sometimes more SCs. SCs usually have eight to ten members who are appointed for fixed periods of time, usually three years, and may be reappointed. SCs meet at least once a year; their tasks include planning SWG activities, reviewing progress, and assessing research proposals submitted by scientists for funding under the Programme. This assessment is based on the relevance of the proposal to the stated plans and objectives of the SWG and on its scientific quality. Table I shows the SWGs and SCs now in operation and their main lines of work.

Research projects under the Programme are conducted by scientists in many countries working within their own institutions, which are funded by the Programme for this purpose. The Programme widely advertises the research plans and priorities of SWGs through its newsletter and other documents as described below, or it may approach scientists directly in order to attract research proposals from them. Thus a scientist active in research in the immunology of malaria may read of the Programme's activities in the newsletter, request more detailed information, and then complete a research proposal form. This proposal would then be reviewed by the SC on the Immunology of Malaria for relevance to the Programme's plans and for scientific quality. If these and certain administrative and ethical requirements are met, the project is funded through a contract with the scientist's institution. Although projects are frequently anticipated to continue for a period of several years, the Programme cannot formally commit itself to funding for more than one year at a time, since its own budget is contributed annually. Annual budgets for research projects vary from a few thousand U.S. dollars to $100,000 or $200,000 for large projects such as those involving field research.

There is an alternative method for funding a limited number of small projects for one year only; this is intended to provide rapid support or support for a line of research which, although relevant to disease control, may not be within current research priorities. Such research is funded under the Director's Initiative Fund and is limited to a single nonrenewable grant of up to $15,000 (U.S.).

The process of policymaking and planning of research and development is a controversial issue. Some research administrators emphasize the key role of the individual, while others favor the idea that a well-informed group will achieve better results. No doubt there are advantages and disadvantages in both procedures. The Special Programme has chosen the group rather than the individual approach, the most compelling reason being the very wide range of expertise required to cover the scope of its research and development activities.

Table I
Scientific Working Groups and Steering Committees Operational in 1982

Component	Scientific working group	Steering committee	Main lines of research
Malaria	Chemotherapy	CHEMAL	New drugs, improved use of existing drugs
	Immunology	IMMAL	Vaccines, immunodiagnostic tests
	Field Research	FIELDMAL	Improvement of control in the field
Schistosomiasis	Schistosomiasis	SCH	Epidemiological studies, fundamental and mode-of-action studies related to drugs, diagnostic tests
Filariasis	Filariasis	FIL	New drugs and improved use of existing drugs, diagnostic tests, epidemiological studies
African trypanosomiasis	African Trypanosomiasis	Epidemiology (EPIAF)	The natural history of disease and its transmission
		Chemotherapy (CHEMAF)	New drugs, and improved use of existing drugs
		Immunology (IMMAF)	Diagnostic tests, mechanisms of immunity
Chagas' disease	Chagas' Disease	Epidemiology (EPICHA)	Distribution and prevalence of different types of disease
		Chemotherapy (CHEMCHA)	New drugs and methods for sterilizing blood for transfusion
		Immunology (IMMCHA)	Improved diagnostic tests, vaccines
Leprosy	Immunology	IMMLEP	Vaccines, diagnostic tests
	Chemotherapy	THELEP	Improved drug regimens and new drugs
Leishmaniasis	Leishmaniasis	Epidemiology (EPILEISH)	Distribution of disease, identification of parasite reservoir hosts, improved vector control
		Chemotherapy (CHEMLEISH)	New drugs, and improved therapeutic regimens
		Immunology (IMMLEISH)	Vaccines, diagnostic tests

Table I   (*Continued*)

Component	Scientific working group	Steering committee	Main lines of research
Epidemiology	Epidemiology	EPD	Design of effective disease control strategies
Biomedical research	Biomedical research	BIOS	Application of advances in basic biology through information exchange and strengthening of research in tropical countries
Biological control of vectors	Biological Control of Vectors	BCV	Biological agents for the control of disease vectors
Social and economic research	Social and Economic Research	SER	Social and economic aspects of disease transmission and control

2.2. Research Strengthening Group

The major responsibility within the Programme for strengthening the research capabilities of tropical countries lies with the Research Strengthening· Group (RSG). This group has some 18 members drawn from each of the regions of the WHO and selected on the basis of their experience in research management and training. They include deans of medical schools, directors of research institutes, and chairmen of national medical research councils. The RSG is responsible for preparing overall plans, for reviewing proposals for specific activities, and for evaluating progress toward the objective of strengthening research capability. The policies and procedures of the RSG differ in important respects from those of SWGs and are described in section 4, below.

Some of the responsibilities of the RSG are delegated to subordinate groups. The Executive Sub-Group (ESG) of the RSG reviews major proposals for institutional strengthening prior to consideration by the RSG. The Research Strengthening Team (RST) is composed of members of the WHO secretariat involved in Programme activities; it reviews and recommends funding for training grants under the policies established by the RSG.

2.3. The Scientific and Technical Advisory Committee

The Scientific and Technical Advisory Committee (STAC) is responsible for an independent scientific and technical review of the entire content, scope, and dimensions of Special Programme activities, including the diseases dealt with by the Programme and the approaches to research and control that are adopted. Thus STAC reviews all activities of SWGs and the RSG and recommends priorities and changes in Programme activities. STAC meets annually and reviews each Programme component in a four-yearly cycle. Much of the detailed work of evaluation is carried out by scientific and technical review committees (STRCs), which are subcommittees of STAC.

In its review, the STAC considers and makes recommendations on the main directions of research under SWGs and of institutional strengthening and training under the RSG, and the relative levels of activities between SWGs and between research on the one hand and the strengthening of research capability on the other. On this basis STAC recommends the financial distribution to different Programme components within the Programme's overall budget. STAC also considers broad issues of importance to the future work of the Programme, such as the development of field research and the Programme's relationship with industry. STAC has some 15 to 18 members who serve in their personal capacities and represent a wide range of scientific disciplines and interests related to research on control of tropical diseases. STAC presents its findings in a report to the sponsoring agencies and to the Programme's Joint Coordinating Board.

2.4. Joint Coordinating Board

The Joint Coordinating Board (JCB) is the top management body of the Programme. Its 30 members include 12 representatives of governments that are financial donors to the Programme, 12 representatives of governments of countries directly affected by the diseases dealt with by the Programme or providing scientific support to the Programme, 3 representatives of governments or agencies selected by members of the Board itself, and representatives of the 3 cosponsoring agencies (the World Bank, the UNDP, and WHO). The JCB reviews all Programme activities, including the report of STAC, and endorses the activities and budget of the Programme for the coming financial period. In a longer-term perspective, the JCB reviews the progress of the Programme toward the achievement of its goals and considers long-term plans of action and their financial implications.

2.5. The Executing Agency

The system represented by the SWGs, RSG, STAC, and JCB provides for very broad cooperation among scientists, governments, and agencies in the operation, evaluation, and funding of the Programme. The Programme was originated and is operated by the WHO. All Programme operations require formal approval by the Director of the Programme under the authority of the Director General of WHO. All Programme activities must meet the requirements of WHO, including ethical approval on experimentation involving human subjects and procedures for collaboration with member states.

2.6. Budget

The total budget of the Programme over a biennial operation period and its allocation to different Programme components is endorsed by the JCB. Governments, agencies, and other donors contribute to the Programme, usually on an annual basis, to provide funds up to the maximum endorsed by the JCB. The Programme carries no financial reserve and is not authorized to borrow, so that activities depend strictly on funds in hand. Figure 2 shows contributions and obligations from 1974 to 1982; Figure 3 shows the obligations by Programme component in 1982.

3. RESEARCH AND DEVELOPMENT

The following sections briefly describe the magnitude of the health problems presented by the six diseases and highlight some of the activities *to the end of 1982*. Progress in research and development is usually a matter of accretion of

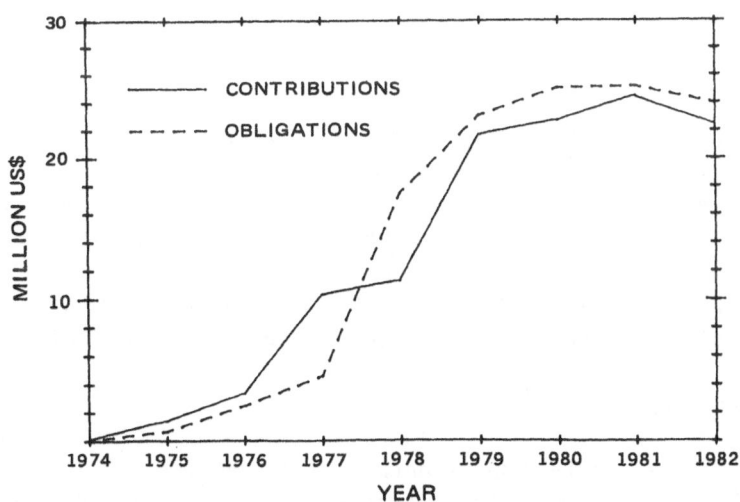

Figure 2.   Financial contributions and obligations of the Programme, 1974–1982.

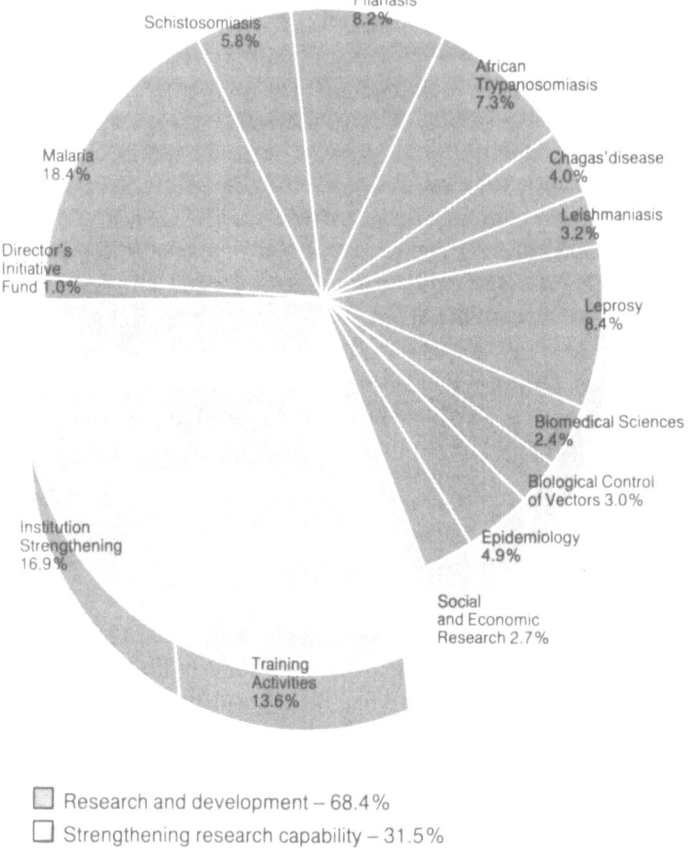

Research and development – 68.4%
Strengthening research capability – 31.5%

Figure 3.   Distribution of financial obligations for Programme operations in 1982.

information acquired from many sources. The main lines of progress described here are derived from Programme activities, but the contribution from research under other auspices has been important and is acknowledged with appreciation. By the end of 1982 the Programme had funded 1655 projects, 1175 under SWGs and 480 under the RSG, and over 1800 publications of research supported by the Programme had appeared in the scientific literature. This account is drawn from Programme reports and from other documents available from the Programme.

3.1. Malaria

Malaria, called the "king of diseases" in ancient India, still retains this status in our day. Substantial gains were made by the large antimalarial campaigns of the 1950s and 1960s, when measures largely based on the use of DDT greatly reduced morbidity in many areas, although with little impact on tropical Africa. Since then malaria has maintained its high incidence in tropical Africa, and it is now increasing in Asia as well as South and Central America. In 1981 some 107 countries were affected by the disease and 1900 million people or 40% of the world's population are now considered to be at risk of infection. Resistance of parasites to drugs and of vectors to insecticides is continuing to spread, and the global situation is expected to deteriorate further over the next few years.

Of all the diseases dealt with by the Programme, malaria has the highest priority; in 1982, 18.4% of the total Programme operations budget was committed to research on this disease. Three SWGs are involved: Chemotherapy (CHEMAL), Immunology (IMMAL), and Field Research (FIELDMAL).

3.1.1. Drug Development

The objectives of CHEMAL are to develop new drugs that will improve malaria control, relieve suffering and save life, prevent infection in individuals and communities, and achieve radical cure of established infections. Research ranges from basic laboratory studies on the host–parasite relationship to clinical and field trials of new compounds. Two major advances made prior to its establishment have formed the basis for much of CHEMAL's work: Trager's method for cultivation of erythrocytic stages of *Plasmodium falciparum*, which paved the way for fundamental studies of the cell biology of parasite and host cells, and the improvement of *in vitro* methods to determine resistance of parasites to drugs. The discovery of the new antimalarial compound mefloquine by the Walter Reed Army Institute of Research (WRAIR) was especially important and timely, in view of the serious and increasing incidence of resistance to 4-aminoquinolines and other antimalarial compounds. CHEMAL has established the effectiveness and safety of mefloquine in tropical populations through trials in collaboration with WRAIR and the pharmaceutical industry in Southeast Asia, Africa, and South America. In 1981 the Steering Committee issued a statement on mefloquine for the guidance of health authorities, indicating that mefloquine "will be safe and effective in the treatment of malaria, particularly infection with chloroquine-resistant parasites." The statement also drew attention to the risk of induction of resistance to mefloquine and emphasized the importance of simultaneous vector control in conjunction with field trials of mefloquine. The advantage of using drug combinations to diminish the risk of emergence of drug resistance was also stressed.

The development of mefloquine is not yet complete; dose-finding studies in infected children as well as trials in adult males with symptomatic malaria and in females of child-bearing age with drug-resistant malaria are in progress. It is expected that this drug will be registered for use in man by early 1984. Combinations of mefloquine with other antimalarials such as primaquine are also being studied. Although it is now expected that mefloquine will be effective for the treatment of chloroquine-resistant malaria, it is anticipated that following its widespread use, resistance will sooner or later appear. It has already been shown that resistance to mefloquine can be induced *in vitro* by repeated exposure of parasites to sublethal drug concentrations.

There is therefore a great need for radically different types of drugs active against malaria. The compound artemisinine (Qing Hao-su) has been identified in China as the active antimalarial ingredient of a herbal remedy prepared from *Artemesia annua*. Artemisinine, lacking nitrogen in its molecule, has a unique structure among known antimalarials and so may be the forerunner of a new generation of compounds. Derivatives of the parent molecule have been prepared, and some of these are significantly more active. Studies in China have shown that the derivative artesunate is fast-acting, effective against chloroquine-resistant infections, and well tolerated. The Programme is assisting with mutagenicity and carcinogenicity testing and with improved procedures for manufacture and standardization.

Other priority areas of research include the development of more effective and less toxic regimens of primaquine for the radical treatment of *Plasmodium vivax* infections, sustained-release systems for blood schizonticidal drugs, new blood schizonticides, and improved laboratory models and hosts for human parasites.

3.1.2. Vaccines

Is it possible to develop vaccines that confer protection against human malaria? This may well be so, since malaria infection itself induces a specific protective immune response in adults in areas of high endemicity. Can vaccines be developed that play a significant role in the control of malaria in populations where disease is endemic? Many additional factors lie behind this question. Aspects such as duration of protection; effectiveness in individuals with current or previous malaria or other potentially immunosuppressive chronic infections and malnutrition; and questions of dosage, delivery, and acceptability must await assessment until vaccine preparations are available for clinical and field trials. Malaria vaccines would be especially valuable for the protection of high-risk groups such as young children and pregnant women in endemic areas. Such considerations form the context of research under IMMAL to develop malaria vaccines.

Like CHEMAL, IMMAL has been able to build from its inception on several antecedant key findings. The *in vitro* cultivation method of Trager has proved indispensable for the production of parasite antigens. The demonstration of immunity to sporozoite challenge in rodents, primates, and man provided a firm basis for further work on immunization against this stage of the life cycle, and there was a model of immunity to blood stages of *Plasmodium knowlesi* in monkeys. Advances in technology have revolutionized research approaches in the last few years. Passive protection by monoclonal antibodies to both sporozoite and blood-stage antigens has identified "protective" antigens and mechanisms of immunity; such antibodies have also served for isolation of antigens. Whereas previously *in vitro* culture represented the most likely, albeit difficult and expensive, approach to antigen production for vaccines, new alternative approaches using genetic engineering or direct synthesis have radically changed concepts of how antigens can be produced in quantity and free from contaminating host material.

Monoclonal antibodies to antigens of several parasite species and developmental stages are now being produced, and several protective antigens have been identified by this means. A monoclonal antibody to a surface protein of *Plasmodium berghei* sporozoites (Pb44) is able to neutralize sporozoites both *in vitro* and *in vivo,* and Pb44 has been shown to be a stage-specific antigen. It appears that a family of analogous molecules occurs in sporozoites of other plasmodial species, including *P. falciparum.* Monoclonal antibodies have also been made to merozoite antigens of several species. Studies in animal models have shown that, depending upon parasite and host species, such antibodies can modify or even terminate infection and block red cell reinvasion. Monoclonal antibodies directed towards certain *P. falciparum* blood-stage antigens have been found to inhibit parasite growth *in vitro;* there is evidence that at least two merozoite surface antigens are involved. Rapid progress may be expected in this most important area. Another approach is based on transmission-blocking immunity; studies on the sexual stage have shown that antibodies from gamete-immunized animals react with surface components of gametes in the mosquito gut, thus preventing fertilization and blocking transmission.

Classical immunochemical methods are also being used for the analysis of malaria antigens, with emphasis on the potentially protective antigens that are bound to cell membranes. Other research under IMMAL includes studies on mechanisms of immunity and immunopathology and the improvement of serodiagnostic methods for malaria. Assays using radioimmunoassay or enzyme-linked immunoassay techniques for antigen detection have been developed for the diagnosis of low-level parasitemia. An assay system based on monoclonal antibodies reactive with circumsporozoite proteins has been developed for the detection of species-specific malaria infection in mosquitos. This assay appears sensitive enough to detect infection in individual mosquitos and has great promise for field studies of vectors.

3.1.3. Research in the Field

Just as the discovery of a vaccine was necessary but not sufficient for the ultimate eradication of smallpox, so discoveries of new drugs, vaccines, and diagnostic tests for malaria will not in themselves be sufficient to achieve improved control. The objective of FIELDMAL is to solve problems related to control of disease in the field and to identify and assess appropriate control methods based on epidemiological principles. Malaria transmission and control measures vary greatly according to climatic, environmental, sociological, and economic factors, so that local conditions must be taken into account in the design and evaluation of control programs. (The importance of field research and its associate problems are further discussed elsewhere in this chapter.) Important areas of research include vector biology, ecology, behavior, and control; the distribution and biology of different malaria species; human aspects (including behavior and attitudes); and the operation of malaria control services.

The spread of resistance of *P. falciparum* to chloroquine and other antimalarial drugs is a matter of great concern at present. Since resistance to chloroquine of *P. falciparum* was first observed in 1959, it has spread widely in Asia and in Pacific countries; resistance is also important in South America, and it has now been documented in four countries in East Africa. Several training courses have been conducted on *in vitro* methods for determining chloroquine sensitivity, and test kits have been distributed under the Programme. Countries in Southeast Asia, the western Pacific, the Americas, and Africa are collaborating in a systematic evaluation; extensive information is now becoming available on severity and geographic distribution. The frequency of chloroquine resistance in some countries in Southeast Asia is alarming; in Thailand, 95% of all cases studied were found to be resistant. Moreover resistance has been demonstrated to other antimalarials, such as the combination of long-acting sulfonamides with pyrimethamine. Resistance is now a severe threat to treatment and control; strategies are being developed to treat resistant cases and to control the spread of malaria. This most serious problem underlines the urgency of the work of CHEMAL in the development of new antimalarial compounds.

FIELDMAL is also concerned with countermeasures to the resistance of vectors to insecticides, and studies have been made on the best ways to use DDT and other insecticides. Very encouraging results have been obtained using larvivorous fish (genus *Tilapia*) in large rainwater reservoirs in Somalia; substantial decreases in numbers of vectors and parasite rates were found in the areas where the fish were introduced. Other studies in progress include the role of community participation in the use of drugs and in indoor spray application; the development of alternative methods for vector control using combinations of chemical, biological, and environmental measures; incrimination of additional mosquito species as vectors and evidence of changed mosquito biting habits after exposure to DDT; and improvement of therapeutic regimens to prevent relapse of *P. vivax* infections.

3.2. Schistosomiasis

This disease in its various forms probably affects some 200 million people; it is associated with poverty, poor housing, and inadequate sanitary facilities. The construction of new water resources in tropical countries, from small ponds to large man-made lakes, is often associated with high rates of infection, as illustrated by the near 100% prevalence around Lake Volta in Ghana. Recently safe and effective oral drugs have been developed, and there have been improvements in diagnostic methods. Nonetheless, control of the disease in most populations has not been achieved, and progress will depend upon both the better use of existing tools and methods and the development of new ones.

The objectives of the SWG on Schistosomiasis are to develop improved methods of control based on research in epidemiology, transmission dynamics, and the biology of snail hosts; improved drugs and diagnostic techniques; and vaccines as well as to elucidate immunopathology. Substantial research on schistosomiasis is in progress outside the Special Programme, including drug screening and development by the pharmaceutical industry and the research programme of the Edna McConnell Clark Foundation. The SWG is especially concerned to bring new advances to the stage of application in the field, but it, like other SWGs, has encountered difficulties due to the lack of scientists trained in field research.

3.2.1. Field Research

Priority topics are chemotherapy delivery systems and their impact on morbidity and transmission dynamics, transmission dynamics in relation to ecology and habitat modification, combined approaches to control involving the above, and evaluation of control activities. The effect of selected population chemotherapy and mollusciciding on disease prevalence in relation to man-made lakes has been studied in an area on the shore of Lake Volta. Studies related to the effectiveness of control strategies are also taking place in Zanzibar, Sudan, Egypt, and China, and a workshop on epidemiology has been held in the Philippines.

3.2.2. Chemotherapy and Biochemistry

In view of the major industrial involvement in drug development and the availability of effective drugs, research is directed toward topics relevant to the development of the modified or new drugs that are likely to be needed in the future. These include the structure–function relationships of established drugs, identification of drug metabolites and the modes and sites of drug action, and the relationship between the host's immune response to the parasite and drug effectiveness. Centers for research and training in clinical pharmacology are being supported in endemic countries.

3.2.3. Immunology and Basic Sciences

Antigens are being isolated and characterized for the purpose of improvement of diagnostic tests and potentially for vaccination studies. A multicenter serological study in collaboration with the Clark Foundation has assessed various antigens and test systems as indexes of infection and morbidity. The presence of antibodies to egg antigens was found to be the most sensitive and specific index of infection but was not correlated with morbidity.

3.3. Filariasis

Eight different types of parasitic worms, including notably *Wuchereria bancrofti, Brugia malayi, Brugia timori,* and *Onchocerca volvulus,* are responsible for the group of filarial infections dealt with by the Special Programme. Hundreds of millions of people are infected. Diethylcarbamazine (DEC) is the most widely used drug, but it can cause severe reactions in patients. No drug generally suitable for the mass treatment of filariasis is available at present; until the advent of the Programme, there was little industrial interest in the development of better drugs. As regards research on onchocerciasis, there are close links with the Onchocerciasis Control Programme (OCP) in West Africa.

The objectives of the SWG on Filariasis are as follows:

1. To improve the use of existing filaricides and to find new ones. The main needs are for safe and practical schedules for the treatment of patients with ocular onchocerciasis who are at risk of blindness, for new macrofilaricides, and for dosage schedules suitable for the large-scale treatment of lymphatic filariasis.
2. To find out how to reduce the inflammatory reaction of the host toward filarial worms and to identify filarial antigens that would be suitable for diagnostic tests and possibly for preventive vaccines.
3. To increase knowledge of the natural history, epidemiology, and vectors of filariasis so as to improve disease control.

Over the past few years a major advance has been achieved by the OCP in the Volta River Basin, where control of vector *Simulium* (blackfly) has resulted in a very substantial reduction in transmission. Therapy of those already infected is a necessary adjunct to vector control, but no suitable macrofilaricidal drug is currently available. Research on drugs is therefore being expanded in a joint effort with the Onchocerciasis Control Programme.

A number of compounds have been tested for microfilaricidal and macrofilaricidal effects in onchocerciasis. Levamisole has been found to be synergistic with mebendazole in reducing the density of microfilaria in the skin, and mebendazole has been found to sterilize adult worms for a period of three to four months. A number of potential new antifilarial compounds have been synthesized, including benzimidazoles, DEC-N oxide (a metabolite of DEC), and various derivatives of suramin and nitroheterocyclic compounds. A screening programme for antifilarial compounds involving 15 investigators in 10 countries, including 7 industrial laboratories, has been established. Six varieties of filaria including *Onchocerca* species in cattle are used in the screens, and several thousand compounds have now been assessed. Three compounds supplied by Ciba Geigy Ltd. have been found to have an important macrofilaricide action against *Onchocerca* in cattle, and further studies are now planned.

Improved diagnostic methods for the assessment of lymphatic filariasis would be valuable. The specificity of tests based on antibody detection is being improved by identification of appropriate antigens, and parasite surface antigens and antigens released during *in vitro* cultivation appear to be more specific in this respect than antigen mixtures from whole parasites. Antibodies of IgE class show evidence of greater species specificity for diagnostic purposes than do IgG antibodies. Monoclonal antibodies are now being studied and may be particularly useful for the detection and measurement of antigens in serum as evidence of active infection and infective load. Recently a relatively simple method for the cultivation of infective larvae of *B. malayi* and *Brugia pahangi* to fourth stage and juvenile adult stages has been developed; this should provide a source of various stage-specific and other parasite antigens for immunological studies.

An important advance related to the control of onchocerciasis has been made under the SWG on Biological Control of Vectors (see below). The spores of *Bacillus thuringiensis* serotype H-14 (*B. t.* H-14) have been shown to constitute a safe and effective larvicide for *Simulium* vectors, and *B. t.* H-14 is now routinely used in the Onchocerciasis Control Programme in areas where *Simulium* has become resistant to chemical insecticides (Figure 4).

3.4. African Trypanosomiases

These diseases constitute a serious threat to some 45 million people living in Africa; some 20,000 new cases are identified each year. Surveillance of the populations at risk plays an important part in control; because of high cost and lack of personnel, however, control is becoming more difficult to achieve in many countries. Neglect of surveillance led to the disastrous outbreaks that occurred recently in Cameroon, Sudan, Uganda, and Zaire. Therapy of infection requires hospitalization, and the only drug that is effective in the late stage of sleeping sickness is melarsoprol, an arsenical compound that causes severe reactions and death in a proportion of cases.

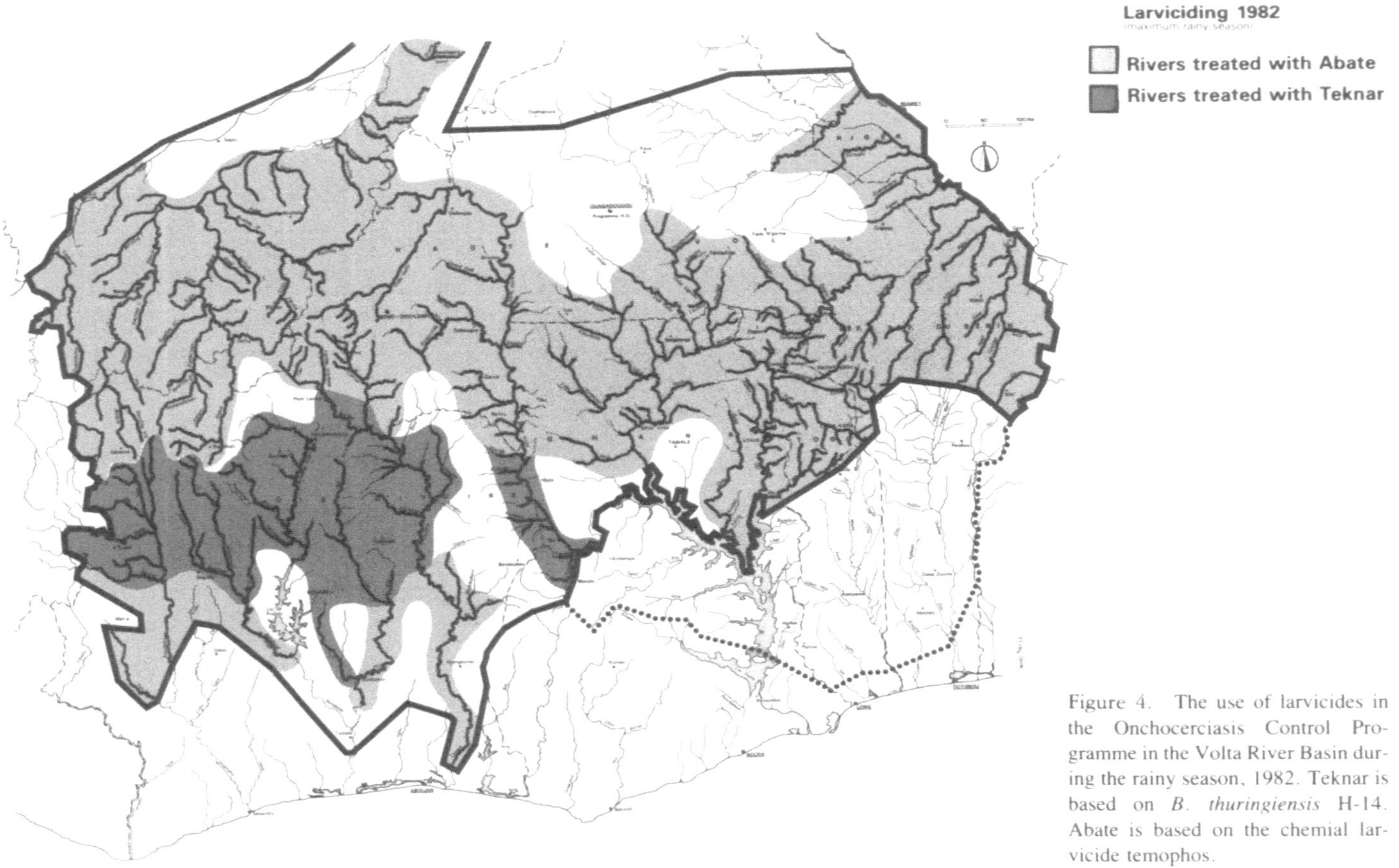

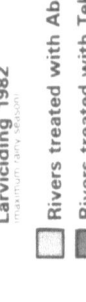

Larviciding 1982
maximum rainy season

☐ Rivers treated with Abate

■ Rivers treated with Teknar

Figure 4. The use of larvicides in the Onchocerciasis Control Programme in the Volta River Basin during the rainy season, 1982. Teknar is based on *B. thuringiensis* H-14. Abate is based on the chemial larvicide temophos.

The SWG on African Trypanosomiasis has three main areas of study: epidemiology, chemotherapy, and immunology.

3.4.1. Epidemiology

The objective is to achieve a better understanding of the natural history of trypanosomiases based on long-term multidisciplinary studies on infection with *Trypanosoma brucei gambiense* (Ivory Coast and Congo) and *Trypanosoma brucei rhodesiense* (Zambia). An important finding related to epidemiology and control has been that tsetse flies are capable of traveling up to 20 km, much further than was previously thought. Simple tsetse traps developed outside the Programme have been found to be remarkably effective in the local control of tsetse flies in West African riverine locations; this method is particularly attractive, since it is nonpolluting and traps can be made in villages. Comparison of isoenzyme patterns and identification by DNA probes suggest that *T. b. gambiense* isolated from domestic and game animals is identical with parasites that cause infection in man.

3.4.2. Chemotherapy

The objectives are to improve therapy through better use of existing compounds and to obtain safer and more effective new compounds. Parasite metabolic pathways and structural sites are being studied as targets for drug action. In laboratories in Kenya and Berlin, over 100 compounds have been screened for activity against trypanosomes. Diamidines have been shown not to penetrate the central nervous system. Naphthoquinone compounds have been found to be trypanocidal *in vitro* but inactive *in vivo,* perhaps due to a very brief half-life in the circulation; chemical modifications and slow-release formulations are being studied in the hope of improving therapeutic effectiveness. Trials with reduced doses of arsenical compounds are planned in the hope of reducing the risk of cerebral complications.

3.4.3. Immunology

The objectives are to improve diagnostic methods and to study immunological and pathological aspects of infection. A simple card agglutination test developed outside the Programme has been found to be valuable for the diagnosis of *T. b. gambiense* infection in endemic areas. The result can be read after a few minutes, and the test can be used for diagnosis in the field as well as for epidemiological studies. Six centers are jointly involved in clinicopathological and epidemiological studies. *Microtus* has been found to be susceptible to infection with *T. b. gambiense* and so may serve for the primary isolation of *T. b.*

gambiense from man and for studies of antigenic variation. Two workshops on antigenic variation have been held and close contact is maintained with several laboratories working on this topic, especially the International Laboratory for Research in Animal Diseases, Nairobi.

3.5. Chagas' Disease

At a conservative estimate, 20 million people in Latin America are now infected with *Trypanosoma cruzi* and are thus at risk of developing Chagas' disease in one of its various clinical forms. Some 65 million people are considered to be at risk of infection. The disease is spread by triatomine insects, whose breeding is favored by the poor construction of dwellings in rural areas and shantytowns. Recently, transmission by blood transfusion has become an increasingly serious problem.

Since the discovery of the disease by Carlos Chagas at the beginning of this century, there has been considerable research interest on Chagas' disease in Latin America. The emphasis of the SWG has been on coordination of research activities, including the standardization of epidemiological, clinical, and serodiagnostic procedures and methods. Most of the projects have been carried out in endemic countries. There are three main areas of study, epidemiology, chemotherapy, and immunology.

3.5.1. Epidemiology of Chagas' Disease

The objectives are to increase knowledge of the geographical distribution, prevalence, and clinical varieties of Chagas' disease and of the distribution of its vectors; to improve diagnostic tests; and to improve methods to reduce man/vector contact. Four courses have been held on standardization of clinical and field procedures for epidemiological studies. Using standardized protocols, long-term population studies have been established in six countries; prevalence studies are in progress in another five. Paints incorporating insecticides have been found to kill vectors for periods up to 12 months. The nature, frequency, and severity of the clinical manifestations and response to chemotherapy of Chagas' disease vary greatly between countries. These differences may be associated with different strains of parasites and a variety of methods is now being used for strain identification, as described below.

3.5.2. Chemotherapy of Chagas' Disease

The objectives are to develop drugs that are effective in eliminating infection at any stage of the disease; to identify more effective substances for the sterilization of blood for transfusion; to improve methods for the detection, cultivation, and harvesting of parasites and to develop a standardized methodology for strain and species detection; and to improve knowledge of mechanisms of recognition and entry of parasites into host cells.

A simple and rapid screen has been devised to test the ability of compounds to kill *T. cruzi* in stored blood; this is now being used to assess the effectiveness of drugs already approved for use in man for other purposes. Some 800 compounds have been tested for suppressive activity against *T. cruzi* in a screen in mice, and a number have shown significant activity. Differences between parasite strains in tissue distribution in host and drug susceptibility are being studied using model infections in mice, and isoenzyme patterns and restriction enzyme analysis of kinetoplast DNA are being used to classify strains.

3.5.3. Immunology of Chagas' Disease

The objectives are to improve knowledge of pathogenesis, especially in relation to the host response and to mechanisms of chronic manifestations of the disease; to improve immunodiagnostic tests; and to develop a safe vaccine and methods for immunotherapy.

It is possible that some features of Chagas' disease are due to an autoimmune reaction induced by cross-reactive parasite antigens. A monoclonal antibody produced following immunization of mice with dorsal root ganglia has been shown to react with *T. cruzi* amastigotes and epimastigotes, pointing to an epitope common to *T. cruzi* and the central nervous system. A model for chronic Chagas' disease has been developed in isogenic rabbits, and a study of potential immunoprotective or immunopathogenic properties of subcellular fragments of *T. cruzi* is in progress. In mice certain subcellular fractions of *T. cruzi* have been found to be partially protective and not associated with the development of pathology. The standardization of serodiagnostic methods, through the establishment of serum collections and common protocols for standard tests, is in progress.

3.6. Leprosy

The number of leprosy cases in the world is now estimated at at least 10.6 million; in some tropical areas the frequency of disease exceeds 10 per thousand. Leprosy can cause severe incapacitating deformities, especially of the hands and feet, and deformed people frequently have to endure the traditional social stigma associated with this disease. The two main areas of study, immunology and therapy, are each handled by an SWG.

3.6.1. Immunology of Leprosy

The lack of any method for *in vitro* cultivation of *Mycobacterium leprae* is a serious obstacle to progress in research. The discovery that *M. leprae* could be obtained in large quantities from infected armadillos made possible for the first time the systematic development of immunological test reagents and vaccines. In 1974 the SWG on the Immunology of Leprosy prepared a plan to develop a leprosy vaccine and tests of the immune response to *M. leprae* in man as well as to increase understanding of immunopathological mechanisms of disease. This plan has been followed in its main features since that time, although some changes have been made. For example, work on transfer factor is no longer included, and work on the development of vaccines based on cross-reactive mycobacteria is given a much lower priority. IMMLEP has made a major investment in the production of *M. leprae* in armadillos, and a stock of some 8 kg of infected armadillo tissues, chiefly liver, is held at the present time. Methods for the separation of *M. leprae* have been carefully devised to obtain good yields of antigenically intact material, free from contamination with armadillo tissue components. A batch of purified, killed *M. leprae* has been produced for human use, and protocols for standardization, potency, and toxicity have been established.

Lepromatous leprosy is the severe, disfiguring form of disease, associated with many bacilli in the tissues; it is the main source of transmission of infection. In this form of leprosy there is a specific deficiency of the cell-mediated immune response to *M. leprae*. Measures to prevent this defect might prevent lepromatous disease, and measures to restore it might cure or prevent the progression of established disease. The immunological basis of vaccine development has been the assessment of *M. leprae* preparations for their ability to induce a specific cell-mediated immune response and, as far as possible, to ensure that all antigens of *M. leprae* are represented in the vaccine preparation. A most encouraging finding has been that killed *M. leprae* without adjuvant induce strong cell-mediated responses and immunity to subsequent challenge with live organisms in animal models. Preparations are now being made for trials of killed *M. leprae* in man. The first step, now beginning, is to conduct sensitization studies in volunteers in nonendemic areas so as to determine whether the preparation can induce a significant delayed hypersensitivity response. Studies on protection in endemic populations will necessarily be long-term, and a number of epidemiological requirements are being considered in their design. A recent claim has been made, based on research outside the Programme, that immunotherapy with killed *M. leprae* and BCG causes skin-test conversion and promotes healing in lepromatous leprosy; studies will be made to confirm this very encouraging and important finding.

3.6.2. Chemotherapy of Leprosy

The objective is to improve leprosy control by chemotherapeutic means. At present, long-term treatment with dapsone is the most frequently used measure, although other drugs are available. There are three main directions of research.

1. *The assessment of the needs for improved chemotherapy.* Surveys of dapsone resistance subsequent to therapy have been conducted in many countries, and resistance has always been found. This secondary form of resistance appears to be worldwide; prevalence rates in treated cases may be as high as 20%. Resistant organisms that persist in treated patients are clearly a likely source of infection for others, hence it is not surprising that primary resistance, before treatment with dapsone, has been found in high prevalence in some areas.

2. *The better use of existing drugs.* Controlled clinical trials are in progress on the effectiveness of different regimens of combined therapy in sterilizing infections. Dapsone, rifampicin, clofazimine, and prothionamide are included in these studies. The persistence of viable *M. leprae* in tissues is detected by injection into immune-suppressed T-cell-deficient rodents, and several laboratories are now capable of undertaking this test. There is now good evidence that chemotherapy need not be continued through the lifetime of the patient; combined regimens which include rifampicin may shorten the time required for cure. Field trials of combined chemotherapy for a limited period followed by a prolonged period of observation are in progress.

3. *The development of new drugs.* Analogues of existing drugs have been screened for activity, and dapsone analogues that are considerably more active than the parent compound in an *in vitro* system have been identified. Patients often take dapsone irregularly; therefore a search is being made for long-acting formulations. Dapsone prepared as crystals of appropriate size is promising.

The development of new compounds is hampered by inability to cultivate *M. leprae in vitro*. Present screening methods are slow and require large amounts of the material under test. A slow-growing cultivable mycobacteria (*Mycobacterium lufu*) found on the banks of a river in Zaire is now being used as a model for screening activity against *M. leprae*.

3.7. Leishmaniasis

The leishmaniases are widespread in tropical and subtropical areas, and some forms occur in temperate zones. They include a wide variety of clinical forms ranging in severity from minor self-healing skin ulcers to severely mutilating lesions and from subclinical infections to disease with high mortality in the absence of treatment. At least 12 different forms of the *Leishmania* parasite are recognized to be implicated in human disease. Until recently the prevalence, extent, and severity of the leishmania were not generally known and their public health importance was largely unappreciated.

3.7.1. Epidemiology

The objectives are to define the geographical distribution and prevalence of the diseases in major endemic areas; to improve methods of isolation and identification of parasites; to study reservoirs and the relative roles of human, canine, and other hosts in transmission; to study the taxonomy and ecology of the sandfly vector; and to improve vector and reservoir control methods.

Studies in many countries have indicated that several different forms of leishmaniasis cause significant public health problems. Animal reservoirs for visceral and cutaneous leishmaniases have been identified and several sandfly species incriminated as vectors in different areas. Methods have been developed for the identification and typing—by serological, isoenzymatic, radiorespirometric, and nucleic acid characterization techniques—of leishmanial isolates.

3.7.2. Chemotherapy

Pentavalent antimonials are presently the compounds of choice for therapy of severe forms of the disease. However, they are not always effective, and limitations imposed by the need for medical supervision, parenteral administration, and prolonged courses of treatment often make their use impracticable. Other drugs are unsatisfactory; hence a more appropriate treatment for less severe forms of the disease is needed. More intensive therapeutic regimens are being developed, and compounds already used in man for other conditions are being assessed for antileishmanial activity. Studies of parasite biochemistry and metabolic pathways are in progress in a search for specific metabolic inhibitors. *In vivo* models have been established for screening and active compounds are now emerging. Studies both outside and within the Programme have shown that the inclusion of antimonial compounds within liposomes increases their effectiveness several hundredfold in animal models.

3.7.3. Immunology

The objectives of this group are to improve diagnostic tests and to develop vaccines. Immunodiagnostic methods are at present not sufficiently specific; improvement is sought by the use of appropriate antigen–antibody systems and of monoclonal antibodies. Healed or cured infection in man usually results in solid, long-lasting immunity to homologous challenge; a form of vaccination against cutaneous leishmaniasis is practiced in some areas by intradermal inoculation of parasites at a site and time of election. A mouse model has shown that nonpathogenic leishmania species afford some cross-protection to infection with pathogenic species and that cross-reactivity between protective and pathogenic species occurs at the level of the cell-mediated immune response. Prospects for vaccine development are considered to be good, and research is now being intensified.

3.8. Epidemiology

The design of disease-control strategies involves the identification and measurement of the critical causal factors contributing to disease, the assessment of the likely impact of possible intervention procedures, and evaluation of the effectiveness of specific tools for control, such as vaccines, drugs, vector-control measures, and human behavioral changes.

The objective of epidemiological research in the Programme is to improve the design of disease control and health strategies. Epidemiological research related to the control of individual diseases takes place under all the disease-oriented SWGs. Research that cuts across and lies beyond the boundaries of the individual diseases is the concern of the SWG on Epidemiology, which also develops new methods and promotes training. The following summary illustrates some of its activities.

Longitudinal multidisciplinary epidemiological studies in populations living in two contrasting ecological areas have been established in Zambia, based at the Tropical Disease Research Centre, Ndola. This facility has research laboratories for parasitology, immunology, biochemistry, hematology, and bacteriology as well as a statistical unit with computer facilities and logistical support capabilities. The research is focused upon investigations into trypanosomiasis (*T. b. rhodesiense*), malaria, and schistosomiasis (*Schistosoma mansoni* and *Schistosoma haematobium*). (The Ndola Centre is described in section 4.) Based on these studies, recommendations are made to national authorities on ways to improve disease-control measures. The studies are also used to develop principles and methods for epidemiological studies of chronic infectious diseases and for postgraduate training. A population-based longitudinal multidisciplinary study of major endemic diseases and their control is also being conducted in Sabah, Malaysia. The main disease problems under study are those of malaria, lymphatic filariasis, leprosy, and malnutrition.

The SWG also develops and disseminates epidemiological methods most appropriate for the study of tropical diseases. Several workshops have been held to explore the potential of new methods for dealing with chronic diseases; for example, case-control studies may obtain answers to key questions in less time and with less expense than previous methods.

Workshops for teachers of epidemiology have been held in the Philippines and the Sudan and are planned in China and Ethiopia in the near future. A field manual for tropical disease epidemiology is being prepared, and computer-assisted simulation exercises based on research on malaria control in Nigeria are used for training purposes.

3.9. Biomedical Sciences

When the Special Programme was established, it was clear that there was great potential for the application of new discoveries in genetics, cell biology, and immunology to the study of parasites and parasitism. Precisely how and when these discoveries would be brought to bear and how they would ultimately relate to disease control were, however, matters more for speculation than prediction at that time. Since then new developments have appeared remarkably quickly. A whole series of methodological advances have been made which are directly applicable to solving some of the problems faced by the Programme. Genetic engineering techniques make possible the production of individual gene products in potentially unlimited amounts; probes are now available to analyze segments of DNA and RNA, providing a powerful method for parasite and vector identification, which helps to solve problems of taxonomy and epidemiology. Monoclonal antibodies can pinpoint epitopes of antigens, identify humoral immune protective mechanisms, and serve for the isolation of antigens; they promise great improvement in immunodiagnosis. In addition, new types of vaccines based on genetic engineering and on direct synthesis are now appearing. Thus fundamental advances in biological sciences are now beginning to make an impact on disease control, and this process seems likely to accelerate over the next few years. The Programme is well placed to keep pace with developments of this type. SWGs draw in the appropriate experts to enable them to exploit new technology and open up new lines of research. Thus all the disease-oriented SWGs use monoclonal antibodies in their research, and registries and banks have been established.

The Biomedical Sciences SWG (BIOS) was established as the generator for this development in the Special Programme. Its objectives were to ensure the full deployment of all promising lines of research in fundamental sciences relevant to improved methods for disease control. BIOS has identified major research topics and promoted them by specific research projects and by exchange of information and contacts between scientists working in different disciplines.

The following list illustrates the nature and scope of research under BIOS:

- An unusual calcium-dependent ribonuclease has been identified in trypanosomes.
- Glycophorin A has been provisionally identified as the site of malaria merozoite attachment to red blood cells.
- A method has been developed for the identification of parasite antigens by labeling the surface of infected macrophages and analyzing immunoprecipitated antigens by two-dimensional gel electrophoresis. A parasite antigen has been identified on the surface of leishmania-infected macrophages by this method.

- The killing of intracellular *T. cruzi* by macrophages has been found to be dependent upon a spleen cell factor requiring T cells for its production.
- Studies on the genetics of hemoflagellates have shown evidence of both haploid and diploid cells.

The following topics have been covered by seminars and workshops:

- The membrane pathobiology of tropical diseases
- *In vitro* cultivation of pathogens of tropical diseases
- Modern genetic concepts and techniques in the study of parasites
- The application of chemical micromethods for the investigation of tropical disease pathogens
- Hybridoma technology and monoclonal antibodies

Reports of these meetings have been published in the Programme's Tropical Disease Research Series, or in paperback form.

The STAC recently reviewed progress in research in fundamental biomedical sciences and concluded that additional efforts were needed to promote research in fundamental biology related to the six target diseases in tropical countries. BIOS is now establishing activities in this area.

3.10. Biological Control of Vectors

There are a wide variety of potential agents for the biological control of vectors and intermediate hosts of parasites. Research on these agents and research on vector ecology and behavior is the responsibility of the SWG on Biological Control of Vectors (BCV). The objectives are to identify, evaluate, and develop biological control agents—with special emphasis on their rapid and practical application in integrated vector control strategies—and to support the needs of institutions in tropical endemic countries for research and training in this area. The agents under consideration include viruses, fungi, bacteria, protozoa, nematodes, insects, and fish. The work is based on a five-stage plan for screening and evaluating the efficiency, safety, and environmental impact of potential biological control agents. A similar plan has been prepared with respect to parasitoids, predators, and competitors. The development of agents is carried through to the stage of proven efficacy and safety in practical application in the field.

The work of BCV is illustrated by the development of the bacterial larvicide *B. t.* H-14. Following its discovery outside the Programme in 1976, this agent has been developed in collaboration with the agrochemical industry to the present stage of application for control purposes in the field. The spores of *B. t.* H-14 have been found to be toxic for mosquito and blackfly larvae with a very large safety margin for mammals and other nontarget organisms, the activity being due to a protein endotoxin. The spores of *B. t.* H-14 are nonreplicating in the field under most circumstances and in this sense can be regarded as similar to a chemical larvicide. Strains of mosquitoes that are resistant to all major types of chemical insecticides have thus far shown no evidence of cross-resistance to *B. t.* H-14. The toxic activity is stable in storage under tropical conditions and is unaffected by salinity and pH within reasonable limits, but it is reduced in polluted water. Assay of *B. t.* H-14 toxicity is based on direct determination of its larvicidal effect; a standard bioassay has been devised and a suitable standard for comparison is available.

Following numerous small-scale field trials, *B. t.* H-14 is now used operationally in the Onchocerciasis Control Programme (OCP) in West Africa. The OCP is largely based on the killing of *Simulium* (blackfly) larvae by the systematic application of insecticides to their breeding sites in rivers and watercourses. In some areas larvae are now becoming resistant to chemical insecticides; *B. t.* H-14 is being successfully used for their control (Figure 4). Present research on *B. t.* H-14 includes the development of strains giving higher yields of toxin as well as improvements of formulation, handling, and application. The effectiveness of *B. t.* H-14 against mosquitoes is being assessed in different environmental conditions.

A number of other promising agents are being studied; there is particular interest in the larvicidal activity of the spores of *Bacillus sphaericus*. This organism replicates more readily in the environment than *B. t.* H-14, and its spores are active in polluted water.

3.11. Social and Economic Research

The success of disease control activities, especially in rural areas, will to a large degree depend upon the understanding of disease and acceptance of control measures by local communities. Economic resources for disease control are often extremely limited, especially in the poor countries and communities where many of the six diseases flourish. The objective of the SWG on Social and Economic Research (SER) is to acquire the knowledge and experience necessary to ensure that social, cultural, and economic factors are given appropriate consideration in the design, conduct, and evaluation of disease control measures. In particular, research focuses on understanding the relationship between social, cultural, and economic factors and disease transmission and control as well as on the design of cost-effective and socially acceptable disease control programs.

These objectives are broad ones, and social and economic circumstances vary greatly between countries and communities. The strategy of the SWG is to develop the required research methodologies and to promote their application to disease control by helping tropical countries to expand their competence in this area. A number of key topics for research have been identified, and all research projects are conducted through institutions in tropical countries. There are at present few trained scientists and institutions in tropical countries with interest in this area, and the Programme assists in the training of scientists to meet this need. Whenever possible, research activities relate directly to national control programs, and results relevant to improvement of control are communicated to national authorities.

The SER carries out its work through the support of research projects and by various promotional and informational exchange activities, including meetings, workshops, and publications. The following are examples of the activities that have taken place.

A study found that malaria control was impeded by peoples' nonacceptance of spraying due to misunderstanding between villagers and the men carrying out the spraying of insecticides. This finding was transmitted to the appropriate authorities so that the training of the spray men could be improved. In an African country it was found that there were many misconceptions in the knowledge and attitudes of primary school children and their teachers toward major local tropical diseases, and the local health education program will be modified accordingly. A study on filariasis in the Philippines found that most people were aware of the disease but did not know how it was transmitted. In Egypt behavioral factors influencing the prevalence of malaria are being studied in a project under the Ministry of Health official responsible for malaria control. This project involves training social and health scientists, and its findings will be incorporated into the design of future malaria control activities. A pioneer study of peoples' knowledge, attitudes, and practices related to leprosy and its control is in progress in the Philippines; it includes psychological testing of patients and their families and study of the social structures of affected communities. The next step will be education to improve the understanding of disease, with the intention of improving control and minimizing the stigma attached to infected people.

Courses and meetings have been held on behavioral aspects of disease control. A meeting on human water contact in relation to the transmission of schistosomiasis emphasized the importance of knowledge on this subject in the design and evaluation of control activities. It recommended appropriate research methods and identified gaps in current knowledge for further study. At a course in Egypt, the participants studied social and economic factors affecting control programs; field visits were used to identify behavioral problems and to stimulate those who attended to identify topics for research. Other topics being developed in a similar way include studies of socioeconomic determinants and consequences of disease, the effects of migration on disease transmission and control, and the role of the community and schools in disease control programs.

Inherent in the operation of the SER SWG is close collaboration with other SWGs and the RSG. There are also links with related activities of WHO and other agencies, including the World Bank.

4. THE STRENGTHENING OF RESEARCH CAPABILITY

The second main objective of the Programme is to strengthen research capability in countries most affected by tropical diseases. This task is the responsibility of the Research Strengthening Group (RSG), whose efforts are entirely directed to this end, and of the SWGs, who—under their prime objective of the development of new tools and methods for disease control—give priority to tropical countries in carrying out their research and training activities.

How can the strengthening of research capability in tropical countries be achieved in a systematic way, considering the magnitude of the task and Programme's limited resources? The initiative and the long-term responsibility lie with the national authorities of tropical countries; without their commitment, nothing of significant and lasting value can be achieved by the Programme acting alone. The principle of all the Programme's activities in this area is therefore to help national authorities to carry out the research training and research needed for the control of diseases. The main feature of the RSG's policies and activities is to provide assistance to strengthen institutions for research related to one or more of the six diseases in a way that, in view of national possibilities and economic resources, is realistic. The objectives of this strengthening are established by the institution and government concerned.

The Programme has established a list of 116 countries that are eligible for support in this way. Institutions within these countries are selected for support on the basis of the geographic distribution of the six target diseases, disease ecologies in different areas, and the needs of countries for research facilities. The policy of the RSG is to provide major support for relatively few institutions at any one time. In a first phase, institutions were selected that were already relatively well advanced, so that after about five years of support they themselves will be able to undertake training for others. Subsequently, less advanced institutions will be supported, with the previously strengthened institutions assisting through collaboration in training and research. In this way the Programme builds on the research capability of developing countries according to the principles of technical cooperation between developing countries.

The RSG provides the following types of assistance to institutions and national authorities: (1) training of scientists and support staff within institutional staff developed plans; (2) organization of collaboration in research and training between institutions; (3) funds for expanding activities, including items such as equipment and supplies but excluding the construction of new buildings; (4) help to national medical research councils or similar bodies for identification of research priorities and for the development of career structures in research; and (5) increasing national capability to translate research findings into improvements in disease control programs. The concept of an "institution" is a broad one, including not only formally established research institutions but also research groups within universities and national disease-control programs.

The Programme awards a variety of different types of grants for training in research and for institutional strengthening, following evaluation of written proposals prepared by scientists and institutions. Individual research training grants are awarded to members of institutions previously identified for strengthening on the basis of a staff development plan submitted by the institution; they range in duration from a few months to sufficient time to acquire a higher qualification, such as a doctoral degree. Such training often involves supervision from another country; in this case arrangements are made so that as much of the work as possible is undertaken in the trainee's home country. Visiting scientist grants enable established scientists to visit other institutions in connection with their research, and reentry grants enable scientists returning home after a period of training abroad to establish research activities. Group training grants support formal courses such as master's courses and ad hoc activities such as seminars, workshops, and scientific meetings directly relevant to the Programme's goals. By the end of 1982, 267 training grants, 42 visiting scientists grants, 55 reentry grants, and 43 group training grants had been awarded.

Institutional grants serve to strengthen national or regional institutions; various types of grants are available. Small grants are intended to initiate research or to support training of research workers within the trainee's country. Short-term support grants are intended to provide institutional support for strengthening which does not clearly fall within other categories. Capital grants serve to increase the research capability of established institutions by providing equipment or other facilities. Long-term support grants are the major form of institutional strengthening; they are awarded in principle for periods up to five years and are reviewed annually. These grants are based on an application that indicates current and planned research and training activities and usually also on the findings of a site visit carried out on behalf of the RSG. By the end of 1982, 35 institutions (11 in Latin America, 12 in Africa, and 12 in Asia) had received long-term support grants. The research areas and disciplines most frequently supported in these institutions were as follows: epidemiology and field research, 17; immunology, 9; entomology and vector studies, 7; clinical research and clinical pharmacology, 3. The location of institutions receiving support under the RSG, including support through training, is shown in Figure 5.

These activities break new ground in the international promotion of research and research training and management, and special attention is given to evaluation of institutional progress. The concept of self-study is a major feature of evaluation and is designed to provide information of value both for the institution and the Programme. Research training grants are evaluated both in terms of the new knowledge and skills acquired by the trainee and of the value of the training in strengthening the trainee's institution.

As noted above, SWGs also play an important role in strengthening research capability in tropical countries. Some types of research under SWGs—such as fundamental biochemical, genetic, and immunological studies—are carried out

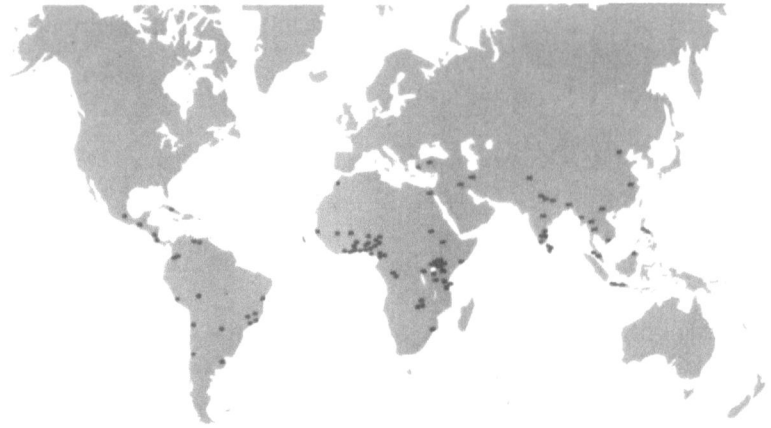

Figure 5. Distribution of research institutions receiving support under the Research Strengthening Group up to December 1982.

wherever in the world there are scientists and resources needed to make rapid progress. Most but not all resources for this work are in developed countries, and this is where the Programme funds most of this research. However, it is the policy of the Programme to promote the transfer of technology of this type, and SWGs assist in this by the award of training grants to scientists from tropical countries to take part in projects and by holding courses in advanced technology. For example two African scientists completed research theses during training as part of a project on folate metabolism of filaria under a senior investigator in the United States, and scientists from tropical countries have attended several seminars and workshops on the application of monoclonal antibodies to research on tropical diseases.

Other types of research under SWGs necessarily take place in tropical countries; for example epidemiological, social, and economic studies and clinical and field trials of new drugs, vaccines, and tests. The studies are undertaken in cooperation with national authorities and with the greatest possible involvement of national scientists, who may, if necessary, receive training for this purpose. Thus clinical trials of mefloquine in Brazil and Thailand take place under national scientists, and all research under the SWG on Social and Economic Research takes place through institutions in tropical countries. In 1982, 35% of all research and development projects were funded to tropical countries.

This description shows that the RSG and SWGs have substantial areas of common interest, and the Programme ensures a close relation between the activities of these groups. Thus the RSG takes the requirements of SWGs into account in the identification of institutions and lines of research that it strengthens, and these institutions are encouraged to apply for project funding under SWGs. At the present time, after less than six years of RSG operations, more than half the institutions that have received grants for strengthening have successfully competed for project funding under SWGs.

The following examples illustrate the activities of some of the institutions strengthened by the Programme.

The Tropical Disease Research Centre, Ndola, Zambia. This center was established in 1975, following a request by the Zambian government. In view of the lack of trained Zambians, it was staffed at that time at the senior level with non-Zambian scientists. Research projects at the center, identified on the basis of national needs and the priorities of the Programme, included longitudinal epidemiological studies on rural populations, studies of the epidemiology of *T. b. rhodesiense* infection, and trials of mefloquine and antischistosomal compounds. The center has trained scientists and technologists, and Zambian scientists are now becoming available for recruitment to senior staff positions. In 1981 the Zambian government assumed administrative responsibility for the center and appointed a Zambian director. The Zambian government has throughout provided substantial support, and as the center has developed, so Programme support is moving from the initial stage of strengthening capability under the RSG toward individual research project funding under SWGs. The center has now developed its own objectives and priorities as a national and international center for research and training in communicable diseases.

The Faculty of Tropical Medicine, Mahidol University, Bangkok, Thailand. This faculty, already a well established institution for the study of tropical diseases, approached the Programme for assistance in modernizing its laboratory facilities and in developing capabilities in field research in the areas of epidemiology, biostatistics, and social and economic research. Support under the RSG has been used to develop collaboration with the London School of Tropical Medicine and Hygiene through a regular exchange of faculty members and collaborative projects with other institutions and national disease-control authorities. The faculty now conducts field research projects in malaria and social and economic research, and scientists are being trained in related disciplines.

The Fundacao Oswaldo Cruz, based in Rio de Janeiro, Brazil. This foundation, which has a long tradition of research in tropical medicine, requested Programme support for developing research and training in Chagas' disease, leishmaniasis, and schistosomiasis especially in relation to immunology. It has received a long-term grant for developing capability in research in the immunology of parasitic diseases; scientists have been trained; and an annual training course is given in basic immunology and the immunology of parasitic diseases. Research in progress includes studies on immunity and autoimmunity, the identification of parasite surface antigens, and the role of macrophages and complement in relation to protection and pathogenesis of disease. Support has been provided under the RSG and by the Schistosomiasis, Filariasis, and Leishmaniasis SWGs.

At the present time, many of the major centers for research in tropical diseases are located in developed countries. These institutions contribute greatly to the Programme by the conduct of research under projects funded under SWGs, by their provision of experienced scientists for planning and evaluation of Programme activities, by the availability of their staff and facilities for the training of scientists, and through collaborative research with institutions in endemic countries. However, in the context of the objective of strengthening research capability in endemic countries, the Programme does not support the strengthening of institutions in developed countries or the training of their scientists.

The ultimate goal of increasing research capability in endemic countries is a long-term one, and success of the Programme's activities will hardly become apparent in a period of less than 20 years. There are, however, encouraging signs. National authorities and institutions are showing enthusiasm for entering into an association with the Programme, which involves a long-term commitment on their part to continue the activity after Programme support diminishes or terminates. There are already examples of increasing national funding as Programme support is reduced.

5. FIELD RESEARCH

Fact-finding studies in epidemiology and sociology and trials of new tools and methods for disease control involve research on populations in the field. Such research is usually expensive and of long duration. The Programme includes an important amount of research of this type. For example, in 1980, 28% of funding under SWGs and 45% of funding under the RSG were for projects that included a component of field research. Nonetheless, there is a severe shortage of scientists and lack of high-quality research projects in this area. This causes difficulties in the implementation of essential field research under the Programme and equally seriously impairs the ability of tropical countries to conduct the research they need to improve disease control. The general solution to this problem lies outside the resources of the Programme; the WHO is drawing the attention of member states to the seriousness of the situation. The Programme is now considering developing a small number of multidisciplinary field research and training programs of high quality; it is also increasing training relevant to field research in epidemiology, parasitology, entomology, malacology, sociology, economics, and biostatistics.

6. COLLABORATION WITH OTHER FUNDING AGENCIES

It is estimated that the Programme currently represents 25–30% of global expenditure on research on major tropical diseases. The Programme's policy on collaboration is to identify research priorities and to ensure that they are met, if not by other sources then by the Programme's own resources. In some areas, such as leprosy vaccine development, the Programme is responsible for nearly all research; in others, such as development of vaccines for malaria, the Programme is responsible for only part of the total world effort and works as closely as possible with other funding agencies, aiming to fill gaps and to avoid the unnecessary duplication of work in progress elsewhere. The final common pathway in the development of all new tools is testing in the field. Operating as it does within WHO, the Programme is well placed to conduct this stage of research in collaboration with the national authorities of tropical countries.

7. COLLABORATION WITH INDUSTRY

Many of the products of research and development under the Programme require the facilities of the pharmaceutical or other industries for certain aspects of research and development and for production. The Programme's policy is to collaborate with industry as necessary to achieve its objectives and in such a way as to preserve public rights related to the products of research, based on equitable assessment of the share of research and development expenditures made by the Programme and by industry respectively. There has been close collaboration over several years with Hoffmann–La Roche in the development of the antimalarial mefloquine. Scientists from industry take part on the basis of their own expertise in meetings of SWGs and as members of steering committees. Nineteen research projects have been funded to industry—for example, screening of potential antifilarial compounds and the preparation of radiolabeled suramin for metabolic studies.

8. INFORMATION ON THE PROGRAMME'S ACTIVITIES

The Programme's policy is to make information on its activities as widely available as possible. All reports of Programme activities other than confidential evaluations are public documents and are available on request from the Director of the Special Programme, World Health Organization, Geneva.

The Programme regularly produces a variety of reports and other documents designed to inform scientists, administrators, and policymakers of activities that are planned or in progress. A newsletter is issued periodically, which summarizes all current Programme activities. Detailed Programme reports, previously issued annually, are now produced biennially. Reports of SWG, RSG, STAC, and JCB meetings are issued. Reviews are prepared on specialized topics such as drug resistance in malaria, parasite cultivation, monoclonal antibodies, and immunodiagnostic techniques; these are published in various ways, according to the subject matter. Publications include the Tropical Disease Research Series, which is available from booksellers in developed countries and free on request to the Programme to scientists in tropical countries; paperback publications for general distribution; and other channels, such as the *Bulletin* of the WHO. The main bulk of research in the Programme is published by investigators in the scientific literature. As noted previously, over 1800 such publications have appeared to the end of 1982. A quarterly bibliography of major tropical diseases, based on the MEDLARS system, is produced in collaboration with the U.S. National Library of Medicine; it provides summaries of publications on the six target diseases. This is available to scientists in tropical countries free of charge, on request. The book *Facts & Figures* lists all projects and principal investigators supported by the Programme and also provides administrative information.

9. AN INTERIM ASSESSMENT

Although at this stage an evaluation in terms of achievement of the stated goals would be premature, it is now reasonable to consider whether or not the Programme is likely to be on the way to achieving them. Certain trends and advances are encouraging.

The Programme has an invaluable asset in the direct involvement of the world's scientific community. The Programme places great emphasis on technical planning and evaluation carried out under SWGs, the RSG, and STAC; many scientists have collaborated enthusiastically in these tasks. Within this framework, the Programme recognizes the importance of individual scientific initiative and of freedom of enquiry. The policy of the Programme is to adapt and incorporate relevant knowledge and technology for its own purposes and to keep flexibility in its planning in order to take advantage of new or unexpected findings. The most important and perhaps the only way by which this can be assured is to charge active scientists with the responsibility for decision making on scientific matters. The evidence that this works is provided in the accounts of progress of the Programme given here and elsewhere.

The Programme links scientists and institutions in different countries to increase the pace of research and development and to strengthen research in disease-endemic countries. Some examples have already been given; others include studies on the clinical pharmacology of drugs for the treatment of onchocerciasis, which are in progress at the Tamale Chemotherapeutic Centre, Ghana. This center is situated in an endemic zone and has access to patients who need treatment. The Tamale Centre is linked to the University of Liverpool, where there is special expertise in research of this type. The effectiveness of therapy of leprosy in therapeutic trials in India is determined by assessment of the presence of living *M. leprae* in lesions. Scientists in Karigiri, India, and in London have collaborated in establishing the methodology for testing in India and in the assessment of material from lesions. Research in malacology is being strengthened by collaboration between the Institute of Public Health, Manila, Philippines, and the Faculty of Science, Mahidol University, Bangkok, Thailand, where there is special expertise in this area.

The Programme uses worldwide scientific resources to further its activities. The only screen known at present for assessment of compounds for activity against onchocerca is provided by infected cattle in Australia. This screen is used within the Programme's development of antionchocercal agents. The Programme obtains rare and important biological materials, such as *M. leprae* and schistosomes, and distributes them to investigators for approved studies in many institutions and countries. The Programme establishes protocols as well as registries and banks for reagents for international studies. For example, protocols have been established for epidemiology of Chagas' disease and chemotherapy of Chagas' disease and leishmaniases. Registries are being established of monoclonal antibodies to antigen of parasites and *M. leprae,* and banks of monoclonal antibodies to malaria antigens are being established and assessed.

The Programme exploits advances made elsewhere to achieve its ends. There are many examples: the rapid development of *B. t.* H-14 to the stage of field use against *Simulium* vectors of onchocerciasis was based on a prior discovery of larvicidal activity; the development of mefloquine is based on the prior demonstration by WRAIR of its antimalarial properties; the demonstration of the effectiveness of traps for tsetse-fly control in certain areas was based on a trap designed outside the Programme. These types of development require international planning and cooperation, which the Programme is well placed to provide.

The Programme identifies research in disease-endemic countries as essential for the improvement of disease control. The Programme works closely with other technical divisions in WHO to identify the types of tools needed to improve disease control and in the testing and application of new tools, as they emerge, in populations in the field. There is now good reason to anticipate that important new tools will be developed over the next decades. Nonetheless, it is not possible to foresee an end to the need for research to improve control. Even given the best tools that can be developed, quite exceptional efforts will be needed to control any of the six diseases on a large scale; eradication of those diseases which have important animal reservoirs will probably not be possible. If drugs are used on a wide scale, parasites will become resistant to them, antigenic changes may render vaccines ineffective, and environmental, social, and economic changes will present new disease control problems. The establishment of field research as a respected discipline and career for scientists and the provision of the facilities and experience needed by tropical countries for the conduct of research are no simple tasks. An international program for research on the control of tropical diseases could more easily achieve its objectives if these tasks were ignored, but then the benefits to be derived would be transient at best.

This account shows how the Programme was established and operates according to the specific guidelines of the 1974 World Health Assembly resolution. Important advances have been made, but as yet these are small in comparison with the great needs for improved disease control. Research on major tropical diseases remains underdeveloped as compared with that on many other diseases afflicting mankind, and the Programme in no way obviates the requirement for other national and international efforts. Viewed in the long term, the Programme's special role and achievement may prove to be the vitalization of research in this neglected area and the mobilization of scientists worldwide, especially in tropical countries, for the task.

ACKNOWLEDGMENT. I am grateful to many of my colleagues on the staff of the World Health Organization who have assisted in the preparation of this account.

2

Infant and Child Mortality in Developing Countries

Tim Dyson

1. INTRODUCTION

Currently there are approximately 50 million annual deaths throughout the world. About 40 million of these deaths occur in less developed countries (LDCs), where roughly 20 million of the victims are individuals under the age of five. In other words about 40% of the people who die each year are infants and young children in the developing world. Framed thus, the title of this paper may be said to point to the world's greatest single health problem. And it is not surprising that international organizations and national governments view the reduction of early-age mortality as a key development goal. The U.N. has adopted as a prime objective the approximate halving of the global level of infant mortality before the year 2000 (U.N., 1981). And the United States Foreign Assistance Act stipulates the reduction of infant mortality as a key criterion by which to assess a country's commitment to the development process.

2. MEASURING EARLY-AGE MORTALITY

In the terminology of health demography, an infant is anyone below the age of 1 (i.e., aged zero), and a child is a noninfant under age 5 (i.e., aged 1–4 years). The infant mortality rate (IMR) is the probability of dying in the year

Tim Dyson • Department of Population Studies, London School of Economics, London WC2A 2AE, England.

immediately following birth. In life-table terms, this is $_1q_0$.* But IMRs are usually expressed per 1000 live births. And a common way to calculate a population's IMR is to divide a year's infant deaths by the same year's live births. The U.N.'s current (1975–1980) estimated IMR for the world's less developed regions as a whole is 100.4 (Bucht and Chamie, 1982). This means that for every 1000 lives births, about 100 are estimated to die before their first birthday. Likewise the child mortality rate is often calculated by dividing a year's child deaths by the estimated number of children aged 1–4 years. This rate is also usually expressed per 1000 population aged 1–4. While infant and child mortality are thus conceptually distinct, we will use the term "early age" to refer to mortality occurring throughout the first five years of life.

Both infant and child mortality rates are simple to compute where satisfactory vital registration and census data exist. But in LDCs this is often not the case. Therefore alternative estimation procedures are employed. These produce alternative, though allied, indexes of mortality. However, these allied measures cannot always be easily translated into conventional infant and child death rates. Among such alternative measures are the life-table probabilities of dying before the second and fifth birthdays ($_2q_0$ and $_5q_0$ respectively).

3. DATA SOURCES

Knowledge of early-age mortality in developing countries comes from a variety of data sources that are sometimes closely related in operation. Three are particularly worth discussing. They are vital registration, censuses and surveys, and surveillance systems.

3.1. Vital Registration

Systems of vital registration are found in some LDCs, but they are often severely deficient as data sources on early-age mortality. Sometimes they are restricted to only parts of a country (e.g., urban areas). More important, in only a minority of LDCs with registration is the coverage of vital events anywhere near complete. Births, and usually to a greater degree deaths, tend to be underreported. The U.N. gives a "C" code to systems that are judged to be "virtually complete" (i.e., 90% or more coverage). But the judgment as to completeness rests with national statistical offices, and many C-coded systems are certainly seriously deficient in coverage.

In general, child deaths are probably better registered than those of infants. Within infancy, neonatal deaths are often especially poorly reported. Given that

*Readers unfamiliar with life-table terminology are referred to Barclay (1958).

registration of births tends to be more complete than that of deaths, IMRs from vital registration are often underestimates. But this is not universally the case. In Colombia the reverse is true, and the resulting infant mortality rate is an overestimate (Palloni, 1981). However, if vital registration and census data are incomplete to an equal degree, then death rates may be estimated satisfactorily despite such deficiencies. Further, even given a different degree of coverage between registration and census data, *trends* in infant and child death rates may be ascertainable so long as the degree of coverage remains constant over time. On the other hand, changes in completeness of coverage, possibly related to changes in registration procedures, can sometimes obscure real trends or produce entirely spurious changes in death rates. Conversely, interpretation of time-series data on early-age mortality from vital registration may be difficult because in actuality annual death rates may fluctuate or be affected in any one year by special conditions, such as a measles epidemic (Heligman *et al.*, 1978). While the production of IMRs from vital registration usually proceeds on an annual basis, child mortality rates tend to be published sporadically, reflecting a common but unfortunate view that they are only of secondary importance. One final limitation of registration data on early-age mortality is that for virtually no country is it cross-classified in any but the most basic of ways (e.g., by urban–rural residence).

3.2. Censuses and Surveys

Probably the single most important body of data on early-age mortality in LDCs stems from special questions included in censuses and surveys. Two sets of questions have been very widely used. These are (1) questions on children ever born and children surviving (CEB/CS) and (2) questions that together constitute a "maternity history." In smaller surveys, both sets of questions may be asked to promote a better response rate. Both sets are usually asked of women aged 15 and over.

3.2.1. CEB/CS Questions

CEB/CS questions have probably been asked at some time in most LDCs. The data they generate can be cross-classified against maternal and household characteristics to give information on mortality differentials. Essentially women are asked (1) How many live births have you ever had? and (2) How many of these infants have subsequently died? Further "probe" questions can be included. To be adequately analyzed, the resulting data must be cross-classified by current age of respondent.

The method of analyzing CEB/CS data was first developed by Brass (see Brass *et al.*, 1968). It has since been marginally improved (e.g., Trussell, 1975).

Table I

Analysis of CEB/CS Data from the 1972 Indian Fertility Survey[a]

Age group of respondent	Proportion of children dead	k factor	Mortality index $({}_nq_0)$	Mortality estimate $({}_nq_0)$	Estimate converted to IMR $({}_1q_0)$	Time reference
15–19	0.141	0.922	${}_1q_0$	0.130	0.130	1.1
20–24	0.134	1.148	${}_2q_0$	0.155	0.119	2.3
25–29	0.150	1.167	${}_3q_0$	0.175	0.121	4.2
30–34	0.166	1.114	${}_5q_0$	0.185	0.119	6.5
35–39	0.178	1.140	${}_{10}q_0$	0.203	0.121	9.0

[a]The proportions of children reported as dead are taken from India (1974). The k factors were derived from the "south"-model life-table regression equations in Trussell (1975). A south-model life table (level 11) was used in obtaining a graduated ${}_2q_0$ value of 0.154 and in converting the ${}_nq_0$ values to values of ${}_1q_0$ (Coale and Demeny, 1966). The time reference column refers to "years prior to the survey" and was obtained using Feeney's (1980) equations. A ${}_2q_0$ value of 0.154 implies an IMR of 118/1000 if a south model is used. But with, for example, a west model, it implies an IMR of 124.

An application to recent data from India—where roughly 30% of the world's early-age deaths occur each year—is summarized in Table I. As can be seen, the technique involves using multiplying (k) factors to translate the proportions of children reported as dead into life-table probabilities of dying $({}_nq_0)$. Specifically, the proportion dead reported by women aged 15–19 is converted into an estimate of the infant mortality rate $({}_1q_0)$; that for women aged 20–24 converts to ${}_2q_0$ and so on.

Unfortunately the ${}_1q_0$ value obtained by this procedure is often suspect, partly because births to women aged 15–19 are usually few in number, and fewer still have died. Also, births to women aged 15–19 tend to be predominantly *first* births; these are unlikely to be representative, in their survivorship, of all births. Estimates of mortality to ages beyond 5 are also often suspect because older women, upon whose responses such estimates are based, tend to be particularly bad at reporting dead children. In view of such considerations, the values of ${}_2q_0$, ${}_3q_0$, and ${}_5q_0$ are often thought to be somewhat more reliable. Yet even these can exhibit pronounced irregularities. In such circumstances a common procedure is to produce an average, "graduated" value of ${}_2q_0$ based on these three preferred values. From this a graduated estimate of the IMR $({}_1q_0)$ can be obtained by extrapolation—provided assumptions are made as to the pattern of early-age mortality prevailing in the population (e.g., see Blacker *et al.*, 1977). In practice this means selecting a set of "model" life tables from among several possible alternatives. Unfortunately, available models are mostly based upon Western rather than developing-country experience (Coale and Demeny, 1966). Yet as we show below, the pattern of early-age mortality in LDCs can be quite different. Thus, where CEB/CS material are analyzed, there exists no really foolproof way

of gauging the two components of early-age mortality separately: in such circumstances estimates of infant mortality are simply extrapolations from data on
early-age mortality as a whole. Further, the accuracy of CEB/CS estimates is
also dependent upon the quality of the raw data. In particular, to the extent that
dead children are omitted by female respondents, estimates will understate true
mortality levels. On the other hand, where early-early age mortality or fertility is
declining, the reverse may be the case (Palloni, 1981).

Important extensions of Brass's method have recently been devised. Provided that the raw CEB/CS data are of satisfactory quality, these enable the
estimation of mortality trends over the years immediately preceding the census or
survey (Feeney, 1980; Palloni, 1981). Table I also outlines this procedure. The
$_nq_0$ values are converted to values of IMR ($_1q_0$), again assuming a particular
model pattern of mortality. The new techniques permit us to "date" the values
so obtained. Responses of younger women give estimates that pertain to the
years immediately prior to the census or survey, while those of older women
relate to earlier periods. However, if older women selectively omit dead children, this can conceal a trend of declining mortality.

Figures 1 and 2 illustrate the time-trending of CEB/CS data from successive
enquiries in Kenya and India. For Kenya, the time-trended estimates from differ-

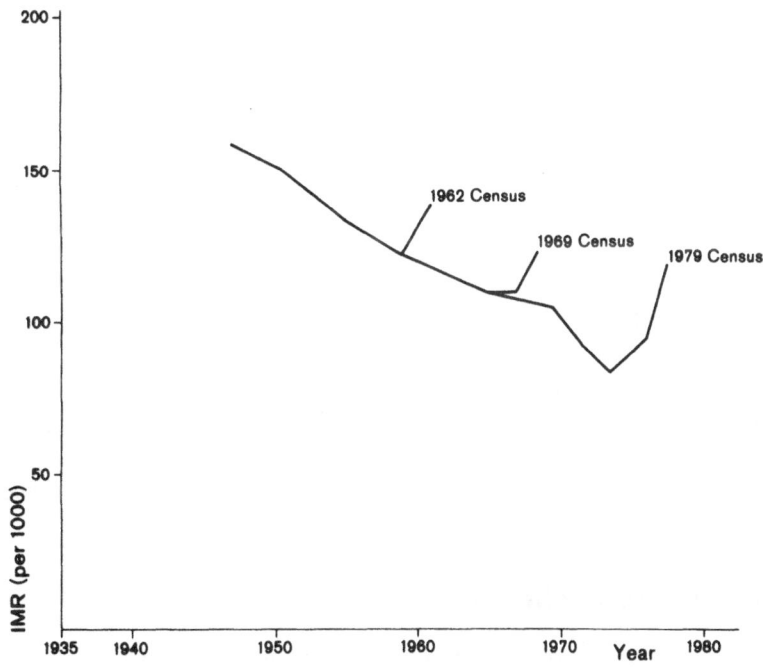

Figure 1.   IMR time-trend estimates from successive censuses in Kenya.

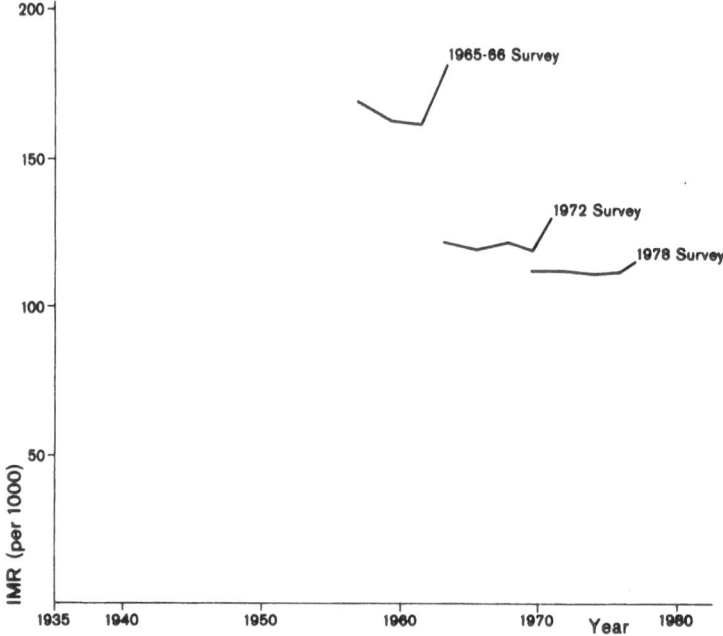

Figure 2.   IMR time-trend estimates from successive surveys in India.

ent censuses interniche very well, especially when, as is the case here, a ''north'' model mortality pattern is used. Indeed, Figure 1 probably constitutes the most convincing evidence available of a sustained improvement in early-age mortality for a black African country. In the Indian case, however, the results are much less satisfactory. The time-located estimates from the three surveys do not over-lap. Indeed, to the degree that the lines are parallel, they indicate constant mortality. Yet comparing the mortality levels implied by the different surveys at different points in time a decline in mortality *is* indicated. It seems very likely that in the Indian case the technique is unsuccessful when it is applied to the results of a single survey (i.e. omission of dead children, particularly by older women, is concealing what comparison between surveys shows to be a real reduction in early-age mortality). Even so, it is likely that the responses of younger women are also deficient, albeit to a lesser extent. Thus the IMRs of 119–121 indicated for women aged 20–29 in Table I are probably also about 10 points too low.

3.2.2. Maternity Histories

Sometimes called "birth histories," these involve asking women detailed questions about each of their live births separately. A minimal list of questions includes the date of each birth, its sex, survivorship status, and, if dead, its date of death. The resulting data can provide detailed estimates of both levels and trends of infant and child death rates separately, so long as it is of satisfactory quality. However, the use of such histories in LDCs is very new. It has largely been confined to the World Fertility Survey (WFS) program, which despite its name also constitutes a partial global survey of early-age mortality. At present, fairly recent WFS estimates of infant and child mortality are available for about 30 LDCs (Hobcraft, 1981; Hobcraft et al., 1982).

But analysis of such material has its problems too. For example, estimates may be affected by dating errors. A tendency for respondents to incorrectly report late infant deaths as occurring at age 1 will, ceteris paribus, lead to an underestimate of infant mortality and an overestimate of child mortality. Also, inaccuracies in dating births and deaths can conceal trends. Again, differential omission of dead children by older women can obscure the extent of early-age mortality decline. Typically, WFS surveys interview only about 5000 women, and sizable sampling errors may attach to estimates when the data are substantially disaggregated, as is the case when trends in infant and child death rates are calculated.

However, WFS surveys have gathered quite a lot of useful background socioeconomic information—for example, on mother's education, place of residence, and work status. Data on breast-feeding have also usually been gathered. The future analysis of WFS early-age mortality data within the context of such information may prove important and, because of its greater detail, methodologically more satisfactory than analogous work with CEB/CS material.* Nevertheless, because WFS surveys were primarily fertility-orientated, the tabulation and analysis of the mortality data collected have hitherto generally received secondary priority. Relatedly, these surveys usually omit questions on topics such as household water and toilet facilities and aspects of infant and child health care.

However, given the great attention and resources devoted to WFS, it is probable that the resulting estimates of infant and child mortality are usually better than those from alternative sources. In Table II we use this to illustrate just how deficient early-age death rates from C-coded vital registration systems can be. The comparison between WFS and registration IMRs for these Latin American countries is only marginally influenced by the differences in dates to which they pertain. Only in Guyana is there a measure of agreement between the two

---

*A major problem with CEB/CS data when they are cross-classified against some other variable (e.g., urban–rural residence) is that they aggregate a woman's *total* lifetime early-age mortality experience against one of her *current* characteristics. For example, a woman currently living in a town may have lost her dead children prior to moving from a rural area. Because WFS surveys ask for more detailed information on the women's past movements, work history, and so on, their data are generally less affected by such problems.

Table II
Comparison of IMR Estimates from Vital Registration and the World
Fertility Survey[a]

Country	Vital registration		World Fertility Survey	
	IMR	Date	IMR	Date
Costa Rica	22.3	1978	53.3	1976
Guyana	50.5	1972	57.6	1975
Trinidad and Tobago	24.4	1978	42.0	1978
Jamaica	16.2	1978	43.0	1975–1976

[a]Vital registration IMRs are taken from U.N. (1980) and Ashworth (1982); WFS estimates are taken from Hobcraft (1981) and Hobcraft et al. (1982). Dates given for WFS relate to year of survey, but WFS estimates themselves pertain to the period 0–4 years prior to the survey.

sources. And even then the difference is greater than 10% (although the WFS results themselves can by no means be regarded as completely error-free). But there can be no doubt that the C classification is entirely unwarranted in the remaining cases.

3.3. Surveillance Systems

By surveillance systems we mean intensive, usually relatively small-scale systems of vital registration which, in addition to recording births and deaths, also collect a great deal of supplementary material over time. Generally a survey establishes the baseline characteristics of the households to be observed. While the total population covered by such an investigation may be large, the number of early-age deaths occurring in the study population each year is unlikely to exceed a few hundred.* Hence very large sampling errors attach to resulting infant and child death rates. On the other hand, because of the fairly continual surveillance of households by study personnel, certain kinds of response errors (e.g., those of dating) may be minimized.

Most important, such studies allow births to be followed through longitudinally and early-age deaths to be examined intensively and contextually. Surveillance studies are really essential for the proper investigation of many of the more proximate variables to an infant or child death—such as birthweight, circumstances at birth, child-care practices, feeding patterns, child morbidity, and causes of death. Hence such studies are vitally important if we are to further our

*For example, if a surveillance system covered a population of 100,000 in which the crude birth rate was 40/1000 and the IMR was 100, only 400 infant deaths would occur in an average year.

understanding beyond the estimation of mortality levels and their relation to a few socioeconomic measures.

Unfortunately, few such systems have operated in LDCs. This is in part because the scope of what can (as opposed to what cannot) be satisfactorily studied with small sample sizes is often insufficiently appreciated. In the latter half of this paper, we necessarily rely heavily upon a few studies that more or less fall into this "surveillance" mold. These include the work of Cantrelle and others in the Sine-Saloum region of Senegal (e.g., Cantrelle and Leridon, 1971); the data collected in Matlab Thana, Bangladesh, by the International Center for Diarrheal Disease Research (e.g., Chen *et al.*, 1980; Chen *et al.*, 1981); material collected by the Keneba project of the UK Medical Research Council in the Gambia (e.g., McGregor *et al.*, 1970; Rowland, 1979). Last, there are several investigations conducted under the aegis of the World Health Organization (WHO); these include the major Inter-American study into patterns of mortality in childhood (Puffer and Serrano, 1973) and other longitudinal studies in Algiers, Algeria (WHO, 1981a); Greater Kabul, Afghanistan, (Dyson, 1981); and Sierra Leone (WHO, 1981b).

At the conclusion of this discussion on data sources, it should be clear that none are without problems. Infant and child deaths tend to be underreported in all forms of enquiry, since people are often understandably reluctant to discuss such matters. As a rule, data tend to be scarcest, most dated, and most defective in exactly those populations where they are most needed (i.e., those with the highest early-age death rates). A recent U.N. review of IMRs in 156 countries found that 17—including such a major nation as Nigeria—had virtually no data on which to base an estimate. Instead, informed guesses had to be used (Bucht and Chamie, 1982). Where data are available they can often be analyzed in a number of ways; the conclusions drawn—for example as to mortality levels and trends—may vary quite substantially according to different interpretations.

4. THE AGE PATTERN OF MORTALITY

Before we examine infant and child death rates for selected developing countries, the issue of their relative level (i.e., age pattern) should be briefly addressed. In many LDCs, little information on this subject is available. Reliable data are scarcest for sub-Saharan populations which, from fragmentary evidence, appear to experience especially unusual patterns. However, it seems that the relationship between the level of infant mortality on the one hand and that of 1–4 mortality on the other can vary substantially both between populations and in the same population over time. Two important features, not well-reflected by available model life tables, are (1) a continuation of high mortality in infancy through into the second year of life and, relatedly, (2) high ratios of child mortality to infant mortality. An early identification of these characteristics came from surveillance data for Sine-Saloum, Senegal (Cantrelle and Leridon, 1971). As Table III shows, the risk of dying during the second year of life ($_1q_1$) was found to be approximately the same as that of dying during infancy ($_1q_0$). Also, the IMR was much lower than the risk of dying between the first and fifth birthdays ($_4q_1$). These features have subsequently been identified in other West African populations (e.g. see Gaisie, 1975).

Table III further compares $_nq_x$ values from three WFS surveys with comparable probabilities of dying derived from model life tables matched at the same infant mortality rates. As in Figure 1, the so-called north-model life table has been used because it is often thought best at reflecting these unusual features. As can be seen, in the WFS Senegalese data, the IMR is lower than in Bangladesh and not much above that for Kenya. But in Senegal, on the other hand, the risk of dying during childhood ($_4q_1$) is much higher than in either Bangladesh or Kenya. This surprising feature is probably real [although detailed WFS results indicate that neonatal deaths may be somewhat underreported in Senegal (Hobcraft *et al.*, 1982)]. In Bangladesh the model fits infant and child mortality quite well, though by no means perfectly. It performs less satisfactorily in matching 1–4

Table III
Comparison of Reported and Model Probabilities of Dying[a]

Country/area	Probabilities of dying			
	$_1q_0$	$_1q_1$	$_3q_2$	$_4q_1$
Sine-Saloum (1962–1968)				
Reported	0.210	0.202	0.190	0.354
Model	0.210	0.070	0.105	0.167
Senegal (1978)				
Reported	0.112	0.074	0.103	0.170
Model	0.112	0.032	0.047	0.077
Kenya (1977–1978)				
Reported	0.087	0.028	0.033	0.061
Model	0.087	0.021	0.033	0.053
Bangladesh (1975–1976)				
Reported	0.135	0.035	0.068	0.101
Model	0.135	0.043	0.062	0.102

[a]Reported probabilities for Sine-Saloum are taken from Cantrelle and Leridon (1971). The remaining reported probabilities are from WFS surveys and are derived from data in Hobcraft *et al.* (1982). For the "north"-model life tables that have been used in matching $_1q_0$, see Coale and Demeny (1966). The probabilities shown are as follows: $_1q_0$ = the probability of dying by age 1 (i.e., the IMR); $_1q_1$ = the probability of dying between the first and second birthdays; $_3q_2$ = the probability of dying between the second and fifth birthdays; and $_4q_1$ = the probability of dying between the first and fifth birthdays (i.e., during ages 1–4).

mortality in Kenya. And for the Senegalese data it performs very badly, in both cases matching the child death probabilities ($_4q_1$) by less than half. Last, it is worth noting that even in the data for Kenya and Bangladesh, the probability of dying in childhood ($_4q_1$) is comparable to, although lower than, the probability of dying in infancy.

So the pattern of early-age mortality in LDCs can be quite variable. Since such variation is not always well captured by models, estimates of levels and trends of infant and child mortality must be viewed that much more tentatively. Clearly too, particularly in populations with high death rates, we cannot differentiate sharply between the stages of infancy and childhood. Nor in such circumstances can we view mortality during the latter period as a matter of secondary importance. It is partly with these considerations in mind that analysts frequently use $_2q_0$ and $_5q_0$ as summary measures of early-age mortality in LDCs, rather than conventional infant and child mortality rates.

5. EARLY-AGE MORTALITY LEVELS

We now present and review selected estimates of early-age mortality for LDCs grouped by region (see Table IV). Inevitably such an excercise is somewhat arbitrary. The recent U.N. (1982) global review systematically employed available data sources and techniques of estimation. For most LDCs it gives IMRs for each quinquennium from 1950–1955 to 2020–2025. However, given its strong temporal framework and the data deficiencies for many countries, the U.N. study inevitably relies heavily upon trend extrapolation and other assumptions. Therefore we have decided to take a somewhat different approach here. The figures presented in Table IV mainly pertain to the latest available period for which, in our view, there exists a fairly plausible estimate. For reasons that should now be clear, we do not confine ourselves to a single index such as the IMR. We will also be much less bold than the U.N. in assessing the scale of past trends. Nevertheless, in some instances we have used figures from the U.N.'s valuable review. We have also employed it as a general "reference standard" to assess the plausibility of individual estimates where alternative consistency checks are unavailable.

5.1. Africa

As can be seen from Table IV, figures for sub-Saharan countries tend to be at least 10 years out of date and are mostly based upon CEB/CS data. Estimates for north African countries are perhaps more reliable; in several cases (e.g., Egypt and Tunisia), they have been derived with reference to not too deficient systems of vital registration. It is clear that early-age mortality is generally very

Table IV
Early-Age Mortality Measures for Selected Countries

Region/country	Source code[a]	Type of data[b]	Date[c]	IMR[d]	Death rate of 1–4/1000	$_2q_0$	$_5q_0$
Africa							
Eastern Africa							
Kenya	1	MH	1977–1978	87	—	0.112	0.142
Madagascar	2	CEB/CS	1966	95	—	0.121	0.142
Malawi	3	—	1975–1980	179	—	—	—
Rwanda	4	CEB/CS	1970	96	—	—	0.147
Tanzania	4	CEB/CS	1969	135	—	—	0.219
Uganda	3	—	1975–1980	100	—	—	—
Zimbabwe	2	CEB/CS	1969	102	—	0.131	0.152
Central Africa							
Central African Republic	2	CEB/CS	1959–1960	222	—	0.274	0.310
Chad	2	CEB/CS	1964	213	—	0.263	0.299
Congo	2	CEB/CS	1960–1961	180	—	0.225	0.257
Zaire	2	CEB/CS	1957–1958	161	—	0.202	0.232
Southern Africa							
Botswana	2	CEB/CS	1971	104	—	0.133	0.155
Lesotho	5	MH	1979	139	—	—	—
Swaziland	6	CEB/CS	1976	162	—	0.192	0.218
Western Africa							
Dahomey	2	CEB/CS	1962	216	—	0.267	0.303
Gambia	3	—	1975–1980	203	—	—	—
Guinea	2	CEB/CS	1954–1955	262	—	0.319	0.358
Mali	2	CEB/CS	1960–1961	256	—	0.312	0.351
Sierra Leone	3	—	1975–1980	215	—	—	—
Senegal	1	MH	1978	112	—	0.178	0.262
Togo	3	—	1975–1980	115	—	—	—
Upper Volta	2	CEB/CS	1960–1961	291	—	0.351	0.393
North Africa							
Algeria	7	—	1970	145	—	—	—
Egypt	3	—	1975–1980	125	—	—	—
Libya	3	—	1975–1980	107	—	—	—
Morocco	7	—	1973	133	—	—	—
Sudan	3	—	1975–1980	131	—	—	—
Tunisia	3	—	1975–1980	106	—	—	—
Latin America							
Caribbean							
Barbados	8	VR	1978	27	2.0	—	—
Cuba	8	VR	1978	22	1.3	—	—
Dominican Republic	5	MH	1975	99	45.0	—	0.128
Guadeloupe	8	VR	1978	21	4.0	—	—
Haiti	5	MH	1977	139	87.0	—	0.191

(*continued*)

Table IV   (*Continued*)

Region/country	Source code[a]	Type of data[b]	Date[c]	IMR[d]	Death rate of 1–4/1000	$_2q_0$	$_5q_0$
Latin America (*continued*)							
Caribbean (*continued*)							
Jamaica	5	MH	1978	43	16.0	—	0.055
Puerto Rico	8	VR	1977	20	1.0	—	—
Trinidad and Tobago	5	MH	1978	42	8.0	—	—
Middle America							
Costa Rica	5	MH	1976	53	19.0	—	0.061
El Salvador	4	CEB/CS	1971	112	—	—	0.173
Guatemala	8	VR	1978	69	—	—	—
Honduras	4	CEB/CS	1971	127	—	—	0.201
Mexico	5	MH	1976–1977	81	36.0	—	0.096
Panama	5	MH	1976–1977	49	17.0	—	0.046
Tropical S. America							
Bolivia	4	CEB/CS	1976	145	—	—	0.239
Brazil	4	CEB/CS	1970	106	—	—	0.157
Colombia	5	MH	1976	73	42.0	—	0.108
Ecuador	9	—	1965–1970	115	—	—	—
Guyana	5	MH	1975	58	17	—	0.077
Paraguay	5	MH	1975–1976	49	17	—	—
Peru	5	MH	1977–1978	112	66	—	0.149
Venezuela	5	MH	1977	45	17	—	0.064
Temperate S. America							
Argentina	9	—	1977	45	—	—	—
Chile	8	VR	1976	60	2.1	—	—
Uruguay	8	VR	1977	48	1.6	—	—
Asia							
East Asia							
China	10	—	1972–1975	56	—	—	0.075
Hong Kong	8	VR	1978	12	0.7	—	—
Southeast Asia							
Indonesia	5	MH	1976	109	80	—	0.158
Malaysia	5	MH	1974–1975	47	14	—	0.050
Philippines	5	MH	1978	57	35	—	0.093
Singapore	8	VR	1978	13	—	—	—
Thailand	5	MH	1975	86	33	—	0.091
Middle S. Asia							
Bangladesh	5	MH	1975–1976	141	87	—	0.222
India	11	CEB/CS	1972	130	—	—	0.185
Nepal	5	MH	1976	166	122	—	0.235
Pakistan	5	MH	1975	136	76	—	0.207
Sri Lanka	5	MH	1975	60	25	—	0.086

(*continued*)

Table IV   *(Continued)*

Region/country	Source code[a]	Type of data[b]	Date[c]	IMR[d]	Death rate of 1–4/1000	$_2q_0$	$_5q_0$
Asia *(continued)*							
Western S. Asia							
Bahrain	3	—	1975–1980	57	—	—	—
Iraq	3	—	1975–1980	84	—	—	—
Jordan	5	MH	1976	74	28	—	0.080
Kuwait	8	VR	1977	39	1.8	—	—
Lebanon	3	—	1975–1980	44	—	—	—
Oman	3	—	1975–1980	135	—	—	—
Qatar	3	—	1975–1980	57	—	—	—
Saudi Arabia	3	—	1975–1980	121	—	—	—
Syria	5	MH	1977–1978	72	25	—	—
Israel	8	VR	1978	17	—	—	—
Turkey	4	CEB/CS	1970	125	—	—	0.196
Oceania							
Fiji	5	MH	1974	51	9	—	0.058
Papua New Guinea	3	—	1975–1980	111	—	—	—

[a]Source codes: (1) Hobcraft (1981); (2) principal source Adegbola (1977), although in fact we present here graduated (west) versions of his estimates based on $_2q_0$, $_3q_0$, and $_5q_0$; (3) U.N. (1982); only average IMRs for the period 1975–1980 are given, the source(s) are unspecified; (4) Palloni (1981); (5) Hobcraft *et al.* (1982); (6) Blacker (1978); (7) estimate cited by Ashworth (1982); (8) U.N. (1980), usually unadjusted vital registration data for which C coding is probably justifiable; (9) Baum and Arriaga (1981); (10) Banister and Preston (1981); (11) Dyson (1982).

[b]VR—vital registration; CEB/CS—children ever born/children surviving estimates; MH—maternity history estimates. In some cases estimates may have been made with reference to several sources.

[c]Date usually refers to date of census, survey, or registration. However this is often only an approximate indicator of the date to which individual estimates relate.

[d]IMRs are given per 1000 and in many cases have been rounded. The same is true for 1–4 death rates. The values of $_2q_0$ and $_5q_0$ are, of course, probabilities of dying. All estimates must be treated as approximate.

heavy in Africa. Within the last 30 years, IMRs over 200 and mortality by age 5 in excess of 30% have been quite common. However, on balance the estimates seem insufficient to support Vallin's (1976) suggestion that the IMR for sub-Saharan Africa as a whole around 1970 exceeded 200. This said, the fairly recent U.N. figures for Malawi and Sierra Leone strongly imply that infant mortality still approaches or exceeds this level in some areas, including, almost certainly, much of the Sahel. The table also sustains Blacker's (1979) suggestion that early-age mortality in west Africa is often substantially heavier than in eastern and southern parts of the continent. Further, it indicates particularly heavy mortality in central Africa, although this whole issue is complicated by differences in dates to which the estimates pertain.

In explaining generally heavier early-age mortality in west and central Africa, the considerations of our previous comparison of Kenya and Senegal in Table III are probably relevant. That is, one suspects that regional mortality differentials within the continent are more pronounced during childhood than during infancy. However this is an issue not easily resolved, given that most of the African estimates in the table are based on CEB/CS data which, as we have already seen, do not readily enable us to separate out levels of infant and child mortality.

Finally, although estimates of infant mortality for countries in north Africa are generally lower than elsewhere in the continent, they are, perhaps somewhat surprisingly, generally higher than IMRs estimated for countries in east Africa.

5.2. Latin America

It is apparent from Table IV that early-age mortality is relatively favorable throughout most of the Caribbean: IMRs in the range 20–40 are common. But Haiti and the Dominican Republic—two of the region's larger countries—have mortality comparable to that in parts of Africa. In Haiti, WFS data indicate that almost 20% of the young die before age 5 ($_5q_0 = 0.191$). An important general point which can easily be illustrated with data for the Caribbean is that at ages 1–4, differences in mortality in percentage terms are more pronounced than they are in infancy. For example, in Haiti the IMR is about five times that in Barbados. But the child death rate in Haiti is over 40 times higher.

A wide range of contrasts also exists in mainland Latin America. The relatively developed countries of the temperate zone have quite low death rates (although not as low as in much of the Caribbean). But elsewhere—for example, in Bolivia, El Salvador, Honduras, and Peru—fairly recent infant and child mortality estimates are comparable to those for African countries such as Kenya or Botswana. Table IV also shows mortality to be quite high in Brazil, which accounts for almost 60% of the population of tropical South America.

5.3. Asia

As we might expect, Asia presents us with an especially varied picture. Recent unpublished surveys in China put the IMR there at slightly over 30, but a figure somewhat above 50 is probably more realistic (Banister and Preston, 1981). In southeast Asia, virtually no reliable estimates exist for Burma, Kampuchea, or Vietnam. But clearly early-age mortality is fairly high in Thailand and Indonesia, although somewhat lower in Malaysia and the Philippines. Small city-states such as Hong Kong and Singapore currently experience infant and child death rates broadly comparable to those of developed countries such as the United Kingdom or the United States.

Within Asia, the bleakest picture is that afforded by the Indian subcontinent. We have already noted the overwhelming importance of India in any world review: it may well be that more infants and children die in that country each year than in the whole of Africa and South America combined. Table IV shows that early-age mortality rates are, if anything, even higher in Bangladesh, Nepal, and Pakistan. Within middle south Asia, the only country with a comparatively low level of early-age mortality is Sri Lanka. But even there almost one child in ten dies before reaching age 5.

Finally, regarding the countries of western south Asia, reliable estimates are fairly scarce. According to the U.N. figures, infant mortality in Saudi Arabia and Oman remains very high. In Turkey, CEB/CS data show a similar picture. But elsewhere, in some of the small oil-rich states such as Bahrain, Kuwait, and Qatar, infant mortality rates appear to be best described as moderate (i.e., in the range 40–60/1000) and child death rates are probably fairly low too.

5.4. Summary

In summary, levels of early-age mortality in the developing world are highest in the Indian subcontinent and Africa. In both these areas, infant and child death rates are probably near or above 130 and 70/1000 respectively. Earlier reviews of the global situation appear to have overestimated infant mortality rates (e.g., Vallin, 1976), but they have also underestimated levels of child mortality in these areas (e.g. Dyson, 1977). Early-age mortality is generally lower in Latin America, but it is lowest in the largest developing region, east Asia, which mainly reflects the presence of China.

6. EARLY-AGE MORTALITY TRENDS

Nearly every developing country has probably experienced some decline in early-age mortality since 1950. Perhaps a little too sweepingly, Bucht and Chamie (1982) write that "since 1950 impressive declines have occurred in the levels of infant mortality throughout virtually every country in the world." Generally speaking, those countries with currently comparatively favorable mortality levels must have experienced substantial improvements over the past three or so decades, whereas slower declines have probably occurred in areas where high early-age death rates still prevail.

6.1. Africa

Little is known about trends in Africa. Comparable data sets for two points in time are rare. Often, time-trended CEB/CS material fails to show clear evidence of declines (Adegbola, 1977). But as we have had cause to note, this does not necessarily preclude their existence. As mentioned earlier, for sub-Saharan Africa perhaps the best evidence of improvement is for Kenya (Figure 1). WFS data for that country confirm CEB/CS material in indicating an IMR decline of around 30% over 1950–1975 (Hobcraft, 1981). For Togo, two independent data sets show a decline comparable to that in Kenya (Bucht and Chamie, 1982). Elsewhere snippets of information suggest marginal or, at best, modest improvements. This is true, for example, for Rwanda and Tanzania according to Palloni's (1981) CEB/CS time-trend analysis. WFS data for Senegal indicate only modest gains between the early 1960s and mid-1970s (Hobcraft, 1981). Only very minor improvements in early-age mortality have been detected for Swaziland (Blacker, 1978). For Sudan, Farah and Preston (1982) remark that early-age mortality "has not improved at anywhere near the pace that has come to be accepted as normal in developing countries"—a conclusion that is probably valid for much of central and western Africa. Where living conditions deteriorate, rises in infant and child mortality may occur. Hence observers such as Eblen (1981) believe that improvements in Africa over the last 10 years may have ceased. In contrast Bucht and Chamie (1982) write that they encountered no evidence of a slowdown in African infant mortality decline. But the evidence for a thorough assessment of the issue simply does not exist.

6.2. Latin America

It is possible to detect substantial postwar mortality improvements in every Caribbean country. For example, the IMR in Barbados was approximately 160 in the late 1940s (Baum and Arriaga, 1981) compared with its present level of about 27. According to WFS data, even Haiti and the Dominican Republic have experienced fairly substantial progress since the early 1960s (Hobcraft, 1981). It is difficult to detect any systematic pattern to changes in the pace of decline of either infant or child mortality. Thus in Puerto Rico, child mortality rates fell by a greater percentage over 1960–1970 than over 1950–1960. But the reverse was true for Jamaica (Baum and Arriaga, 1981).

Postwar declines in early-age mortality have also occurred throughout mainland Latin America. In the temperate countries, these began in the early decades of this century. More recently, a diversification of trends appears to have taken place. Baum and Arriaga (1981) write that some countries "continued to have a rapid decline, while others experienced a progressive reduction in the rate of decline." Also there seems to be no easily identifiable relationship between the recent rate of decline and the level of early-age mortality. Countries with pronounced declines over the past 20 years include Costa Rica, Colombia, Panama, Venezuela, and—with still high infant and child mortality levels—Peru. But in Guyana, Argentina, and Chile, where death rates are already quite low, recent

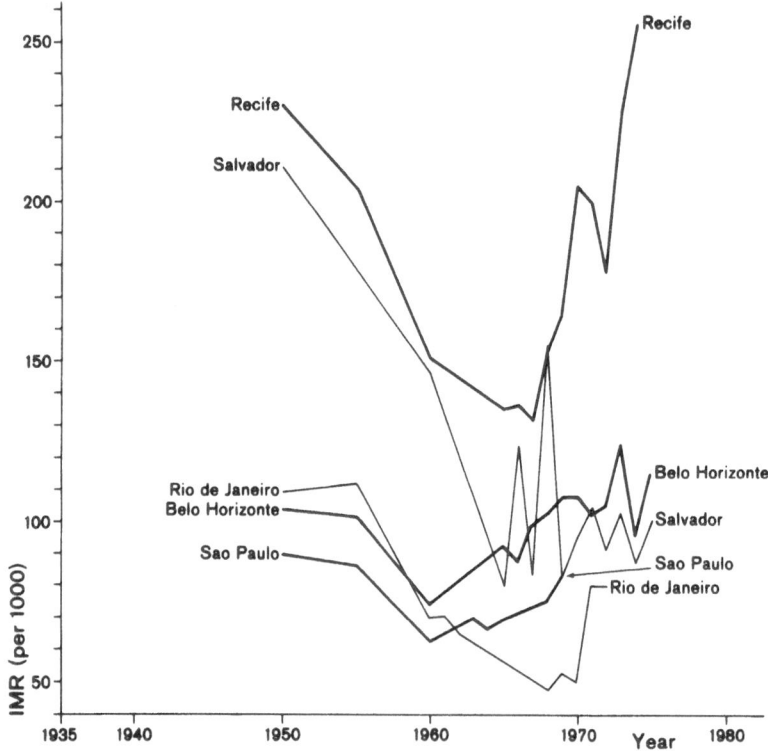

Figure 3.   Registered IMRs for the five largest urban areas of Brazil.

declines are harder to detect. Disturbingly, only slow recent improvements are estimated for Honduras, Bolivia, and Brazil (Baum and Arriaga, 1981; Palloni, 1981).

Many writers have pointed to rises in registered IMRs since 1960 for major urban areas of Brazil and have linked them with worsening income distribution, rapid urban growth, and declines in real wages of the urban poor (Yunes, 1981; Carvalho and Wood, 1978). However, as Figure 3 shows, the registered IMRs for these areas exhibit a considerable degree of annual fluctuation. Such erratic data should be treated with great caution and do not by themselves warrant the firm attribution of an upward trend. Recently CEB/CS data from the 1980 census have become available. They imply that there was a moderate decline in early-age mortality in Brazil during the 1970s. Nevertheless, stagnation in some urban areas of the country cannot be entirely ruled out.

6.3. Asia

In Asia, Sri Lanka and Singapore illustrate the spectacular infant and child mortality declines that have occurred in quite a few of the world's relatively small national populations (Figure 4). Until recently, such dramatic improvements were thought to be ungeneralizable to large LDCs. But for China both raw data and U.N. estimates suggest a similar pace of decline (Figure 4), although the U.N. figures probably correctly imply continual underestimation of the level of infant mortality in the raw figures. However since the early 1950s China probably has the best record of any major developing country or region in reducing early-age mortality.

Elsewhere in Asia the picture is less encouraging. According to U.N. guesstimates (U.N., 1982), between 1965–1970 and 1975–1980 IMRs increased by 102% and 30% in Kampuchea and East Timor, respectively. The U.N. also considers recent improvements in Afghanistan unlikely. Perhaps most worrying is the situation in the subcontinent. In Nepal and Pakistan, WFS indicates at best modest progress over the past two decades (Hobcraft, 1981). WFS data also show little positive change in Bangladesh—a finding consistent with surveillance data from Matlab Thana, which show increases in both infant and child death rates during years of severe social disruption in the early 1970s (Chowdhury and Chen, 1977). For India itself, while there appear to have been major improvements during the 1950s and early 1960s, CEB/CS data suggests something of a reduction in the recent pace of decline (Figure 2). Data from the Sample Vital Registration System (SRS) in India actually imply that infant mortality rose slightly between 1970–1972 and 1975–1976 (see Table V). This is unlikely, given a recorded reduction in the 0–4 death rate as a whole, and probably reflects improvements in the level of coverage together with better reporting of age at

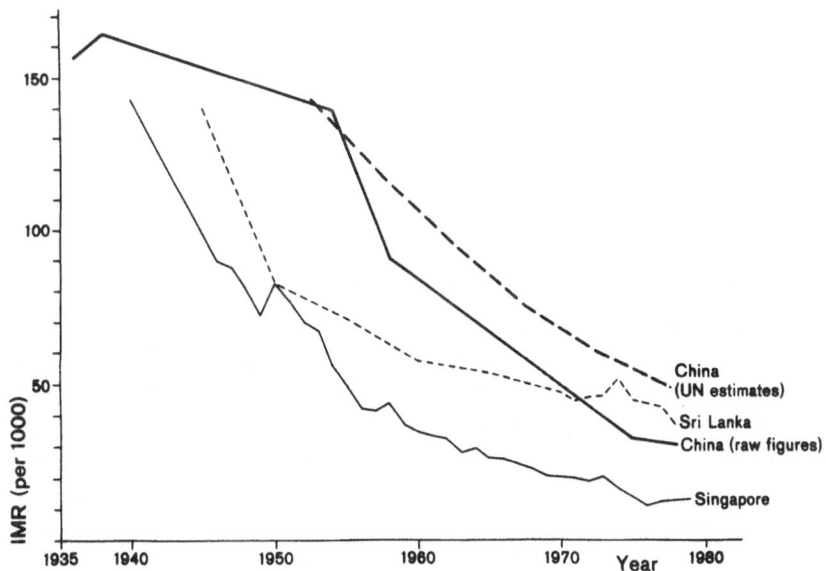

Figure 4.   Estimates of IMR decline for Sri Lanka, Singapore, and China.

Table V
Recent Trends in Early-Age Mortality in India according to
the Sample Registration System[a]

	Period		
	1970–1972	1975–1976	Percentage change
IMR	132	135	+2
Death rate, ages 0–4	54.6	51.0	−7

[a]Death rates for the two periods are annual means. They are taken from India, *Sample Registration Bulletin* (various years).

death. Nevertheless, on balance, SRS data also suggests some reduction in the pace of improvement of early-age mortality in India. And it also alerts us to the possibility that infant and child mortality improvements do not always occur in parallel.*

Last, in western south Asia, the picture appears to be somewhat more encouraging. According to the U.N. (1982) fairly dramatic postwar developments have occurred in Kuwait, Bahrain, Qatar, and the United Arab Emirates. In the larger countries of the region, including Turkey, declines have also occurred, although at a slower pace (Bucht and Chamie, 1982).

6.4. Summary

Our review of trends reveals a picture of considerable diversity. In LDCs where infant and child death rates are already quite favorable, absolute reductions in death rates are generally becoming smaller over time. In such circumstances, minor rises in death rates may occur in any one year, but they do not necessarily mean either the reversal or cessation of long-term downward trends (see, e.g., Sri Lanka in Figure 4), as commentators (e.g., Gwatkin, 1980) sometimes infer. More worrying are populations, such as Bangladesh and India, where the pace of reduction seems to have waned in absolute or percentage terms since the late 1960s while the overall level of early-age mortality remains high. In LDCs experiencing severe socioeconomic dislocation, often consequent on war, substantial rises in death rates have almost certainly occurred. However, the evidence generally contradicts Newland's (1981) assertion that since 1950 "in most of Africa and South Asia infant death rates have been static." In Africa among those few countries with data, in some such as Swaziland, recent progress

---

*England and Wales, during the latter half of the 19th century, exemplify a well-documented case where child mortality improved while infant mortality remained relatively constant.

may have been slow, but in others such as Kenya and Togo improvement has been quite substantial and sustained. In Latin America and Asia, it is encouraging that only two WFS surveys—those for Bangladesh and Guyana—found no real evidence of some decline since the late 1960s. And in many countries the declines implied by WFS were moderate to substantial (Hobcraft, 1981).

7. EARLY-AGE MORTALITY AND LEVELS OF PER CAPITA INCOME

Since early-age death rates and specifically infant mortality rates are often taken to be key indicators of "development," Figure 5 plots, for some countries with better recent data, estimated IMRs against estimated per capita incomes. Despite the difficulties involved in such a comparison, it is clear that the relationship is fairly weak, especially when the few higher-income LDCs shown in

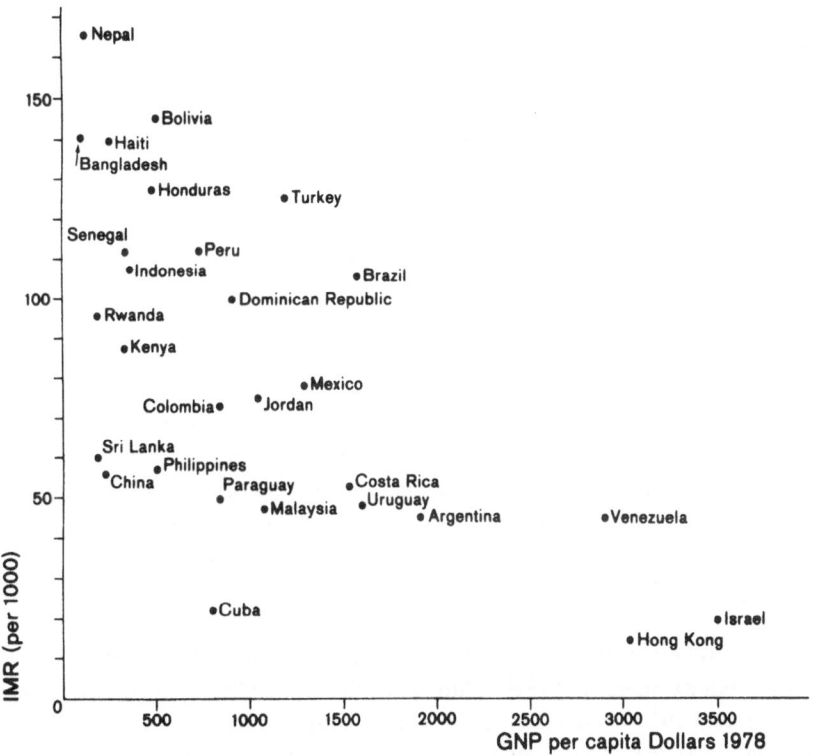

Figure 5.   Infant mortality plotted against per capita income for selected countries.

Figure 5 are excluded. For example, taking countries with per capita incomes below $250, we can compare China and Sri Lanka, with IMRs at or below 60, with Nepal, which has an estimated IMR of 166. Some very poor African countries almost certainly have higher levels of infant and child mortality than Nepal. Alternatively, comparing IMRs across income, Brazil experiences comparable infant mortality levels to Rwanda, but their estimated per capita incomes are $1500 and $180 respectively. If we were to introduce some of the newly oil-rich countries into the comparison, the exercise becomes almost bizarre. For example, for Saudi Arabia, the U.N. (1982) estimates the IMR at 121, while per capita income levels exceed $7500 (World Bank, 1980). Thus while, on balance, rising levels of living may engender lower early-age death rates, these benefits do not always appear to have yet fully translated through in some of the newly rich states. Taking income as a yardstick, the two centrally planned societies of China and Cuba perform well. So too does Sri Lanka and, perhaps more surprisingly, Paraguay and the Philippines. On the other hand, Costa Rica, which is often forwarded as a "superachiever" in health, performs less well on this criterion.

So while high incomes, well distributed throughout a population, probably do eventually ensure comparatively favorable early-age death rates, the relationship has clearly been short-circuited in some cases. To a considerable extent this is possible because, as will become apparent below, by any reasonable criteria the bulk of infant and child deaths in LDCs must be classified as technically preventable, and at relatively low cost.

8. INTRACOUNTRY VARIATION

We now consider variation in early-age mortality within LDCs. We begin by considering regional and urban–rural variation and go on to examine the influence of factors that may be more directly involved in the causal chain leading to an infant or child death. For the most part, we will consider variation in infant and child mortality together. Later, however, we briefly deal with circumstances in which these two components of mortality under age 5 do not necessarily vary either to the same degree or in the same direction.

8.1. Regional Variation

Geographic disparities in early-age mortality within LDCs can be very great indeed. For example, in Brazil estimates of the probability of dying before age 2 ($_2q_0$) around 1970 ranged from 0.055 in the south to 0.208 in the northeast region (Carvalho, 1974). The latter figure is comparable to many for countries in Africa. Again, both infant and child death rates tend to be much higher in northern than in southern India. To take the extremes, recent estimates of $_2q_0$ vary from 0.085 in Kerala to 0.236 in Uttar Pradesh (Dyson, 1982). Adegbola (1977) presents estimates for Tanzania, Mozambique, Zaire, Gabon, and Chad, all of which indicate very substantial areal variation.

It would be quite wrong to think that marked regional differentials are found only in large countries. Thus a comparable degree of areal variation has been found within the small territory of western Gambia (Samateh, 1981). On the other hand, within a fairly large country such as Bangladesh, levels of early-age mortality are high and fairly invariant across most districts (Blacker *et al.*, 1977).

It is increasingly felt that such regional variation may sometimes be of long standing and may often reflect the geographic distribution of ethnic groups—for example, tribes in Africa or indigenous peoples in some areas of Latin America (Behm, 1979). Obviously many factors may be relevant in explaining such differentials, including differences in natural environment. But whatever the causes, it is important to bear such variation in mind. For example, WFS results give an IMR of 79 for the Sudan (Hobcraft *et al.*, 1982). Such a figure appears implausibly low, but it transpires that, unusually, the WFS survey in Sudan was conducted only in certain parts of the country.

8.2. Urban–Rural Variation

Early-age death rates by urban–rural residence almost always show lower mortality in urban areas. But this relationship is little explored and probably more complicated than is often entertained. Examining Algerian data, Tabutin (1976) found that the really significant differential was between a few large cities on the one hand, in which the IMR averaged 100, and the remainder of the country (rural plus smaller urban areas) on the other, where infant mortality was 50% higher. Relatedly, where they can be measured, early-age death rates in Africa's major cities (e.g., Freetown or Nairobi) are often substantially lower than a simple urban–rural cross-tabulation for the country as a whole would imply (Vallin, 1976). Similarly the usual aggregation of data for all urban areas combined may hide the fact that mortality in the appalling slum conditions of large cities may sometimes actually be higher than that in rural areas. Primary towns, particularly capital cities, usually house a nation's rich and educated elite, whose early-age mortality may approach that of more developed populations. Typically such cities contain a concentration of medical facilities. These benefit most of those sections of the population for whom they are accessible—generally the middle classes. Primary cities also usually have much better provision for piped water and sanitation.

Some of these complexities have been documented for Brazil. There, in several states, both 1970 and 1980 census CEB/CS data shows higher urban than rural early-age mortality. Carvalho and Wood (1978) have shown that for middle and upper income groups in Brazil, early-age mortality is lower in urban areas. But for the bulk of the population on lower incomes, the reverse is true.* The urban poor often have very limited access to medical services, suffer from crowding as well as poor toilet and water facilities, and may also practice less breast-feeding than rural populations. As already noted, some writers connect apparent IMR rises in Brazilian cities with declining real incomes.

Data from elsewhere in Latin America—El Salvador, Puerto Rico, and Haiti—also hint at roughly comparable levels of urban and rural child mortality (U.N., 1980; Hobcraft *et al.*, 1982). This may be related to the particularly rapid urban growth experienced in this region.

8.3. Maternal Education

Maternal education has been found to be by far the most important of household socioeconomic characteristics in explaining variation in levels of early-age mortality. The relationship is almost universally negative and generally seems to be somewhat stronger at educational levels beyond just 2 or 3 years of schooling.† Studies tend to indicate that for a given amount of maternal education, levels of early-age mortality drop faster in urban than in rural areas (Baum and Arriaga, 1981). Relatedly, many surveys indicate a much greater degree of health service utilization among more educated mothers (e.g., see, Caldwell and Orubuloye, 1975).

Multivariate analysis almost always confirms the primacy of maternal education among socioeconomic variables. Thus WFS material shows that level of maternal education usually precedes paternal education in order of importance in explaining variation in early-age mortality (except, interestingly, in a few patriarchal Asian societies where the order is reversed). But both paternal and maternal educational level appear to be much more influential than, say, the employment status of the mother (Hobcraft *et al.*, 1982). Perhaps this should be not surprising, since the nature of any expected relationship between early-age mortality and maternal work status is not clear: work may give women some independent income and perhaps broaden their horizons, but it can also impede mother–child contacts. More remarkable is the implication from analysis of Mexican data (Hobcraft, 1981) that maternal education can have an even more important effect on a youngster's life chances than the presence or absence of proper toilet facilities. As Caldwell (1979) has written of an analogous study of

---

*Again, however, CEB/CS material requires careful interpretation. Also, real incomes in rural areas may be higher than money values indicate.

†In fact, this may not be the case. The implication (found in many instances) may be spurious if response errors—particularly failure to record dead children—are greater among those women with no schooling than among those with only 2 or 3 years.

Nigerian data, in explaining early age mortality "a woman's education is a good deal more important than even her most immediate environment."

In view of the potential policy significance of such findings, surprisingly little effort seems to have been made to explore the nature of the relationship involved. For example, is maternal education itself the important factor, or does it merely reflect more fundamental differences between women in their overall status? To what extent is the specific health content of education operative—for example, as regards teaching the importance of breast-feeding, cleanliness, and diet? Alternatively, is education working through increased levels of female literacy? Caldwell (1981) forwards three interrelated explanations. First, more educated women are less fatalistic about their children's illnesses. Second, they are more capable of manipulating available health facilities and personnel. And certainly many studies do show that better-educated women in LDCs are much more likely to have received antenatal care, to have given birth with some medical attendance, and to have taken their children at some time to see a physician (e.g., see WHO, 1981a, 1981b; Dyson, 1981). Finally and, according to Caldwell, probably most important, female education has profound effects on child care inasmuch as it alters the traditional balance of intrafamily relationships. For example, a woman with several years of schooling is much more likely to challenge her mother-in-law or family patriarch. Hence she can better exercise her natural indulgence toward her children or see that they receive attention should they fall ill.

8.4. Birth Order, Birth Interval, and Maternal Age

Data from several countries in the inter-American study, such as those for El Salvador in Table VI, indicate that infant mortality increases with birth order (when age is controlled) and decreases with age (when birth order is controlled). Both effects tend to be more pronounced the higher the level of early-age mortality prevailing in the population. As can be seen, the combined effect is usually a U-shaped relationship of IMR with maternal age.

The importance of birth interval may be even greater than that of either birth order or maternal age. The WFS Nepalese survey showed that the IMR for births occurring after an interval of 34–60 months was less than half that of births occurring after an interval of only 8–23 months (Thapa and Retherford, 1982). Similar work on Ecuadorean data led Wolfers and Scrimshaw (1975) to write that infant mortality in such circumstances might be halved if birth intervals shorter than 27 months could be avoided. Such an assessment is probably too optimistic, since it neglects the fact that women experiencing short birth intervals probably also have other characteristics making for higher infant mortality. Nevertheless, the magnitude of IMR variation by birth interval and birth order certainly supports their suggestion that postpartum prescription of contraception might be-

Table VI
IMR by Birth Order and Mother's Age, El Salvador[a]

Birth order	Age of mother					Total mothers (all ages)
	Under 20	20–24	25–29	30–34	35+	
1	90	44	31	27	43	61
2	162	69	40	24	18	72
3	335	102	53	46	42	81
4		196	68	37	45	87
5		318	86	57	75	97
6			204	74	79	127
7			349	131	61	137
8				292	110	220
9 and over					301	427
Total	117	84	73	81	94	88

[a]Source: Puffer and Serrano (1975).

come routine. And the fact that, Africa aside, fertility is declining in most LDCs is one encouraging sign for the future course of early-age mortality trends.

8.5. Breast-Feeding

Shorter durations of breast-feeding tend to result in shorter birth intervals (Jain *et al.*, 1970). And, of course, the death of an infant or child that is still breast-feeding can bring forward the date of the next live birth. But clearly there are other reasons why shorter durations of breast-feeding may increase the risk of death for those youngsters already alive. A mother's milk is nutritious, passes antibodies to the feeding infant, and helps avoid exposing it to bacteriologically hazardous or insufficient foods. On the other hand, beyond 4 to 6 months of age, breast milk by itself becomes nutritionally inadequate for the child—sooner if the mother is malnourished (Ashworth, 1982). Interestingly, in several LDCs where breast-feeding is widespread, rates of weight gain lag behind international growth standards by several months (Waterlow *et al.*, 1980).

Really satisfactory studies of the relationship between early-age mortality and breast-feeding are practically nonexistent. Complex two-way interactions are involved in which, for example, an early-age death may partly result from or partly bring about an early cessation of breast-feeding. Also, large numbers of observations are required and, particularly in rural Africa and Asia, breast-feeding tends to be both almost universal and prolonged.*

*Yet as we have seen, early-age death rates in these areas can still be very high indeed.

Newland (1981) cites a number of small studies, in Papua New Guinea, Chile, and the Philippines which suggest that death rates tend to be higher among youngsters that are weaned earlier. In Kabul, children who had completed breast-feeding and died before age 5 had a mean duration of breast-feeding of 14.4 months, compared with 16.9 months for those who survived (Dyson, 1981). The inter-American study showed that diarrheal disease was far more prevalent among children who were artificially fed (Puffer and Serrano, 1973). But in Sine-Saloum, Senegal, contrary to expectation, the average age of weaning for children who died was greater than for surviving youngsters—the figures were 25.6 and 24.3 months respectively (Cantrelle and Leridon, 1971). The researchers speculate that breast-feeding may be prolonged for offspring of delicate health.

An alarming finding of the inter-American study was an unexpectedly widespread failure to breast-feed as well as its early termination in several Latin American countries (Puffer and Serrano, 1973). Elsewhere in the developing world, studies generally indicate that the length of time women breast-feed increases with maternal age. But it is not always clear whether this means that breast-feeding patterns are deteriorating among younger women, although one fears that this is often the case.

On balance there can be little doubt that widespread and lengthy breast-feeding keeps early-age death rates in many LDCs lower than they would otherwise be. Especially for the first few months of infancy, breast-feeding partially insulates a baby from some harmful environmental influences. As we elaborate briefly below, to some degree this reduces the extent to which we find differentials in infant as opposed to child mortality in LDCs. Relatedly, the period around weaning is a time of special susceptibility. In some societies, cessation of breast-feeding can occur very abruptly. Also, weaning diets are often contaminated and inadequate. Hence the age at which children are weaned from the breast can influence the age pattern of mortality. Thus in west Africa, heavy child mortality—especially in the second year of life—relative to mortality in infancy, may partly reflect lengthy breast-feeding. Conversely, the relatively early age of weaning found in Latin America has been cited to explain the high levels of infant mortality found there relative to mortality at ages 1–4 (Palloni, 1981).

Finally, to complete the circle, since one factor precipitating the end of breast-feeding is the arrival of a new baby, we might expect the survival chances of the first child of a pair to be reduced when the arrival of a new baby interrupts breast-feeding—again, especially if the birth interval is short. After all, kwashiorkor is often thought of as a malady affecting the elder of two such children. This effect has been little studied. But it has been detected by Wolfers and Scrimshaw (1975) in data from Ecuador.

8.6. Birth Weight

Turning to consider early-age mortality according to the characteristics of the infants and children themselves, an infant's survival chances in particular are almost certainly highly influenced by its birth weight. However, again, large-scale, well-designed studies on the subject are rare. Particularly valuable was the Algiers study (WHO, 1981a). This found that the proportion of infants weighing less than 2½ kg at birth was five times higher among under-5 deaths than among children that survived.

In developing countries the problem is not so much one of premature births as of low-birth-weight full-term babies (Petros-Barvazian and Behar, 1978). In parts of India and Bangladesh about 50% of all live births weigh less than 2½ kg. A figure of about 10% seems to be applicable in Latin America (WHO, 1980). Low birth weights may result from maternal malnutrition and possibly shorter birth intervals (although average birth intervals in the Indian subcontinent are not particularly short). According to Ashworth (1982), most studies indicate that food supplementation during pregnancy can increase average birthweights and reduce the proportion of low-weight births. She calculates that modest supple-mentation in Bangladesh might reduce infant mortality by up to 30%. However, again, we cannot really be sure that such a major improvement would result. Low birth weights almost certainly occur differentially to particularly deprived mothers, and the IMR differentials by birth weight assumed in Ashworth's calculations may reflect the influence of a complex of other factors that are also associated with low birth weights. However, this said, both the general promi-nence accorded by Ashworth to low birth weights in explaining high early-age mortality in LDCs and her call for more research seem fully justified.

8.7. Single or Multiple Births

In LDCs as elsewhere, the great majority of deliveries result in the birth of one infant. But many studies show that multiple births in developing countries are markedly more at risk of death than are singletons. For example in rural Senegal, Cantrelle and Leridon (1971) found that the probability of a twin dying in the first three months after birth was a staggering 0.294, compared with 0.073 for a single birth.

8.8. Sex of Child

Early-age death rates in LDCs vary according to the sex of the child. In sub-Saharan Africa and most of Latin America, the differential is slightly to the advantage of females. This is consistent with the general view that the biological risk of dying is higher among males. However, currently or in the fairly recent past, a marginal differential in the opposite direction has prevailed in North Africa and, less certainly, parts of Latin America [e.g., Mexico (U.N., 1980) and Ecuador (Scrimshaw, 1978)]. In large areas of western south Asia—stretching across through Pakistan and the northern states of India to Bangladesh—current early-age death rates are often very much higher for females, especially in rural areas. For example, in the north Indian state of Uttar Pradesh, $_2q_0$ has been estimated at 0.249 for males and 0.311 for females (Dyson, 1982).

Several surveillance studies throw light on the causes of this phenomenon. Using Matlab data, Chen *et al.* (1981) found that much higher percentages of girls were moderately or severely malnourished. Female calorie and protein consumption levels were found to be well below those of males. And female intake levels were poorer even allowing for sex differentials in biological requirements. Interestingly, differentials in morbidity by sex (e.g., the number of diarrheal or respiratory disease episodes experienced) were almost nonexistent. But when male offspring fell sick, they were nearly twice as likely to be taken for treatment. Similar findings on sex differentials in intrafamilial food distribution and provision of medical care were detailed for the Punjab by the classic Khanna study (Wyon and Gordon, 1971).

Such results are suggestive of the importance, at some level, of social preferences in the nexus of factors conditioning early-age death rates in some LDCs. In Scrimshaw's (1978) controversial view, early-age mortality is often either an unconscious or even overt way by which people in very difficult circumstances attain a given family size or composition. In her words, "every possible effort may not be made to prevent some child deaths"—for example, of female births, multiple births, or births at higher orders.

9. CAUSES OF EARLY-AGE DEATHS

Infectious and parasitic diseases play the major role in accounting for high early-age death rates in LDCs. Indeed, the presence or absence of these two broad cause-of-death categories has been shown to largely differentiate between countries with high and low early-age mortality, (Preston, 1972). Those LDCs with favorable infant and child death rates have cause of death mixes comparable to developed countries. Thus in Hong Kong and Singapore accidents, congenital defects and neoplasms dominate (Arriaga, 1979). In Louwan district of Shanghai in 1978, over 35% of infant deaths were attributed to congenital defects (Jiang and Karkal, 1981).

In countries with heavy early-age mortality the importance of individual infectious and parasitic diseases appears to be quite variable. But everywhere varieties of diarrheal disease are major killers. It has been estimated that about one of every ten children born in less developed regions dies of diarrhea before reaching age 5 (Parker *et al.*, 1980). Pneumonia is another major cause of death. Together enteritis and pneumonia account for about 40% of infant deaths registered in Brazil (Yunes, 1981). Gastritis–enteritis was found to be the major underlying cause of death in both infancy and childhood in the inter-American study areas (Puffer and Serrano, 1973). A similar picture emerges from the other WHO studies (WHO 1981a, 1981b, Dyson 1981). Matlab data on child morbidity shows that both infants and 1-year-olds can expect to suffer about five episodes of diarrhea and ten episodes of respiratory infection annually (Chen *et al.*, 1981). But while diarrheal disease and pneumonia are always important, they do not always predominate. In Uttar Pradesh one study attributed 43% of infant deaths to neonatal tetanus (Simmons *et al.*, 1978). And a recent nation-wide investigation in India ascribed 15% of infant deaths to this cause (Padmanabha, 1982).* In many LDCs measles can be the most common cause of death. In Kabul it was the major underlying cause of 1–4 deaths, accounting for 31 of 122 deaths observed (Dyson, 1981). A similar finding arose from the WHO survey in Sierra Leone (WHO, 1981b). Likewise in 6 of the 22 Latin American areas of the inter-American study, measles surpassed diarrheal disease in accounting for child deaths (Puffer and Serrano, 1973). Other important causes of early-age deaths include malaria, influenza, bronchitis, whoopingcough, tuberculosis, diphtheria, and accidents.

In addition, causes of death in infancy often reflect the circumstances of birth as well as the usual context of high levels of fertility. Thus tetanus is a major cause of infant and as opposed to child deaths. Likewise categories such as "immaturity," "other perinatal causes," and "asphyxia" tend to be prominent in infant as opposed to child deaths. In Kabul these causes combined were the underlying cause of death in 22% of infant deaths, but none at ages 1–4 (Dyson, 1981).

10. SYNERGISTIC INTERRELATIONS WITH MALNUTRITION

Although deaths due to "malnutrition" alone are comparatively rare, infectious and parasitic diseases often interact with nutritional deficiencies to bring about an early-age death. To appreciate this really requires a multiple cause-of-death classification. The inter-American study used such an approach. It showed that for all project areas combined, malnutrition or, relatedly, immaturity was implicated in some way in 57% of deaths under age 5 (Puffer and Serrano, 1973). In contrast, however, the recent Indian investigation gives virtually no

---

*Undoubtedly unhygienic birth practices among traditional birth attendants are responsible in large part.

idea of the likely importance of nutritional deficiency because it adopted only a single cause-of-death classification (Padmanabha, 1982).

Studies imply that the role of nutritional deficiency is marginally more important in early childhood than in infancy. To some extent this probably reflects the relative insulation provided by breast-feeding. The components and precise nature of the synergistic interrelationships involved can vary, although diarrheal disease is always an important part in the syndrome. A recent Matlab study assessed the nutritional status of children and their subsequent mortality (Chen et al., 1980). It found that mortality risks accompanying mild and moderate forms of malnutrition were similar to those experienced by normally nourished children. However, the death rate for those severely malnourished was 3.2 times higher than that for all other children. Indeed, if severely malnourished children were excluded, the overall child death rate dropped by some 45%. The risks of dying from diarrheal disease and measles were 3.7 and 2.3 times higher among the severely malnourished children than among the remainder.

While malnutrition may reduce a youngster's ability to cope with a disease attack, such disease episodes themselves constitute a major factor precipitating (or in the case of low-birth-weight babies, essentially sustaining) conditions of severe malnourishment. Again, many mechanisms are involved. Sick children lose their appetites and may have their food adversely changed or withdrawn altogether by well-meaning but ignorant parents. Infections may raise the body's demand for dietary protein; diarrheal diseases in particular tend to reduce the capacity to absorb nutrients while also leading to fluid and salt loss. Studies in Latin America (Drasar et al., 1981) have identified marked increases in numbers of children suffering from malnutrition after outbreaks of diarrhea (see also Morley et al., 1968). Related considerations may partly explain the very high levels of 1–4 mortality in West Africa. Thus Rowland (1979) compares Keneba data from Gambia with that for an east African community. The diet of the Gambian children is actually superior, but the incidence of diarrheal disease is much greater in Keneba. Largely as a consequence, the nutritional status of Keneba children is worse than that of their counterparts in East Africa at ages beyond 6 months. The greater incidence of diarrheal disease may be partly explained by more compact village structures, and more intimately shared (i.e., more polluted) water supplies. Perceptively, Rowland also notes that the agricultural labor demands of the east African women were less seasonal and hence less disruptive of patterns of child care.

11. FURTHER FACTORS

We have dealt with some of the more important variables generally associated with higher probabilities of early-age death. Many other factors are relevant but cannot be detailed here. For example, in Bangladesh mortality has been

found to be markedly higher in households living in more crowded and struc-
turally inferior dwellings (Chen *et al.*, 1980; Blacker *et al.*, 1977). In interpreting such findings, one must remember that dichotomous comparisons do not
necessarily imply causality. Thus those living in more crowded conditions are
also likely to be less educated and probably have above-average fertility. Moreover as we have seen, many factors may mediate between environmental conditions and an early-age death. However, several further aspects of the environment are particularly germane.

11.1. Water and Toilet Facilities

Several studies have found higher risks of early-age death in households
with poor water and toilet facilities. For example in the inter-American study the
incidence of diarrheal disease was lowest in households having piped drinking
water and flush toilet facilities (Puffer and Serrano, 1973). The recent Indian
study estimated the IMR at 63 in urban households where drinking water came
from a tap compared with 93 when water came from a well (Padmanabha, 1982).
In multivariate analysis of WFS data for Mexico and Sri Lanka, current access to
proper toilet facilities was found to influence infant mortality, especially beyond
the postneonatal stage (Hobcraft, 1981).

11.2. Health Service Availability

The increasing provision of health services by LDC governments has undoubtedly been a major factor behind the postwar reduction in early-age death
rates. Yet specific evaluations of their effectiveness are few. However, there is
little doubt that even in quite adverse conditions the introduction of health services of good caliber can result in quite sizable reductions in mortality. But such
services are often concentrated in urban areas and may have little effect outside
their immediate localities. In Nigeria, Caldwell and Orubuloye (1975) compared
two similar communities, one with and one without a health center. Women in
the community without a center had lost 39% of their ever-born live births,
compared with only 23% lost in the community with a health center.

11.3. Climatic Seasonality

Afflictions such as diarrheal disease, respiratory infections, malnutrition,
and malaria can be highly seasonal in character. So too, often, are relevant social
factors such as patterns of female employment, weaning, and diet. As a result
early-age deaths often tend to be concentrated at certain times of year [see the
various contributions in Chambers *et al.*, (1981)]. In Kabul, 20 of the 124 child
deaths observed happened in September, as did 30% of under-5 deaths where the

underlying cause was nutritional deficiency (Dyson, 1981). For Sine-Saloum, Cantrelle and Leridon (1971) show that the annual IMR might be 140 instead of 210 if a 3-month high-risk period could be eliminated. It seems likely that different degrees of seasonality play a role in explaining regional variations in early-age mortality in Africa (Rowland, 1979) and elsewhere.

12. INFANT VERSUS CHILD MORTALITY

While infant and child mortality are closely related, it should be clear that important distinctions remain. To reiterate, infant mortality, and especially neonatal mortality, is particularly conditioned by the circumstances of childbirth and the influence of breast-feeding. Hence general environmental factors probably play a slightly smaller role in infant than in child deaths—although, of course, neonatal mortality is also conditioned by the environmental circumstances of the mother prior to birth. We have noted that to some extent it is considerations of this kind that underlie the fact that the age pattern of mortality in LDCs can be quite variable.

These general conditions are important when one is examining early age mortality differentials. Vis-à-vis several of the variables we have discussed, mortality differentials may be of a different order in childhood than in infancy. Indeed, they may even be reversed. To list just a few examples, we have noted that regional mortality differentials within Africa are more pronounced at ages 1–4 than in infancy. During and after the Bangladesh war of independence, child death rates rose substantially, whereas neonatal mortality rates were relatively unaffected (Chowdhury and Chen, 1977). The seasonal distribution of infant deaths may be quite different to those aged 1–4 because the timing of the former can be highly affected by the seasonal distribution of births (e.g., see Becker and Sardar, 1981). In some areas, sex differentials in neonatal mortality may favor females, while the reverse is true for postneonatal and child mortality (WHO, 1981a). Analysis of WFS data tends to show that environmental influences such as maternal education or the presence or absence of good sanitary facilities are easier to identify when mortality during the first few months of life is set aside (Hobcraft *et al.*, 1982).

Finally a word is in order regarding the distribution of deaths by age. This is affected not only by the age pattern but also by the overall level of early-age mortality. In LDCs with very low death rates (e.g., Hong Kong, Singapore) early-age deaths overwhelmingly occur within infancy; within infancy, the vast majority (usually 70% or more) occur during the first month of life. But where death rates are high, a much smaller proportion of early-age deaths generally occur within either infancy or the neonatal period. For example in the remarkable data from Sine-Saloum, only 35% of infant deaths occurred during the first 3 months of life (Cantrelle and Leridon, 1971). Elsewhere in Africa, a majority of infant deaths occur during the postneonatal stage (ECA, 1979). However, as has recently been noted (Ashworth, 1981), there are exceptions, especially where neonatal tetanus is common. In this context recent Indian data indicate that a staggering 62% of infant deaths occur during the first month of life (Padmanabha, 1982).

13. CONCLUSION

Early-age mortality in LDCs is a very complex phenomenon; much remains to be learned. To some extent the complexities involved may have been obscured by the variable-by-variable approach we have adopted here. Let us therefore underscore the fact that the variables we have identified as making for high early-age death rates tend to be highly correlated in individuals—especially poor rural people. Many downward, "vicious circle," synergistic interactions are involved. To pinpoint just two: (1) diarrheal disease promotes malnutrition, which promotes diarrheal disease, and (2) high fertility promotes high early-age mortality, which promotes high fertility. Unraveling such complexities requires careful longitudinal studies, of which there are comparatively few.

Nevertheless, our understanding is improving. Within the last 5 to 10 years new data sets and new techniques have enabled us to better analyze levels, trends, and patterns of infant and child mortality. And our view of what factors condition and bring about a reduction in early-age mortality has become wider and more informed. We now know that some measure of postwar improvement has been well nigh universal in the developing world. And in many LDCs progress has been substantial. Further, we now appreciate that the attainment of low levels of early-age mortality does not necessarily require "development" in the narrow economic sense. In particular, there is considerable evidence to suggest that more widespread female education coupled with a greater provision of basic health services could be an especially potent combination. Specific low-cost simple interventions such as oral rehydration therapy, routine vaccination, maternal food supplementation, and the promotion of methods of fertility control can also be powerful weapons. However, introduced by themselves they may have an impact below their full potential, given the complex synergistic interrelationships involved. Indeed, one suspects that the emergence of maternal education as an important variable partly reflects the fact that it can potentially influence behavior in many aspects of both infant and child care.

But while most early-age deaths in the developing world must be considered preventable, at least from a technical viewpoint, the promotion of the necessary kinds of social and health policies required for really substantial improvement has evidently not been forthcoming in some LDCs. In such countries the future reduction of infant and child death rates may prove much more difficult than did any past progression. And in this light, the attainment of the U.N. objective of halving the infant mortality rate in the developing world by the end of the century must be considered unlikely.

REFERENCES

Adegbola, O., 1977, New estimates of fertility and child mortality in Africa south of the Sahara, *Popul. Stud.* 31:467–486.

Arriaga, E. E., 1979, Infant and child mortality in selected Asian countries, in: *Proceedings of the Meeting on Socioeconomic Determinants and Consequences of Mortality*, El Colegio de Mexico, Mexico City, June 1979, p. 98.

Ashworth, A., 1982, International differences in infant mortality and the impact of malnutrition: A review, *Hum. Nutr. Clin. Nutr.* 36:7–23.

Banister, J., and Preston, S. H., 1981, Mortality in China, *Popul. Dev. Rev.* 7:98–110.

Barclay, G. W., 1958, *Techniques of Population Analysis*, Wiley, New York.

Baum, S., and Arriaga, E. E., 1981, Levels, trends, differentials and causes of infant and early childhood mortality in Latin America, *World Health Stat. Q.* 34:147–167.

Becker, S., and Sardar, M. A., 1981, Seasonal patterns of vital events in Matlab Thana, Bangladesh, in: *Seasonal Dimensions to Rural Poverty* (R. Chambers, R. Longhurst, and A. Pacey, eds.), Frances Pinter (Publishers) Ltd., London, p. 149.

Behm, H., 1979, Socioeconomic determinants of mortality in Latin America, in: *Proceedings of the Meeting on Socioeconomic Determinants and Consequences of Mortality*, El Colegio de Mexico, Mexico City, June 1979, p. 139.

Blacker, J. G. C., 1978, *Report on the 1976 Swaziland Population Census*, vol. 1, Central Statistical Office, Mbabane, Swaziland.

Blacker, J. G. C., 1979, Mortality in Tropical Africa: the Demographer's Viewpoint, paper presented to the Conference on Medical Aspects of African Demography, Peterhouse, Cambridge, England, September 1979.

Blacker, J. G. C., Devis, T. L. F., Hill, K. H., Dyson, T., and Khan, M. A., 1977, *Report on the 1974 Bangladesh Retrospective Study of Fertility and Mortality*, Population Bureau, Ministry of Overseas Development, London.

Brass, W., Coale, A. J., Demeny, P., Heisel, D. F., Lorimer, F., Romaniuk, A., and Van de Walle, E., 1968, *The Demography of Tropical Africa*, Princeton University Press, Princeton, N.J.

Brazil, 1979, *Anuario Estatistico do Brazil*, Secretaria de Planejamento da Presidencia da Republica, Fundacao Instituto Brazileiro de Geografia e Estatistica.

Bucht, B., and Chamie, J., 1982, Estimates and Projections of Infant Mortality Rates, paper presented to the 1982 Annual Meeting of the Population Association of America, San Diego, Calif., May 1982.

Caldwell, J. C., 1979, Education as a factor in mortality decline: An examination of Nigerian data, in: *Proceedings of the Meeting on Socioeconomic Determinants and Consequences of Mortality*, El Colegio de Mexico, Mexico City, June 1979, p. 172.

Caldwell, J. C., 1981, Maternal education as a factor in child mortality, *World Health Forum* 2:75–78.

Caldwell, J. C., and Orubuloye, O., 1975, Impact of public health services on mortality, *Popul. Stud.* 29:259–272.

Cantrelle, P., and Leridon, H., 1971, Breastfeeding, mortality in childhood and fertility in a rural zone of Senegal, *Popul. Stud.* 25:503.

Carvalho, J. A. M., 1974, Regional trends in fertility and mortality in Brazil, *Popul. Stud.* 28:401–421.

Carvalho, J. A. M., and Wood, C. H., 1978, Mortality, income distribution, and rural-urban residence in Brazil, *Popul. Dev. Rev.* 4:405–420.

Chambers, R., Longhurst, R., and Pacey, A., 1981, *Seasonal Dimensions to Rural Poverty*, Frances Pinter (Publishers) Ltd., London.

Chen, L. C., Chowdhury, A. K. M., and Huffman, S. L., 1980, Anthropometric assessment of energy-protein malnutrition and subsequent risk of mortality among preschool aged children, *Am. J. Clin. Nutr.* 31:1836–1845.

Chen, L. C., Huq, E., and D'Souza, S., 1981, Sex bias in the family allocation of food and health care in rural Bangladesh, *Population and Development Rev.* 7:55–70.

Chowdhury, A. K. M., and Chen, L. C., 1977, The dynamics of contemporary famine, in *Proceedings of the International Population Conference*, Mexico, published by the International Union for the Scientific Study of Population, Liege, Belgium.

Coale, A. J., and Demeny, P., 1966, *Regional Model Life Tables and Stable Populations*, Princeton University Press, Princeton, N.J.

Drasar, B. S., Tomkins, A. M., and Feachem, R. G., 1981, Diarrheal diseases, in: *Seasonal Dimensions to Rural Poverty* (R. Chambers, R. Longhurst, and A. Pacey, eds.), Frances Pinter (Publishers) Ltd., London, p. 102.

Dyson, T., 1977, Levels, trends, differentials and causes of child mortality—A survey, *World Health Stat. Q.* 30:282–311.

Dyson, T., 1981, Infant, child and maternal mortality and associated conditions of health in the Greater Kabul region of Afghanistan, *World Health Stat. Q.* 34:14–43.

Dyson, T., 1982, India's Regional Demography, Department of Population Studies, London School of Economics, London (Mimeographed).

ECA (Economic Commission for Africa), 1979, Mortality differentials and their correlates in Africa, in: *Proceedings of the Meeting on Socioeconomic Determinants and Consequences of Mortality*, El Colegio de Mexico, Mexico City, June 1979, p. 208.

Eblen, J. E., 1981, Current Assessments and Prospects for Mortality Decline in Africa, prepared at the Division of Health Statistics, World Health Organisation, Geneva (Mimeographed).

Farah, A. A., and Preston, S. H., 1982, Child mortality differentials in Sudan, *Popul. Dev. Rev.* 8:365–383.

Feeney, G., 1980, Estimation of mortality trends from child survivorship data, *Popul. Stud.* 34:109–128.

Gaisie, S. K., 1975, Levels and patterns of infant and child mortality in Ghana, *Demography* 12:21–34.

Gwatkin, D., 1980, Indications of change in developing country mortality trends: The end of an era? *Popul. Dev. Rev.* 7:615–644.

Heligman, L., Finch, G., and Kramer, R., 1978, *Measurement of Infant Mortality in Less Developed Countries*, International Research Document No. 5, Bureau of the Census, U.S. Department of Commerce, Washington, D.C.

Hobcraft, J., 1981, Use of Special Mortality Questions in Fertility Surveys—The WFS Experience, paper presented to a UN/WHO Working Group on Data Bases for Measurement of Levels, Trends and Differentials in Mortality, Bangkok, October 1981.

Hobcraft, J., McDonald, J., and Rutstein, S., 1982, Socioeconomic Factors in Infant and Child Mortality: A Cross-national Comparison, World Fertility Survey, London. (Mimeographed)

India (various years), *Sample Registration Bulletin*, published biannually by the Office of the Registrar General, New Delhi.

India, 1974, *Fertility Differentials in India, 1972*, published by the Office of the Registrar General, New Delhi.

Jain, A. K., Hsu, T. C., Freedman, R., and Chang, M. C., 1970, Demographic aspects of lactation and postpartum amenorrhea, *Demography* 7:255–271.

Jiang, Z., and Karkal, M., 1981, Mortality decline in China, in: *Dynamics of Population and Family Welfare, 1981* (K. Srinivasan and S. Mukerji, eds.), Himalaya Publishing House, Bombay.

McGregor, I. A., Rahman, A. K., Thomson, A. M., Billewicz, W. Z., and Thompson, B., 1970, The health of young children in a West African (Gambian) village, *Trans. Roy. Soc. Trop. Med. Hyg.* 64:48–77.

Morley, D. C., Bicknell, J., and Woodland, M., 1968, Factors influencing the growth and nutritional status of infants and young children in a Nigerian village, *Trans. Roy. Soc. Trop. Med. Hyg.* 62:164–199.

Newland, K., 1981, Infant Mortality and the Health of Societies, Worldwatch Paper 47, Worldwatch Institute, Washington, D.C.

Padmanabha, P., 1982, Mortality in India: A note on trends and implications, *Economic and Political Weekly (Bombay)* 17:1285–1290.

Palloni, A., 1981, A review of infant mortality trends in selected underdeveloped countries: Some new estimates *Popul. Stud.* 35:100–119.

Parker, R. L., Rinehart, M. P. H., Piotrow, P. T., and Doucette, L., 1980, *Oral Rehydration Therapy (ORT) for Childhood Diarrhea,* Population Reports, series L, number 2, The Johns Hopkins University, Baltimore.

Petros-Barvazian, A., and Behar, M., 1978, Low birth weight—A major global problem, *Ambio* 7:157–167.

Preston, S. H., 1972, Influence of cause of death structure on age-patterns of mortality, in: *Population Dynamics* (T. N. E. Greville, ed.), Academic Press, New York.

Puffer, R. P., and Serrano, C. B., 1973, *Patterns of Mortality in Childhood,* PAHO Scientific Publication No. 262, Washington, D.C.

Puffer, R. P., and Serrano, C. B., 1975, *Birthweight, Maternal Age, and Birth Order: Three Important Determinants in Infant Mortality,* PAHO, Washington, D.C.

Rowland, M. G. M., 1979, Dietary and Environmental Factors in Child Mortality in the Gambia and Uganda, paper presented to a Conference on Medical Aspects of African Demography, Peterhouse, Cambridge, England, September 1979.

Samateh, L., 1981, Demographic Variation in the Gambia, M.Sc. dissertation, London School of Economics, London.

Scrimshaw, S. C. M., 1978, Infant mortality and behavior in the regulation of family size, *Popul. Dev. Rev.* 4:383–403.

Simmons, G., Smucker, C., Misra, B. D., and Majumdar, P., 1978, Patterns and causes of infant mortality in rural Uttar Pradesh, *J. Trop. Pediatr.* 24:207–216.

Singapore, 1979, *Report on the Registration of Births, Deaths and Marriages,* The Republic of Singapore.

Sri Lanka, 1981, *Statistical Pocket Book of the Democratic Socialist Republic of Sri Lanka,* Ministry of Plan Implementation, Colombo.

Tabutin, D., 1976, *Mortalité infantile et juvenile en Algérie,* Institut National D'Etudes Demographiques, Paris.

Thapa, S., and Retherford, R. D., 1982, Infant mortality estimates based on the 1976 Nepal fertility survey, *Popul. Stud.* 36:61–80.

Trussell, T. J., 1975, A re-estimation of the multiplying factors for the Brass technique for determining childhood survivorship rates, *Popul. Stud.* 29:97–107.

U.N., 1980, *Demographic Yearbook, 1979,* Department of International Economic and Social Affairs, United Nations, New York.

U.N., 1981, *International Development Strategy for the Third United Nations Development Decade,* United Nations, New York.

U.N., 1982, Infant Mortality: World Estimates and Projections, 1950–2025, *Popul. Bull. U.N.* 14:31–53.

Vallin, J., 1976, World trends in infant mortality since 1950, *World Health Statistics Report,* 29:646–674.

Waterlow, J. C., Ashworth, A., and Griffiths, M., 1980, Faltering in infant growth in less-developed countries, *Lancet* 2:1176–1177.

WHO, 1980, The incidence of low birth weight: a critical review of available information, *World Health Stat. Q.* 33:197–224.

WHO, 1981a, Infant and juvenile mortality at Algiers, *World Health Stat. Q.* 34:44–63.

WHO, 1981b, Summary of the ad hoc survey on infant and early childhood mortality in Sierra Leone, *World Health Stat. Q.* 34:220–238.

Wolfers, D., and Scrimshaw, S., 1975, Child survival and intervals between pregnancies in Guayauil, Ecuador, *Popul. Stud.* 29:479–496.

World Bank, 1980, *World Development Report,* 1980, The World Bank, Washington, D.C.

Wyon, J., and Gordon, J. B., 1971, *The Khanna Study: Population Problems in the Rural Punjab,* Harvard University Press, Cambridge, Mass.

Yunes, J., 1981, Evolution of infant mortality and proportional infant mortality in Brazil, *World Health Stat. Q.* 34:200–219.

3

Oral Rehydration Therapy

DILIP MAHALANABIS

1. INTRODUCTION

Acute diarrheal diseases are among the leading causes of childhood mortality and morbidity in developing countries and contribute significantly to malnutrition. A critical review (Snyder and Merson, 1982) of 27 active surveillance studies conducted for a year or more suggests that about 750 million children below 5 years of age in Asia, Africa, and Latin America suffer from acute diarrhea and between 3 and 6 million of them die annually.

The scientific development of oral rehydration therapy (ORT) for the treatment of acute diarrhea is a major therapeutic advance. Since the demonstration (Phillips, 1964) in a few actively purging adult cholera patients that an orally administered glucose-containing electrolyte solution induced significant absorption of sodium and water from the small bowel lumen, leading to their net positive balance, a series of careful studies in the late 1960s and 1970s in adults and children with acute diarrhea established the practical usefulness of ORT and defined the optimum composition of glucose or sucrose based oral rehydration solutions (ORSs). ORT has emerged as a powerful therapeutic tool and is capable of doing away with the need for I.V. therapy in 80–90% of those clinically dehydrated patients with acute diarrhea of diverse etiology who would have received I.V. therapy if treated according to conventional criteria.

Furthermore, the World Health Organization (WHO) in 1971 began recommending a specific ORS (see section 2.4.1. below). This ORS has been successfully adapted and extensively tested, under controlled hospital conditions as well

DILIP MAHALANABIS • Kothari Centre of Gastroenterology, The Calcutta Medical Research Institute, Calcutta-700027, India.

as in the field, to meet the varying needs of rehydration therapy in patients of all ages—infants, children, and adults—suffering from acute diarrheas due to many etiologic agents (e.g., rotavirus, enterotoxigenic *Escherichia coli*, *Vibrio cholerae*, *Shigella* and *Salmonella* species, and others). In the vast majority of patients it is effective in spite of vomiting when given in small amounts at short intervals, the amounts absorbed being a good deal more than the amounts usually lost. ORT has been identified as one of the few technically simple and widely applicable therapeutic interventions that can substantially reduce mortality from diarrhea in infants and children; it has emerged as a powerful public health weapon.

ORT has made it possible for WHO to undertake an immediate and global diarrheal diseases control program (CDD) with the immediate or short-term objective of reducing deaths from acute diarrhea and diarrhea associated malnutrition. Furthermore, ORT serves as an effective entry point for the promotion of appropriate child-care and environmental health practices for reducing morbidity, which is the long-term goal of this program. Readers are referred to a few recent reviews (Hirschhorn, 1980; Anonymous, 1980a; Mahalanabis, 1981b).

2. EVOLUTION OF ORT

2.1. Early Empirical Use of ORT

In 1949 Darrow suggested that an electrolyte solution containing glucose and given by mouth could supplement parenteral therapy of infantile diarrhea. Harison (1954) documented the composition of the ORS that was in use for some time in the hospitals of Baltimore, in the United States, to treat milder cases of diarrhea at the outpatient level. Its composition was Na^+, 64; K^+, 20; Cl^-, 54; lactate, 30; and glucose, 167—all in millimoles per liter of water. In Calcutta, India (Chatterjee, 1953), 186 adult cholera patients with relatively mild dehydration were successfully treated with an oral glucose electrolyte solution. The rationale for adding glucose at that time was to prevent ketosis and to provide some calories. These early workers did not critically evaluate how well the salts and water administered orally are absorbed from the small intestine during active diarrhea. Subsequently, numerous commercial formulations were used in the 1950s and 1960s for oral replacement therapy in mild diarrhea in infants and small children. Many of them had high concentrations of glucose and/or other sugars (for palatability), which are liable to cause osmotic water loss and predispose infants and small children to hypernatremia (discussed below). *The foregoing studies predate any deliberate application of the relevant discoveries*

*in basic science, such as glucose-linked enhanced sodium absorption which are
the basis of modern ORT.*

2.2. Glucose-Linked Enhanced Sodium Absorption and Its Early
     Application in ORT

As early as 1902, studies by Reid using dog intestinal loops demonstrated
that intraluminal glucose enhances sodium absorption from the mammalian small
intestine. These findings were confirmed by Barany and Sperber (1939). Riklis
and Quastel (1958) showed that sodium ion was essential for *in vitro* absorption
of glucose. Subsequent detailed studies on the effects of different sodium concentrations on the kinetics of glucose absorption have been reviewed (Czaky,
1963; Crane, 1965). *In vitro* studies also demonstrated that glucose stimulated
sodium transport across the small intestinal mucosa (Schultz and Zalusky, 1964;
and Barry *et al.*, 1965). Schedl and Clifton (1963) demonstrated a dramatic
improvement in sodium, chloride, and water absorption from Ringer's solution
by adding 1% glucose in both jejunum and ileum of normal human subjects,
using transintestinal intubation techniques.Subsequent *in vivo* studies in normal
human small intestine further defined the quantitative relationships of glucose-
linked enhanced sodium and water absorption (Malawar *et al.*, 1965; Levinson
and Schell, 1966; Fordtran *et al.*, 1968).

The first evidence that glucose-linked enhanced sodium and water absorption remains largely intact in humans during acute diarrhea was first produced by
Phillips (1964) in a few severely purging adult cholera patients. Further definitive studies of great practical usefulness (Pierce *et al.*, 1968b; Hirschhorn *et al.*,
1968; Nalin *et al.*, 1968, Pierce *et al.*, 1969) showed that even in the severest
form of watery diarrhea such as cholera, fluid and electrolyte losses could be
adequately replaced by an optimally constitued oral electrolyte solution containing glucose. Carpenter *et al.* (1968) showed that, in canine jejunal and ileal
Thiry-Vella loops challenged with crude cholera toxin, net sodium and water loss
was reduced when glucose was added to the perfusion electrolyte solution.
Radioactive tracer studies in patients with cholera showed that 2% glucose induced net absorption of sodium and water (Taylor *et al.*, 1968) from the small
intestine.

A series of carefully controlled clinical trials established ORT as a powerful
therapeutic tool in treating diarrheal dehydration in children with cholera (Mahalanabis *et al.*, 1974; Sack *et al.*, 1980a); in infants and small children with
rotavirus-induced and enterotoxigenic *E. coli*-induced (Nalin *et al.*, 1978, 1979,
1980; Patra *et al.*, 1982a,b) diarrhea and in infantile diarrhea of multiple
etiologies (Hirschhorn *et al.*, 1972; 1973; Chatterjee *et al.*, 1977, 1978; Patra *et
al.*, 1982b,c). A crucial demonstration of the effectiveness of ORT was provided

by its successful use under the most difficult field conditions in a study among the 10 million Bangladesh refugees who crossed the border during the 1971 civil upheaval (Mahalanabis *et al.*, 1973).

2.3. A Critical Look at the Scientific Basis of ORT

Almost all water-soluble molecules that are absorbed from the small intestine enhance the absorption of sodium (Schultz, 1977). Examples are D-hexoses, amino acids, dipeptides, tripeptides, and some water-soluble vitamins. *In vivo* perfusion studies in human volunteers (Fordtran, 1975) as well as in animals (Patra *et al.*, 1982a) suggest that the faster the absorption of an organic molecule, the greater is the absorption of sodium, water movement being dictated purely by osmotic forces. As explained earlier, unabsorbed solutes in the gut lumen hinder absorption of water and thus limit the extent to which organic compounds can enhance a balanced absorption of sodium and water (Mahalanabis and Patra, 1983).

The intestinal lavage technique used by radiologists and immunologists (Sack *et al.*, 1980b) illustrate this powerful mechanism whereby water-soluble organic nutrients are associated with enhanced sodium absorption. In this procedure, the patient, after an overnight fast, drinks a balanced salt solution (containing no nutrients) at a rapid rate (250 ml/10 min) up to 4 hr. This large volume of fluid overwhelms the absorptive capacity of the intestine and diarrhea results (more than 50% of the ingested volume is purged). If, however, the patient "cheats" and takes a breakfast some time before the procedure, it fails to produce diarrhea. Instead, all the water is passed in the urine, the organic nutrients from the breakfast having presumably enhanced absorption of the salt solution.

The jejunum absorbs sodium (and water) at an enhanced rate when glucose or a similar organic nutrient (such as an amino acid) is present (Fordtran, 1975; Patra *et al.*, 1982a). The closer the sodium concentration is to its plasma level, the higher is its net absorption (Sladen and Dawson, 1969). In duodenum and jejunum, isosmolality is quickly attained in the ingested fluid by the flow of water/solutes; hence an isosmotic oral fluid should create a minimal disequilibrium (Fordtran and Dietschy, 1966; Sladen and Dawson, 1969). Bicarbonate is actively absorbed from the jejunum against a steep electrochemical gradient and enhances sodium (and water) absorption independently (Turnberg *et al.*, 1970a,b; Fordtran *et al.*, 1968), even when glucose-linked enhanced sodium absorption is maximized (Mahalanabis and Patra, 1983). Potassium is absorbed passively from a higher concentration to a lower one; its absorption occurs when its concentration is higher than that of plasma. The ileum actively absorbs sodium and chloride against a steep electrochemical gradient even in the absence of

Table I
Formulation of the ORS Currently
Recommended by the WHO

Ingredients
Sodium chloride, 3.5 g
Sodium bicarbonate, 2.5 g
Potassium chloride, 1.5 g
Glucose, 20.0 g
Water, 1.0 liters
Composition (mmol/liter of water)
Sodium, 90
Potassium, 20
Chloride, 80
Bicarbonate, 30
Glucose, 111

glucose. Glucose and similar nutrients, however, also enhance absorption of sodium from the ileum.

2.4. Oral Rehydration Formulation

2.4.1. WHO Complete Formula

The formulation for the ORS now recommended by the WHO is shown in Table I.

These ingredients are distributed by UNICEF in aluminum foil packets labeled ''Oral Rehydration Salts.'' This complete WHO formula is regarded as the physiologically most appropriate single formulation for worldwide use.

ORT has been identified by the diarrheal disease-control program of the WHO as an eminently suitable tool for application at the primary health care level and an excellent entry point for appropriate health education activities. Given the constraints of the health care delivery systems in the developing countries, there is a generally recognized need for a composition that can be used for the treatment of dehydration in all age groups and in acute diarrheas of all causes. Because of the need to supply ORS packets to many different parts of the world, it would probably be advisable to make the same formulation available everywhere.

2.4.2. Recommended Use of the Single ORS Formula in Diarrheal Illness

One major theoretical criticism of this approach is that its relatively high sodium concentration may predispose an infant to hypernatremia. In the following paragraphs we briefly discuss the basis of this single solution, how it has been adapted to meet the needs of fluid therapy in infants as well as in older children and adults, and the accumulated experience in its use.

ORS is used to replace the salt and water deficit, usually within 6–12 hr, that has already occurred in a dehydrated child (i.e., for rehydration). For this purpose the composition of the WHO ORS is felt to be optimal (Darrow, 1946; Darrow *et al.*, 1949, Mahalanabis *et al.*, 1970). The ORS is then used to replace ongoing diarrheal stool losses; it is not meant to be used to meet the normal water and salt needs of the body while the patient is being treated.

The variable stool sodium losses are met by administering the ORS in quantities to meet the sodium deficit; additional water need, if any, is met from other sources. In infants, water as well as nutrient needs are met from breast milk, which is continued during rehydration therapy, and from water, dilute foods, and other fluids (commenced as soon as clinical dehydration is corrected and without waiting for the diarrhea to stop). This regimen adequately meets normal water needs as well as additional need for water due to ORS ingestion in excess of the need.

Justification for this approach has been critically evaluated in an earlier report (Mahalanabis, 1981b). Details of treatment methods for acute diarrhea incorporating optimum use of the ORS and its scope and limits have been given in a recent WHO publication (Anonymous, 1980b) and will not be discussed in this review.

2.4.3. Optimum Concentration of Organic Compounds in ORS and Use of Compounds Other Than Glucose

2.4.3a. Glucose and Sucrose. Early balance studies in adult cholera patients (Pierce *et al.*, 1968b; Hirschhorn *et al.*, 1968) indicate that a glucose concentration of 2–3 g/100 ml in the ORS induces optimal absorption without inducing osmotic problems due to unabsorbed glucose. Conventional wisdom suggests that a substantial increase in the concentration of glucose in the ORS will lead to osmotic water loss. Paucity of data in clinical diarrhea led to a controlled clinical trial (Mahalanabis and Patra, 1983) using 4 g in place of 2 g/100 ml of glucose in the ORS designed for use in infants and children with acute diarrhea and moderate to severe dehydration. The trial was abandoned due to profuse diarrhea in many and a failure rate of 50% in the study group.

Sucrose, on hydrolysis by the brush-border enzymes, produces equimolar quantities of glucose and fructose. Absorption of either enhances absorption of sodium (Fordtran, 1975). Fructose, however, is absorbed more slowly and hence is potentially capable of inducing osmotic water flow into the gut lumen. Several studies have firmly established sucrose as a valuable alternative to glucose when twice the amount (40 g sucrose in place of 20 g glucose/liter) was used and was shown to be nearly as effective as glucose containing ORS (Sack *et al.*, 1979;

Palmer *et al.*, 1977) except in patients with a high purging rate (more than 10 ml/kg per hr), in whom the failure rate was slightly higher. The latter may be explained by the osmotic drag of slowly absorbed fructose liberated from sucrose, as demonstrated by a marker perfusion study in rat small intestine (Patra *et al.*, 1982a). This study showed marked increase in sodium absorption with paradoxical decrease in water absorption from a sucrose-based ORS. It also lends support to the view that high sugar concentrations in an ORS may contribute to hypernatremia. One study in infantile diarrhea (Chatterjee *et al.*, 1977) achieved a high degree of success (with no failures) using a hypoosmolar sucrose ORS (260 mosm/kg of water).

   2.4.3b. Glucose Polymer. Use of an ORS containing a very high concentration of a commercial glucose polymer in infants with diarrheal dehydration (Sandhu *et al.*, 1982) led to hypernatremia in 1 out of 7 patients, presumably due to osmotic water loss. It is conceivable that a lower concentration of the glucose polymer in the ORS could achieve a higher degree of success.

   2.4.3c. Rice. Rice on digestion yields glucose, amino acids, dipeptides, and tripeptides, all of which could enhance absorption of sodium from the small intestine. Rice is eaten by 60% of world pupulation; replacing the glucose or sucrose in an ORS with rice offers a great potential advantage. A recent case-control study (Molla *et al.*, 1983) in adults and older children (>5 years) with cholera and enterotoxigenic *E. coli* diarrhea compared a rice-based ORS (30 g rice in place of 20 g glucose per liter) with a sucrose-based one. This study showed that both solutions were equally effective. A randomized controlled study (Patra *et al.*, 1982a,b) in infants and small children with diarrhea and moderate to severe dehydration used 50 g rice powder in place of 20 g glucose and reported substantial and significant reduction in diarrheal stool output, duration of diarrhea, and volume of ORS required. In addition, the patients on rice ORS received 40 calories and 1 g protein/kg body weight from the rice in the ORS during a mean period of 30 hr, thus offering substantial nutritional benefit.

   2.4.3d. Amino Acids. An early study in adults with cholera-like diarrhea used a mixture of glycine (an amino acid) and glucose in its ORS and reported a marked reduction in stool output compared with the control group, which was treated with a glucose ORS (Nalin and Cash, 1970). A recent controlled clinical trial investigated the efficacy of the WHO-recommended glucose-based ORS with added glycine (111 mmol/liter) in diarrheal dehydration of infants and small children; it demonstrated a marked reduction in the duration and volume of diarrhea as well as the amount of ORS required. These findings point to the formulation of an improved ORS (as discussed below).

2.4.4. ORS and Hypernatremia in Infantile Diarrhea

   A major theoretical criticism of the ORS recommended by the WHO is its relatively high sodium concentration (90 mmol/liter), which, it is feared, may encourage the development of hypernatremia in infants. It cannot be over-emphasized that the ORS is designed to counter existing salt and water deficits in the dehydrated child (e.g., during first 6–8 hr) and to replace ongoing losses due to diarrhea. It is not intended to supply the body's normal water and salt require-ments during treatment. In infants, additional requirements for water are filled by breast milk (unrestricted during therapy), water, dilute foods, and other fluids given soon after rehydration but before diarrhea stops.

ORT using the WHO-recommended formula has met with uniform success in treating infants with hypernatremic dehydration. As examples, Nalin *et al.* (1978, 1979, 1980) used the ORS in treating 23 infants with hypernatremia; all recovered uneventfully. In two separate studies, Pizarro *et al.*, 1979a; 1983) treated 24 bottle-fed neonates with hypernatremic dehydration and demonstrated highly successful outcomes. The foregoing studies either used the ORS and plain water sequentially in a 2:1 volume ratio or achieved complete clinical hydration initially with the ORS followed by ingestion of half the volume of plain water. Several studies (Chatterjee *et al.*, 1977, 1979; Hirschhorn *et al.*, 1972, 1973) involving varying numbers of dehydrated and hypernatremic infants treated them on admission with the ORS and all the infants made uneventful recoveries. In a recent study in Egypt (Cleary *et al.*, 1981), 16 infants with moderate to severe hypernatremia were treated with ORS. All, including one who had a brief focal seizure at 24 hr, made complete recoveries without any neurological sequelae.

The results of treating hypernatremic dehydration with an ORS compares favorably with the best clinical results reported with intravenous therapy (Rosen-field *et al.*, 1977).

3. ORT IN THE COMMUNITY

It is postulated that if ORT is applied early in the course of illness as a primary health care activity, it should prevent the development of severe de-hydration and thus reduce the need for intravenous therapy and hospitalization. In a limited study in Bangladesh (Chen *et al.*, 1980), home delivery of oral rehydration solution by trained village health workers resulted in a reduction of 29%, over a 4-month period, in the number of cases seeking therapy in a treatment center. Another study in Bangladesh carried out in remote rural areas (Rahman *et al.*, 1979) and over a longer period showed a significant reduction in case fatality rates when ORS packets were made easily available through trained village-based volunteer workers after a short promotional campaign had been conducted to inform the village population. Studies conducted in urban environ-ments in Costa Rica (Pizarro *et al.*, 1979b) and Jamaica (D. E. C. Ashley, 1979, unpublished) showed that oral rehydration can be carried out successfully in the home. In these studies, nurses' aids instructed and enlisted the help of mothers in the oral rehydration of their acutely ill infants during visits to a hospital emergency room. Mothers were then taught to mix and administer the ORS at home and to assess dehydration from skin elasticity. In both studies 85–90% were satisfactorily managed at home by their mothers. Half the 10–15% infants brought back to emergency room were again successfully managed with the ORS alone.

Incomplete ORS Formula

Some public health workers have attempted to simplify the composition of the ORS and its method of delivery in the field. Use of ordinary teaspoons for the preparation of incomplete formula containing common salt and domestic sugar only have been shown to result in dangerously high concentrations as well as low, ineffective levels of sodium in the fluids so prepared. Estimation of the amount of salt (with a two-finger-and-thumb pinch) and of sugar (with a four-finger scoop), as is practiced for cooking purposes, has also been found to produce large variations in the concentrations of the ingredients. To solve this problem, a number of two-ended special plastic measuring spoons have been devised. Although these are more accurate, they imply a dependence on centralized supplies. Shortcomings in the preparation of home-made (and therefore incomplete) oral rehydration formulations that are both safe and effective have not yet been overcome. These facts have been recently reviewed (Mahalanabis *et al.*, 1980).

In a large field program in Punjab, India, the use of a salt–sugar solution by village health workers and mothers for the early treatment of diarrhea led to a reported 50% decrease in diarrhea mortality (Kielmann and McCord, 1977). Additional studies on the safety and efficacy of the simplified procedures in the home are being conducted.

4. ORT AND FEEDING PRACTICES

A recently published WHO manual (Mehalanabis *et al.*, 1980) on the treatment of acute diarrhea advocates a policy of early feeding (i.e., as soon as the signs of dehydration are corrected and before diarrhea stops) as well as unrestricted breast-feeding from the onset of rehydration therapy with an ORS. This policy is based on the highly successful general outcome in many studies on acute diarrheas in which ORT with such liberal feeding practices were followed, as judged by duration of diarrhea, weight gain in the acute phase, and early end to fluid therapy. Hirschhorn and Denny (1975) compared the discharge weight of a group of Apache Indian infants treated with ORT and liberal food intake during the acute phase of recovery with a comparable group treated with I.V. fluids and a slow return to normal diet; a better weight gain in the former group was shown. Since a large part of the food ingested during the acute phase of diarrhea is absorbed (Chung 1948; Mahalanabis, 1981a), this favorable outcome was probably due to better nutrition. An international study by WHO in the Philippines (1977) showed that, over a seven-month period of observation, infants who received oral rehydration therapy together with proper dietary management during and after the diarrhea had a better appetite and gained significantly more weight than the controls. Several other studies showing a similar trend of weight gain have been reviewed (Mahalanabis *et al.*, 1981).

5. ORS AS AN ABSORPTION-PROMOTING DRUG

The present WHO-recommended oral rehydration formula is a powerful therapeutic tool that can adequately replace the deficits of moderately severe dehydration due to acute diarrhea and repair the ongoing losses due to diarrhea with rates not exceeding 10 ml/kg per hr (Mahalanabis *et al.*, 1974; Chatterjee *et al.*, 1977, 1978). As compared with I.V.-treated controls, ORT neither reduces nor increases diarrheal stool loss in infants and children with rotavirus diarrhea (Sack *et al.*, 1978) or cholera (Mahalanabis *et al.*, 1974). In adults with cholera, diarrheal stool output may even increase by 15–20% as the result of treatment with ORS (Pierce *et al.*, 1969; Hirschhorn *et al.*, 1968).

As has been pointed out, almost all water-soluble organic molecules that are absorbed from the small intestine enhance the absorption of sodium and water; examples are D-hexoses, amino acids, dipeptides, and tripeptides (Schultz, 1977). Also, *in vivo* perfusion studies (Fordtran, 1975; Patra *et al.*, 1982a) suggest that net sodium absorption is linked to the absolute molar quantity of organic solute absorbed (expressed in terms of monomers). The concentration of water-soluble organic compounds cannot, however, be increased substantially, as this would raise the solution's osmolality far above that of plasma. As a result, osmotic backflow of water from plasma to gut lumen (due to unabsorbed organic compounds) would negate the beneficial effects of increased absorption unless the organic molecules were sufficiently absorbed to eliminate the adverse osmotic effect. Furthermore, bicarbonate independently enhances the absorption of sodium and water from the small intestine (Fordtran *et al.*, 1968; Turnberg *et al.*, 1970a, 1970b; Mahalanabis and Patra, 1983) and is additive to glucose-linked absorption.

We postulate that an ORS containing polymers (e.g., rice starch and proteins or a mixture of organic molecules such as glucose and amino acids) that are absorbed quickly through independent carrier mechanisms aided by bicarbonate-linked enhanced absorption of sodium can not only replace the diarrheal losses of water and electrolytes but also lead to reabsorption of sodium and water secreted into the small bowel lumen, thus reducing the magnitude and duration of diarrhea. Such an oral rehydration solution could then be regarded as an absorption-promoting drug.

5.1. Clinical Studies Supporting the Postulate

An early study in adults with severe cholera-like diarrhea used a mixture of glucose and glycine in ORS. This study showed marked reduction in diarrheal stool output in the treated patients as compared with controls given a glucose-based ORS. A recent controlled trial in infants and small children with diarrhea and moderate to severe dehydration involved the use of an ORS in which 20 g glucose was replaced by 50 g of cooked rice powder. The results showed a significant and substantial reduction in mean diarrheal stool volume (49%), mean duration of diarrhea (30%), and mean volume of ORS required (36%) by comparison with controls (Patra *et al.*, 1982). These results are superior to those achieved with antisecretory drugs in studies with humans (Rabbani *et al.*, 1979; Burke *et al.*, 1980). A similar controlled study using the standard WHO-recommended ORS fortified with glycine showed comparable improvement in magnitude and duration of diarrhea as well as in the volume of ORS required (Mahalanabis and Patra, 1983).

5.2. Future Prospects

Although absorption of larger quantity of water-soluble organic compounds from the small intestine induces larger absolute quantity of sodium absorption (Fordtran, 1975; Patra *et al.*, 1982a), unabsorbed organic molecules inside the gut lumen lead to osmotic water loss and a dissociation between sodium and water absorption (Mahalanabis and Patra, 1983). There is no simple way of balancing the absorption of organic molecules and the osmotic loss of water due to malabsorption. It is of interest to note that dipeptides and tripeptides are absorbed faster and presumably by different mechanisms than are their constituent amino acids. The possible beneficial role of organic molecules in an ORS has not yet been explored. A series of *in vivo* animal and human studies is being conducted in the author's laboratory to define the optimum composition of an ORS with maximum absorption-promoting capability.

REFERENCES

Anonymous, 1980a, Oral rehydration therapy (ORT) for childhood diarrhoea, *Popul. Rep.* 1(2):624.
Anonymous, 1980b, A manual for the treatment of acute diarrhoea. Document WHO/CDD/SER/80.2, World Health Organization, Geneva.
Barany, E. H., and Sperber, E., 1939, Absorption of glucose against a concentration gradient by the small intestine of the rabbit, *Scand. Arch. Physiol.* 81:290.

Barry, R. J. C., Smyth, D. H., and Wright, E. M., 1965, Short circuit current and solute transfer by rat jejunum, *J. Physiol.* 181:410–431.

Burke, V., Gracey, M., Suharyono, and Sunoto, 1980, Reduction by aspirin of intestinal fluid loss in acute childhood gastroenteritis, *Lancet* 1:1329–1330.

Carpenter, C. C. J., Sack, R. B., Feeley, J. C., and Steenberg, R. W., 1968, Site and characteristics of electrolyte loss and effects of intraluminal glucose in experimental canine cholera, *J. Clin. Invest.* 47:1210–1220.

Chatterjee, H. N., 1953, Control of vomiting in cholera and oral replacement of fluid, *Lancet* 2:1063.

Chatterjee, A., Mahalanabis, D., Jalan, K. N., Maitra, T. K., Agarwal, S. K., Bagchi, D. K., and Indra, S., 1977, Evaluation of a sucrose/electrolyte solution for oral rehydration in acute infantile diarrhoea, *Lancet* 1:133–135.

Chatterjee, A., Mahalanabis, D., Jalan, K. N., Maitra, T. K., Agarwal, S. K., Dutta, B., Khatua, S. P., and Bagchi, D. K., 1978, Oral rehydration in infantile diarrhoea, *Arch. Dis. Child.* 54:284–289.

Chen, L. C., Black R. E., Sarder, A. M., Merson, M. M., Bhatia, S., Yonus, M., and Chakraborty, J., 1980, Village-based distribution of oral rehydration therapy packets in Bangladesh, *Am. J. Trop. Med. Hyg.* 29:285–290.

Chung, A. W., 1948, The effect of oral feeding at different levels on the absorption of foodstuffs in infantile diarrhoea, *J. Pediatr.* 33:1–13.

Cleary, T. G., Cleary, K. R., Dupont, H. L., El-Maligh, G. S., Kordy, M. I., Mohieldin, M. S., Shoukry, I., Shurky, S., Wyatt, R. G., and Woodward, W. E., 1981, The relationship of oral rehydration solution to hypernatraemia in infantile diarrhoea, *J. Pediatr.* 99:739–741.

Crane, R. K., 1965. Sodium dependent transport in the intestine and other animal tissues, *Fed. Proc.* 24:1000–1006.

Czaky, T. Z., 1963, A possible link between active transport of electrolytes and non-electrolytes, *Fed. Proc.* 22:3–7.

Darrow, D. C., 1946. The retention of electrolyte during recovery from severe dehydration due to diarrhoea, *J. Pediatr.* 28:515.

Darrow, D. C., Praft, E. L., Flett, J., Jr., Gamble, A. H., and Wiese, H. F., 1949, Disturbances of water and electrolytes in infantile diarrhoea, *Pediatrics* 3:129.

Fordtran, J. S., 1975, Stimulation of active and passive sodium absorption by sugars in the human jejunum, *J. Clin. Invest.* 55:728–737.

Fordtran, J. S., and Dietschy, J. M., 1966, Water and electrolyte movement in the intestine, *Gastroenterology* 50:263.

Fordtran, J. S., Rector, F. C., and Carter, N. W., 1968, The mechanism of sodium absorption in the human small intestine, *J. Clin. Invest.* 47:884–900.

Harison, H. E., 1954, The treatment of diarrhea in infancy, *Pediatr. Clin. N. Am.* 1:335–348.

Hirschhorn, N., 1980, The treatment of acute diarrhea in children: An historical and physiological perspective, *Am. J. Clin. Nutr.* 33:637–663.

Hirschhorn, H., Kinzie, J. L., Sechar, D. B., Northrup, R. S., Taylor, J. O., Ahmad, S. Z., and Phillips, R. A., 1968, Decrease in net stool output in cholera during intestinal perfusion with glucose containing solutions, *N. Engl. J. Med.* 279:176–181.

Hirschhorn, N., Cash, R. A., Woodward, W. E., and Spivey, G. H., 1972, Oral fluid therapy of Apache children with acute infectious diarrhoea, *Lancet* 2:15.

Hirschhorn, N., McCarthy, B. J., Ranney, B., Hirschhorn, M. A., Woodward, S. T., Lacapa, A., Cash, R. A., and Woodward, W. E., 1973, Ad libitum glucose electrolyte therapy for acute diarrhoea in Apache children, *J. Pediatr.* 83:562–571.

Hirschhorn, N., and Denny, K. M., 1975, Oral glucose electrolyte therapy for diarrhea a means to maintain or improve nutrition? *Am. J. Clin. Nutr.* 28:189–192.

Kielmann, A. A., and McCord, C., 1977, Home treatment of childhood diarrhoea in Punjab villages, *Environmental Child Health* 23(4):197–201.

Levinson, R. A., and Schedl, H. P., 1966, Absorption of sodium, chloride, water, and simple sugars in rat small intestine, *Am. J. Physiol.* 211:939–942.

Mahalanabis, D., 1981a, Nitrogen balance during recovery from secretory diarrhea of cholera in children, *Am. J. Clin. Nutr.* 34:1548–1551.

Mahalanabis, D., 1981b, Rehydration therapy in diarrhoea, in: *Acute Enteric Infections in Children: New Prospects in Treatment & Prevention* (T. Holme, J. Holmgren, M. H. Merson, and R. Mollby, eds.), Elsevier–North Holland, pp. 303–318.

Mahalanabis, D., and Patra, F. C., 1983, In search of a super oral rehydration solution: Can optimum use of organic solute mediated sodium absorption lead to the development of an absorption promoting drug? *J. Diarrh. Dis. Res.* 1:76–81.

Mahalanabis, D., Wallace, C. K., Kallen, R. J., Mondal, A., and Pierce, N. F., 1970, Water and electrolyte losses due to cholera in infants and small children: A recovery balance study, *Pediatrics* 45:374.

Mahalanabis, D., Chowdhury, A. B., Bagchi, N. G., Bhattacharya, A. K., and Simpson, T. W., 1973, Oral fluid therapy of cholera among Bangladesh refugees, *Johns Hopkins Med. J.* 132(4):197–205.

Mahalanabis, D., Sack, R. B., Jacobs, B., Mondal, A., and Thomas, J., 1974, Use of an oral glucose electrolyte solution in the treatment of pediatric cholera: A controlled study, *J. Trop. Pediatr. Environ. Child Health* 20(2):82–87.

Mahalanabis, D., Merson, M. H., and Barua, D., 1981, Oral rehydration therapy—recent advances, *World Health Forum* 2(2):245–249.

Malawar, S. J., Enton, M., Fordtran, J. S., and Ingelfinger, F. J., 1965, Interrelation between jejunal absorption of sodium glucose and water in man, abstract, *J. Clin. Invest.* 44(6):1072.

Molla, A. M., Sarkar, S. A., Hossain, M., Molla, A., and Greenough, W. B., III, 1982, Rice powder electrolyte solution as oral therapy in diarrhoea due to *Vibrio cholerae* and *Escherichia coli*, *Lancet* 1:1317–1319.

Nalin, D. R., and Cash, R. A., 1970. Oral or nasogastric maintenance therapy for diarrhea of unknown aetiology resembling cholera, *Trans. Roy. Soc. Trop. Med. Hyg.* 64:769–771.

Nalin, D. R., Cash, R. A., Islam, R., Molla, M., and Phillips, R. A., 1968, Oral maintenance therapy for cholera in adults, *Lancet* 2:370–373.

Nalin, D. R., Levine, M. M., Mata, L., de Cespedes, C., Vargas, W., Lizano, C., Loria, A. R., Simhon, A. and Mohs, E., 1978, Comparison of sucrose with glucose in oral therapy of infant diarrhoea, *Lancet* 2:277–279.

Nalin, D. R., Levine, M. M., Mata, L., de Cespedes, C., Vargas,W., Lizano, C., Loria, A. R., Simhon, A., and Mohs, E., 1979, Oral rehydration and maintenance of children with rotavirus and bacterial diarrhoea, *Bull. W.H.O.* 57:453–459.

Nalin, D. R., Harland, E., Ramlal, A., Swaby, D., McDonald, J., Gangarosa, R., Levine, M., Akierman, A., Antoinee, M., Mackenzie, K., and Johnson, B., 1980. Comparison of low and high sodium and potassium content in oral rehydration solution, *J. Pediatr.* 97:848–853.

Palmer, D. K., Kostar, F. T., Islam, A. F. M. R., Rahman, A. S. M. M., and Sack, R. B., 1977, Comparison of sucrose and glucose in the oral electrolyte therapy of cholera and other severe diarrhoea, *N. Engl. J. Med.* 297:1107–1110.

Patra, F. C., Mahalanabis, D., and Jalan, K. N., 1982a, Stimulation of sodium and water absorption by sucrose in the rat small intestine, *Acta Pediatr. Scand.* 71:103–107.

Patra, F. C., Mahalanabis, D., Jalan, K. N., Sen, A., and Banerjee, P., 1982b, Can acetate replace bicarbonate in oral rehydration solution for infantile diarrhoea? *Arch. Dis. Child* 57:625–627.

Patra, F. C., Mahalanabis, D., Jalan, K. N., Sen, A., and Banerjee, P., 1982c, Is rice electrolyte solution superior to glucose electrolyte solution in infantile diarrhoea? *Arch. Dis. Child* 57:910–912.

Phillips, R. A., 1964, Water and electrolyte losses in cholera, *Fed. Proc.* 23:705–712.

Pierce, N. F., Banwell, J. G., Mitra, R. C., Caranos, G. J., Keimowitz, R. I., Mondal, A., and Manji, P. M., 1968a, Oral maintenance of water-electrolyte and acid-base balance in cholera, a preliminary report, *Ind. J. Med. Res.* 56:640–645.

Pierce, N. F., Banwell, J. G., Mitra, R. C., Caransos, G. J., Keimowitz, R. I., Mondal, A., and Manji, P. M., 1968b, Effect of intragastric glucose electrolyte infusion upon water and electrolyte balance in Asiatic cholera, *Gastroenterology* 55:333–343.

Pierce, N. F., Sack, R. B., Mitra, R. C., Banwell, J. G., Brigham, K. L., Fedson, D. S., and Mondal, A., 1969, Replacement of water electrolyte losses in cholera by an oral glucose-electrolyte solution, *Ann. Int. Med.* 70:1173.

Pizarro, D., Posada, G., Mata, L., Nalin, D., and Mohs, E., 1979a, Oral rehydration of neonates with dehydrating diarrhoeas, *Lancet* 2:1209.

Pizarro, D., Posada, G., Mohs, E., Levine, M. M., and Balin, D. R., 1979b. Evaluation of oral therapy for infant diarrhoea in an emergency room setting: The acute episode as an opportunity for instructing mothers in home treatment, *Bull. W.H.O.* 57:983–986.

Pizarro, D., Posada, G., and Mata, L., 1983, Treatment of 242 neonates with dehydrating diarrhoea with an oral glucose-electrolyte solution, *J. Pediatr.* 102:153–156.

Rabbini, G. H., Greenough, W. B., Holmgren, J., and Lonroth, L., 1979, Chlorpromazine reduces fluid loss in cholera, *Lancet* 1:410.

Rahman, M. M., Aziz, K. M. S., Patwariy, and Munhi, M. H., 1979, Diarrhoeal mortality in the Bangladeshi villages with and without community based oral rehydration therapy, *Lancet* 2:809–812.

Reid, E. W., 1902, Intestinal absorption of solutions, *J. Physiol. [London]* 28:241.

Riklis, E., and Quastel, J. H., 1958, Effects of cations on sugar absorption by isolated surviving guinea pig intestine, *Can. J. Biochem. Physiol.* 36:347–362.

Rosenfield, W., DeRomano, G. L., Jleinman, R., and Finberg, L., 1977, Improving the clinical management of hypernatremic dehydration: Observations from a study of 67 infants with this disorder, *Clin. Pediatr.* 16:411.

Sack, D. A., Chowdhury, A. M. A. K., Eusof, A., Ali, M. A., Merson, M. H., Islam S., Black, R. E., and Brown, K. H., 1978, Oral hydration in rotavirus diarrhoea: A double blind comparison of sucrose with glucose electrolyte solution, *Lancet* 2:280.

Sack, D. A., Islam, A., Holmgren, J., and Svennerhalm, A., 1980a, Development of methods for determining the intestinal immune response to *Vibrio cholera* antigens in humans in: *Proceeding of the XV Joint Conference on Cholera,* Bethesda, Maryland, pp. 423–439.

Sack, D. A., Islam, S., Brown, K. H., Islam, A., Kabir, A. K. M. I., Chowdhury, A. M. A. K., and Ali, M. A., 1980b, Oral therapy in children with cholera: A comparison of sucrose and glucose electrolyte solution, *J. Pediatr.* 96:20–25.

Sack, D. A., Islam, S., Merson, M. H., Brown, K. H., Black, R. E., Rahman, M., Chowdhury, M. A. K. A., and Ali, M. A., 1979, Sucrose or glucose—which sugar to use in oral rehydration solution: A summary of four clinical trials, in: *Symposium on Cholera* (K. Takeya and Y. Zinnaka, eds.), Karatsu, Japan, 1978 (Proceedings of the Fourteenth Joint Conference, U.S.–Japan Co-operative Medical Science Program, Cholera Panel), Japanese Cholera Panel, Tokyo, pp. 154–164.

Sandhu, B. K., Jones, B. J. M., Brook C. G. D., and Silk, D. B. A., 1982, Oral rehydration in acute infantile diarrhoea with a glucose-polymer electrolyte solution, *Arch. Dis. Child* 57:152–154.

Schedl, H. P., and Clifton, J. A., 1963, Solute and water absorption by the human small intestine, *Nature [London]* 199:1264–1267.

Schultz, S. C., 1977, Sodium-coupled solute transport by small intestine: A status report, *Am. J. Physiol.* 223:E249–254.

Schultz, S. C., and Zalusky, R., 1964, Ion transport in isolated rabbit ileum: II. The interaction between active sodium and active sugar transport, *J. Gen. Physiol.* 47:1043–1059.

Sladen, G. F., and Dawson, A. M., 1969, Interrelationships between the absorption of glucose, sodium and water by the normal human jejunum, *Clin. Sci.* 36:119–132.

Snyder, J. D., and Merson, M. H., 1982, The magnitude of global problem of acute diarrhoeal disease: Review of active surveillance data, *Bull. W.H.O.* 6:605–614.

Taylor, J. O., Kinzie, J., Hare, R., and Hare, K., 1968, Measurement of sodium flexure in human small intestine, abstract 0964, *J. Clin. Invest.* 27:386.

Turnberg, L. A., Bieberdorf, F. A., Morawski, S. G., and Fordtran, J. S., 1970a, Interrelationships of chloride, bicarbonate, sodium and hydrogen transport in the human ileum, *J. Clin. Invest.* 49:557–567.

Turnberg, L. A., Fordtran, J. S., Carter, N. W., and Rector, F. C., Jr., 1970b, Mechanisms of bicarbonate absorption and its relationship to sodium transport in the human jejunum. *J. Clin. Invest.* 49:548–556.

4

Functional Consequences of Iron Deficiency
Nonerythroid Effects

R. K. CHANDRA AND DEVHUTI VYAS

Iron undernutrition is the most common single nutrient deficiency worldwide. Socioeconomically underprivileged groups, young children, women during the reproductive period, and the elderly are the most common victims of the deficiency. Nutrition surveys in the early 1970s have shown that marginal to moderate iron deficiency is prevalent in 15–20% of the population under the age of 18 years in United States. A national nutrition survey in Canada revealed that, in different age groups, the incidence of iron deficiency varied from 2.3–12.7% (Nutrition Canada, 1973). The effect of reduced iron availability on hemoglobin levels and other hematopoietic indices has been well recognized for a long time. It is only recently that the association between iron deficiency itself, with or without anemia, on immunocompetence, cognition, physical work capacity, and other functions has been documented (Chandra, 1976a,b; Jacobs, 1982; Vyas and Chandra, 1983a,b). Anemia, commonly considered to be synonymous with iron deficiency, is a late manifestation of iron undernutrition which is preceded by the earlier stages of depleted iron stores of the body, reduced serum iron concentration, and lower transferrin saturation. A number of organs and systems often show variable changes in structure and function before any drop in hemoglobin occurs. This is not surprising, because iron is an integral component or an

R. K. CHANDRA • Department of Pediatrics, Janeway Child Health Centre, Memorial University of Newfoundland, St. John's, Newfoundland, Canada A1A 1R8.   DEVHUTI VYAS • Health Sciences Centre, Memorial University of Newfoundland, St. John's, Newfoundland, Canada A1B 3V6.

essential cofactor of several enzymes that play an important role in metabolic processes and cell proliferation. These include aconitase, catalase, cytochrome C, cytochrome C reductase, cytochrome oxidase, formiminotransferase, monoamine oxidase, myeloperoxidase, peroxidase, ribonucleotidyl reductase, succinic dehydrogenase, tyrosine hydroxylase, tryptophan pyrrolase, and xanthine oxidase (Higashi *et al.*, 1967; Wrigglesworth and Baum, 1980). These enzymes are involved in a number of key pathways such as DNA synthesis, mitochondrial electron transport, and catecholamine metabolism. It is not unexpected, then, that iron deficiency results in a variety of functional abnormalities.

1. IMMUNOCOMPETENCE AND INFECTION

Iron is essential to the normal development and function of lymphoid tissues. Thus iron dficiency may be expected to impair immune responses mediated by lymphocytes and granulocytes, thereby increasing susceptibility to infection.

1.1. Immune Responses

An important nonspecific first-line defense mechanism is the phagocytic system. The bactericidal potential of leukocytes depends upon optimum opsonization, ingestion, chemotaxis, and intracellular digestion. In iron deficiency, opsonization and ingestion of bacteria by neutrophils were reported to be normal but intracellular digestion was reduced (Figure 1) (Chandra, 1973; Chandra and Saraya, 1975; MacDougall *et al.*, 1975; Prasad, 1979; Srikantia *et al.*, 1976). Likhite *et al.*, (1976) observed some impairment of phagocytosis also. The one report showing normal bacterial killing function in iron deficiency (Kulapongs *et al.*, 1976) was based on a small number of subjects with severe anemia due to hookworm disease. Moreover, the ratio of leukocytes to bacteria was not optimum. We observed impaired reduction of nitroblue tetrazolium by neutrophils estimated by a quantitative spectrophotometric method in patients with iron-deficiency anemia compared with healthy controls (Chandra, 1973), while others (MacDougall *et al.*, 1975; Van Heerden *et al.*, 1981) by counting the number of neutrophils with the reduced dye, have reported this parameter to be within the normal range. The apparent discrepancy in the results might be due to the differences in the methods. The nitroblue tetrazolium test used as a qualitative measure detects the number of neutrophils capable of reducing the dye. If it is used as a quantitative measure, the amount of dye reduced by a unit number of cells can be compared, which may reveal the impaired metabolic ability of each cell to reduce the dye. The molecular mechanism underlying the reduced micro-

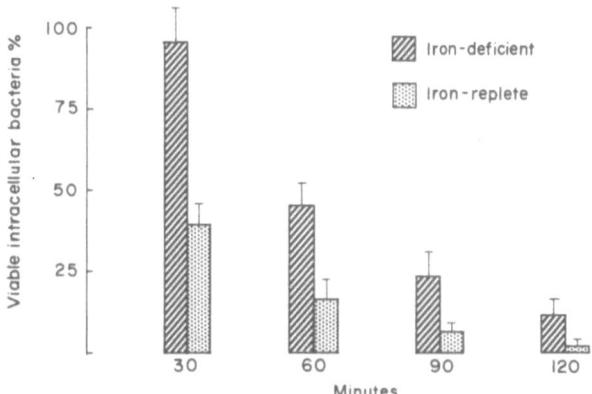

Figure 1.   Bacterial killing capacity of neutrophils. *Staphylococcus aureus* and polymorphonuclear cells were mixed in a ratio of 5:1 in the presence of 10% plasma. Aliquots of cells were lysed for viable intracellular bacterial count at different time intervals.

bicidal function of leukocytes in iron deficiency is not clear, but it might be the result of reduced myeloperoxidase-mediated halogination of bacterial cell wall. In fact, decreased myeloperoxidase activity in polymorphs of iron-deficient children was reported by Higashi *et al.* (1967) and Prasad (1979). The defects in bacterial killing and the nitroblue tetrazolium reduction test were corrected within 4 to 7 days of iron administration, before any appreciable change in hemoglobin took place (Chandra, 1973).

Iron is essential for the morphologic maintenance and functional integrity of the lymphoid apparatus. Iron depletion by a chelating agent, desferoxamine mesylate, resulted in a reduction of the weight of the thymus and depletion of mononuclear cells (Chandra *et al.*, 1977). Reduction in thymus weight was recently observed by Kuvibidila *et al.* (1983) in mice on an iron-deficient diet. The majority of the studies show impaired cell-mediated immune response in iron-deficient subjects, judged by the slightly reduced number of circulating T cells (Figure 2), impaired delayed cutaneous hypersensitivity (Table I), and attenuated lymphocyte transformation response to mitogens (Figure 3) and antigens (Figure 4). Iron-deficient subjects show slightly reduced numbers of T lymphocytes, whereas B cells are normal in number. Thus, a proportionate increase in null cells is seen, which may have functional implications in the modulation of immune response (Chandra, 1977). Decreased T-cell number has been confirmed by Bhaskaram and Reddy (1975) and MacDougall *et al.* (1975) However, Van Heerden *et al.* (1981) found no change in circulating T- and B-cells counts. A significantly low lymphocyte transformation response to phytohemagglutinin observed in iron-deficient subjects was corrected after iron administration (Chandra and Saraya, 1975). Similar observations of reduced [3]H

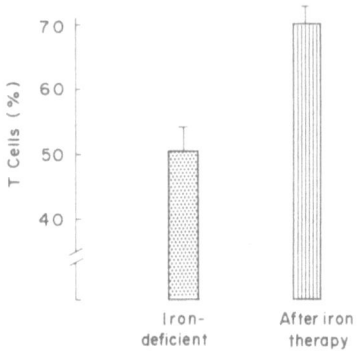

Figure 2. Rosette-forming T cells before and after treatment with iron.

thymidine incorporation by lymphocytes in response to phytohemagglutinin (Bhaskaram and Reddy, 1975; Srikantia *et al.*, 1976; MacDougall *et al.*, 1975; Van Heerden *et al.*, 1981), concanavalin A (Van Heerden *et al.*, 1981), purified protein derivative (Joynson *et al.*, 1972) and *Candida* (MacDougall *et al.*, 1975) have been reported. Impaired response is seen also in those with latent iron deficiency without anemia. Animal studies also showed decreased blastogenic response of lymphocytes to concanavalin A and phytohemagglutinin (Kuvibidila *et al.*, 1983; Soyano *et al.*, 1982). In contrast, Kulapongs *et al.* (1974) and Gross *et al.* (1975) did not observe impaired blastogenic response of lymphocytes to mitogens. The failure to find any impairment in blastogenic response of peripheral blood lymphocytes may be due to differences in study subjects and methods used. For example, in one study (Kulapongs *et al.*, 1974), the small group of patients examined had anemia from chronic blood loss due to hookworm disease. In another report (Gross *et al.*, 1975), only 5 patients were investigated and iron deficiency was marginal (mean serum iron concentration, 54 μg/dl, range up to 88 μg/dl). Even then, the 2 subjects restudied after iron therapy showed a 44–55% increase in lymphocyte response to phytohemagglutinin. Hershko *et al.* (1970) showed that in chronic iron deficiency the incorporation of radiolabeled thymidine into DNA was reduced; decreased content of cellular DNA and impaired utilization of iron and glycine for heme and protein

Table I
Cutaneous Delayed Hypersensitivity

Group	Candida	Trichophyton	Streptococcus	Mumps	Purified protein derivative
Healthy (*n* = 40)	32	29	33	22	11
Iron-deficient (*n* = 40)	17	13	17	9	7

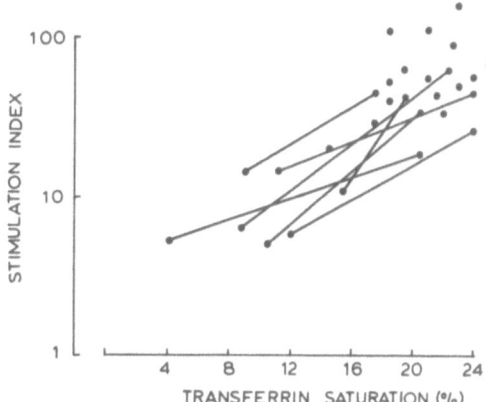

Figure 3. Lymphocyte proliferation response to an optimum dose of phytohemagglutinin. In some subjects, the test was repeated after several weeks of iron therapy.

synthesis were also noted. The production of lymphokines—for example, macrophage migration inhibition factor (MIF)—in response to previously experienced antigens is reduced (Joynson *et al.*, 1972). Iron-deficient individuals may respond less often to recall antigens like *Candida, Trichophyton,* streptokinase–streptodornase, mumps, and purified protein derivative (PPD), as seen in Table I (Chandra and Saraya, 1975); however, it must be emphasized that it is rare to encounter complete anergy in this group as opposed to patients with protein–energy malnutrition (Chandra, 1980). Others (MacDougall *et al.*, 1975; Joynson *et al.*, 1972) have also observed impaired delayed cutaneous hypersensitivity in iron-deficient subjects using antigens like *Candida,* diphtheria toxoid, and PPD.

Kuvibidila *et al.* (1981) reported decreased inflammatory response in anemic mice measured by ^{125}I-deoxyuridine incorporation at the site of din-

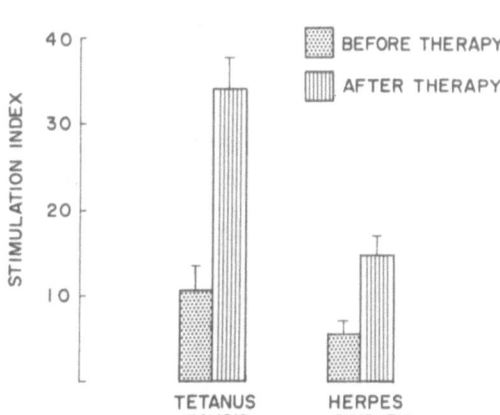

Figure 4. Lymphocyte stimulation response to tetanus toxoid and herpes simplex antigen.

Table II
Serum Immunoglobulin and Complement C3 Levels[a]

Group	No. of children	IgG (mg/dl)	IgA (mg/dl)	IgM (mg/dl)	Complement C3 (mg/dl)	Number showing C3 conversion products
Healthy	50	1080 ± 192	110 ± 29	88 ± 21	136 ± 31	0
Iron-deficient						
Without infection	16	1163 ± 215	98 ± 36	80 ± 29	121 ± 42	0
With infection	4	1870 ± 203	148 ± 27	131 ± 39	92 ± 27	2

[a]Means and standard deviations are presented.

itrofluorobenzene application five days after the primary sensitization with the same antigen, which was restored after a single intraperitoneal injection of Imferon (100 µg Fe) 24 hr prior to recall antigen application. In contrast, Gross *et al.* (1975) did not find any impairment in the delayed cutaneous hypersensitivity test after 2,4,-dinitrochlorobenzene application. Splenocytes of iron-deficient mice had low cytotoxic activity against mastocytoma tumor cells as measured by ^{51}Cr release (Baliga *et al.*, 1982).

Serum immunoglobulins are within the normal range in iron-deficient subjects and increase after infection (Table II). The number of B lymphocytes and serum complement levels were also found to be comparable in iron-deficient and healthy children (Chandra and Saraya, 1975; MacDougall *et al.*, 1975, Van Heerden *et al.*, 1981). Serum antibody responses after challenge with tetanus toxoid and *Salmonella typhi* was within the normal range (Table III). Although salivary IgA level may be normal, specific IgA antibody to measles virus was reduced in a small group of iron-deficient subjects (Chandra *et al.* 1977; Chandra, 1983a); this may be due to changes in mucosal epithelium (Guha *et al.*, 1968) and consequent decreased synthesis of secretory component (Chandra, 1983b). Iron-deficient rats produced significantly less antibody to tetanus toxoid (Nadler *et al.*, 1972). In mice, iron-deficiency was shown to impair the shift from IgM to IgA production (Baliga *et al.*, 1982). These changes in immune responses occur early in the evolution of iron depletion (Chandra, 1981; MacDougall *et al.*, 1975). Similarly, in those with iron-deficiency anemia, treatment with iron improves immunocompetence prior to increase in hemoglobin levels (Chandra, 1973). These observations indicate that reduction in tissue and cellular iron concentration, and not the anemia, is the primary cause of altered immunity associated with lack of iron.

The differences in the results of various studies on immune responses in iron

Table III
Specific Serum Antibody Response

Immunizing antigen	Iron-deficient subject	Healthy subject
Tetanus antitoxin (U/ml):		
Primary	0.096	0.073
Booster	0.230	0.269
Salmonella agglutinins (reciprocal titer):		
Primary 'O'	16	32
'H'	16	16
Booster 'O'	512	1024
'H'	1024	2048

Source: Chandra, 1975.

deficiency may well be due to a number of confounding variables, including variations in methodology of various immunity function tests such as dose of antigen or mitogen, number of microorganisms, and so on (Buckley, 1975; Chandra, 1976a,b). In some reports, the numbers of subjects examined was very small—five or eight (Kulapongs *et al.*, 1974; Gross *et al.*, 1975). A second important variable is the presence of concomitant or recent infection and parasitic disease. Third, the cause of iron deficiency is a significant factor; reduced dietary intake of iron produces more prominent effects on immunity than deficiency resulting from blood loss, including hookworm disease. The diagnosis of iron deficiency in some reports was suspect, and appropriate controls may not always be used.

1.2. Iron Status and Incidence of Infections

1.2.1. Observations in Man

Iron deficiency generally predisposes the subject to infection (Bünger *et al.*, 1982). A WHO Expert Group (1968) commented that individuals with nutritional anemia tend to have more frequent infection, but no definitive data were presented. Beneficial effect of iron supplementation in terms of reduction in episodes of bronchitis, gastroenteritis, diarrhea, and upper and lower respiratory tract infections have been observed in a number of studies (Mackay, 1928; Andelman and Sered, 1966; Stekel and Heresi, 1982; Chandra, 1983b). However, Burman (1972) and James and Combes (1960) did not find such an effect.

The association of iron undernutrition with certain chronic or recurrent infections is of considerable interest. For example, iron deficiency and impaired cellular immunity are common findings in patients with chronic mucocutaneous candidiasis (Higgs and Wells, 1973). The skin lesions as well as immunologic abnormalities reversed rapidly on administration of iron. Fletcher *et al.* (1975) reported *Candida albicans* infection in the mouth lesions seen in iron-deficient individuals; the patients' saliva supported fungal growth better than control samples. A local factor, such as changes in microflora consequent to iron lack, was postulated to be important.

Our observations on a group of medical students with recurrent cold sores due to herpes simplex infection showed a higher prevalence of iron deficiency in them compared with other students without herpes (Chandra *et al.*, 1977). Moreover, the response of lymphocytes to herpes simplex antigen and tetanus toxoid improved significantly four weeks after oral iron therapy and was associated with clinical remission monitored over a period of 1 year.

The association of iron and infection must be carefully examined. The assertion that "iron deficiency protects against infection" is not supported by a critical analysis of observations. The data of one report (Masawe *et al.*, 1974) often cited as evidence for this hypothesis are reviewed here in detail so that valid conclusions can be drawn. This study looked at the presence of infection on admission among 110 adults with hemoglobin below 10 g/dl; of the 67 with severe iron-deficiency or dimorphic anemia, 5 (7%) were diagnosed as having bacterial infection and 16 (24%) malaria. It was stated that the "malarial attacks in the iron-deficiency group usually developed after iron treatment was started." The workers concluded that "the low frequency of bacterial infections in the iron-deficient group suggests that patients with iron-deficiency anemia are not as vulnerable to infections as has hitherto been suspected, but they are susceptible to malaria." These conclusions are not justified on the basis of the observations reported. First, no control group of nonanemic subjects was examined. What was being compared was the prevalence of infection among patients with different etiologic types of anemia. Second, those with positive bone marrow iron included patients with sickle cell disease and sickle cell trait as well as other pathologic conditions known to change susceptibility to infectious disease. Third, the diagnosis of iron deficiency was based on blood and bone marrow smears; serum iron and transferrin saturation were not examined. Fourth, blood cultures to document bacterial infection were set up only in those patients (34 of 110) who had fever. It is well known that protein–calorie malnutrition, possibly present in many of the study subjects, can suppress febrile response. In others, bacterial infection was diagnosed on the basis of response to antibiotics; the self-limited course of many infectious illnesses, especially viral ones, makes the therapeutic response an unsatisfactory diagnostic criterion. Similarly, malaria was diagnosed by demonstration of the parasite in only 6 patients; in the remaining 12, it was based on response to chloroquine. Also, the nature of iron supplements and their duration are not stated, and posttherapy data are provided for malaria but not for bacterial infections. The impact of other associated nutrient deficiencies (for example, 33 had swelling of the legs, which may imply the presence of protein deficiency, and ? malarial nephrotic syndrome) was not considered. These limitations of the reported data detract seriously from the conclusions reached. Similarly, the observation (Murray *et al.*, 1978) that symptomatic disease was evident more often in a group of African people after a period of iron supplementation may mean that the prevalence of clinical diseases in which cell-mediated immunity plays a role in *clinical expression* may be more apparent because iron therapy has improved cellular immunity, but these data do not imply that the *incidence* or the *outcome* of infectious illness is adversely affected by treatment of iron deficiency. Lack of documentation of infection, effects of season, overcrowding, and other variables present major difficulties in the interpretation of these data.

Infection in certain pathologic conditions (like destruction of the liver in viral hepatitis, silent or overt hemolytic anemia, and thalassemia) is often held to be due to a hyperferremic state. In thalassemia, however, severe infections occur after splenectomy and may be due to the asplenic condition rather than increased transferrin saturation. Similarly, in sickle cell anemia, there are more infections during the first five years of life, when increased serum iron concentration does not ordinarily occur.

Some reviews on the topic (Lukens, 1975; Gross and Newberne, 1980) have failed to emphasize these limitations of reported data, implying that iron deficiency protects people from infections. There is little objective evidence that this is indeed true.

1.2.2. Observations in Animals

Laboratory animals provide an excellent opportunity to study the relationship between iron status and susceptibility to infection. The infectious consequences of dietary iron deficiency have been evaluated in several animal models and the data have been reviewed (Chandra, 1976a,b; 1980; Gross and Newberne, 1980; Vyas and Chandra, 1983). In young swine rendered iron-deficient and exposed to *Escherichia coli* endotoxin, the mortality in the experimental anemic group was extremely high. Antibody production in response to tetanus toxoid immunization was significantly reduced in rats that received inadequate dietary iron. The susceptibility to infective challenge with *S. typhi* or *Streptococcus pneumoniae*, assessed by morbidity and mortality, was enhanced in iron-deficient animals. Preweaning iron deprivation impaired the rats' ability to resist the stress of infection, even if a period of nutritional rehabilitation had intervened. Inability to produce and deliver myeloperoxidase-containing cells was considered to be the pathogenesis of vulnerability to *S. typhi*. There is some evidence, on the other hand, that the *parenteral* administration of iron compounds reduces the number of bacteria necessary to produce disease or death. For instance, the growth of nonpigmented mutants of *Pasteurella pestis* was enhanced by injections of iron. In an experimental mouse model, changes in iron status secondary to administration of endotoxin or iron mediated the susceptibility of animals to challenge with *C. albicans*. Thus the route of administration and the nature of the iron compound used may be important in host–bacteria interactions. Recently, the effect both of oral iron and intramuscular iron– dextran on the incidence of pneumonia and diarrhea in calves has been reported. Iron–dextran administration reduced the frequency of anemia and drastically reduced the development of crowding disease; oral iron produced a more distinct benefit than intramuscular therapy, the effect being more evident in the duration of pneumonia compared with that of diarrhea.

1.3. Iron Administration, Bacterial Growth, and Infection

Plant and animal as well as microbial cells with the exception of lactobacillus require iron for their growth. A variety of mammalian sera and milk have been shown to have a bacteriostatic effect due to the presence of iron-binding ligands (transferrin and lactoferrin), which avidly bind the metal and render it unavailable to the microbes (Figure 5). Bacteria, on the other hand, synthesize siderophores to sequester iron from the immediate environment. Fever, a host-protective mechanism, suppresses the ability of pathogens to synthesize iron ligands. Each molecule of transferrin can bind two atoms of iron and, under normal conditions in the serum at 25% transferrin saturation, free ionic iron in the environment would be far less than what is required to support microbial growth.

Several *in vitro* experiments have demonstrated the ability of added iron to reduce the microbiostatic function of serum (Weinberg, 1974). Extrapolation of the results of such *in vitro* experiments aroused concern and raised questions about the beneficial effect of iron treatment. The notion that an iron-rich environment predisposes the host to infection by increasing the virulence of pathogens is misleading and holds true only for *in vitro* experiments. First, the absorption of iron from the gut is regulated except in chronic hemolytic conditions like thalassemia, sideroblastic anemia, and pyruvate kinase deficiency, in which plasma iron concentration and transferrin saturation are normal or even elevated and still a high rate of absorption continues. Thus, oral iron should not increase the ionic iron required for bacterial growth. Moreover, during infection there is further inhibition of intestinal absorption of iron. *In vitro* experiments show that to reduce the bacteriostatic action of serum, transferrin saturation in excess of

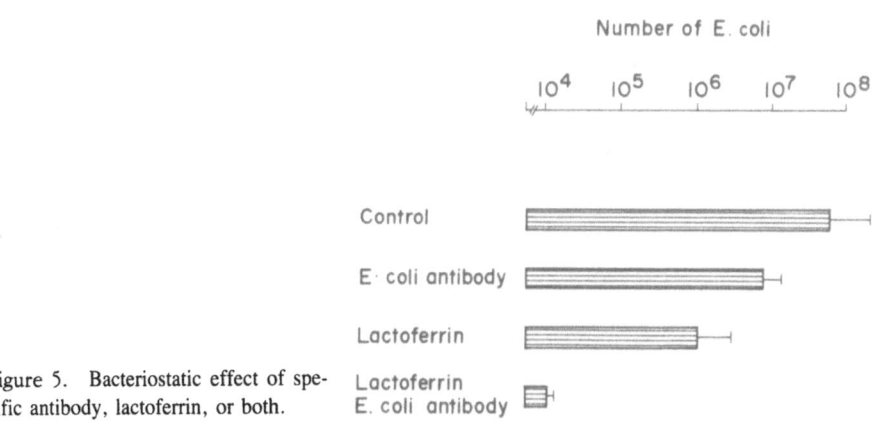

Figure 5. Bacteriostatic effect of specific antibody, lactoferrin, or both.

70% is generally required, which seldom occurs in clinical practice. Moreover, even at 100% transferrin saturation in thalassemic serum, Baltimore *et al.* (1982) did not find any increase in the growth of *E. coli*. Increased transferrin saturation obtained *in vitro* by adding inorganic ferric or ferrous salts is not an identical condition to iron-transferrin formed during the assimilation of iron *in vivo* (Hegenauer and Saltman, 1975), wherein iron is tightly bound to the ligands and is not easily extracted. It should be clearly mentioned that oral iron treatment or iron fortification of food neither saturates the circulating transferrin *in vivo* nor increases the availability of free ionic iron needed for microbial growth.

However, the administration of iron by intravenous, intraperitoneal, or intramuscular injection, depending upon the dose used and levels of iron-binding proteins of the individual, may equal or exceed the total iron-binding capacity and accordingly may increase the virulence of pathogen. Children suffering from protein–energy malnutrition present a special problem, since they have reduced levels of iron-binding proteins (Antia *et al.*, 1968); this reduction correlates with chances of survival. However, the risk is minimized if iron administration is delayed for a few days, allowing for the repair of transferrin synthesis (Table IV). A report of high incidence of gram-negative septicemia in Polynesian neonates given a series of iron–dextran injections (Barry and Reeve, 1977) has evoked concern about the use of iron in the prevention of iron deficiency in infants. However, neonates may have a relatively inefficient mechanism for dealing with large quantities of complexed iron. Macrophage blockade may impair host defense. The use of moderate doses of iron–dextran after the neonatal period did not predispose infants to infections (Hesse, 1981). However, the degree of hyperferremia after parenteral iron administration greatly exceeds that which occurs in ordinary oral therapy. Certainly, the use of the conventional preventive or therapeutic doses of oral iron has not been associated with increased risk of infection; if at all, this may decrease such common illnesses as otitis and upper and lower respiratory tract infections (Chandra, 1983b).

Table IV
Timing of Iron Therapy and Mortality in Well-
Nourished and Malnourished Children with Iron
Therapy

Group	After 72 hr of admission	Within 72 hr of admission
Well-nourished	2/50[a]	1/41
Kwashiorkor	3/18	5/12
Marasmus	2/35	1/16

[a]Number of deaths/total number of patients.

2. GASTROINTESTINAL SYSTEM

Iron deficiency is associated with a variety of clinical manifestations pertaining to the gastrointestinal tract. Histological studies have shown changes in epithelial morphology, including metaplasia of the buccal and esophageal mucosae. Surface epithelial cells in tissues obtained from iron-deficient subjects have a reduced content of cytochrome and other enzymes. Hypo- and achlorhydria may occur. Impaired fat, D-xylose, and vitamin A absorption as well as steatorrhea are observed. Variable degrees of duodenal and jejunal atrophy—ranging from partial to subtotal villous atrophy, focal fusion and blunting of villi, decreased villous/crypt ratio, increased depth of crypts, and cellular infiltration in the lamina propria—were reported (Naiman et al., 1964; Guha et al., 1968). Partial or complete recovery of gastrointestinal structure and function was observed after appropriate therapy. Fecal occult blood is detected more often in iron-deficient subjects than in controls. Iron-deficient subjects have a higher incidence of beeturia; iron treatment often reduces the absorption of the red pigment. The functional significance of this observation is not clear. Iron deficiency in young puppies and rats was associated with reduced activity of sugar-splitting enzymes, but the mucosal architecture was preserved (Hoffbrand and Broitman, 1969; Sriratanaban and Thayer, 1971). The subject of small intestinal structure and function in nutritional deficiency has been recently reviewed (Vyas and Chandra, 1983).

3. THERMOREGULATION

The maintenance of normal body temperature depends on a complex set of interacting mechanisms, including hormones, diet, amount and type of adipose tissue, and hypothalamic control. It has been reported that iron-deficient rodents cannot maintain normal core body temperature when stressed with cold, the conversion of T4 to T3 is impaired (Dillman et al., 1980), and there may be an increase in reverse T3 (Chandra, 1983b). The serum and urinary levels of catecholamines are increased. Iron deficiency alters mitochondrial electron transport systems both in adipose tissue and brown fat. Body insulation is not changed, since hair thickness is unaltered and cutaneous vasoconstriction is intact. Oxygen consumption at 4°C is reduced. Treatment with iron resulted in reversal to normal T3 levels in one week. The modulating influence of thyroid dysfunction in thermoregulation was shown also by the observations that thyroidectomized iron-deficient rats injected with T3 did not show cold-stress-induced hypothermia, whereas T4 administration failed to prevent hypothermia and increased catecholamines at 4°C (Dillman et al., 1980).

4. PHYSICAL WORK CAPACITY

Studies of the distribution of iron in adult males have shown that 70% of the body's iron resides in hemoglobin; 25% in ferritin, hemosiderin, and transferrin; and 4% in myoglobin. Iron content or myoglobin concentration of muscle in adult anemic subjects does not differ from that in normal subjects. However, iron deficiency in children is associated with growth retardation, and serum myoglobin concentrations also show changes that parallel the level of hemoglobin concentration in the blood. It seems that the myoglobin content of adult muscle is much more resistant to iron deficiency than is that of children's muscle, probably because during growth the requirement of iron for myoglobin synthesis must be higher in children.

4.1. Respiratory and Cardiovascular Adjustments

Physical work performance is an energy-demanding task, and tolerance depends upon the individual's maximum aerobic capacity (VO_2 max). That is, aerobic capacity, or efficiency in delivering oxygen to the skeletal muscle, determines the maximum work capacity. When iron deficiency is severe enough to cause anemia, the oxygen-carrying capacity of the blood falls concomitantly with the reduction in hemoglobin levels. In such a situation, in order to deliver the required amount of oxygen to the muscle, a physiological adaptation depending upon the energy cost of the work is required. For a sedentary worker, even a low level of hemoglobin- and oxygen-carrying capacity is sufficient and no physiological adjustment may be needed. But when physical work demands more energy, additional compensatory adaptations are called for to improve oxygen delivery to the required site. Due to its reduced hemoglobin level, the blood acquires low buffering capacity. Moreover, anemic blood has a relatively higher proportion of plasma and hence a greater capacity to carry carbon dioxide in solution. Loss of buffering capacity and high carbon dioxide tension in anemia during muscular work reduces the pH of the blood, which, in turn, decreases the affinity of oxygen to hemoglobin; as a result, more oxygen is dissociated and supplied to the tissues. Want of oxygen in an anemic subject is also fullfilled by an increase in pulmonary ventilation which, however, places additional demands on respiratory muscle. In addition, VO_2 max also increases due to the increase in cardiac output caused by the increased heart rate. All these increase the energy cost of the given exercise. Even at a submaximum level of exercise, anemic individuals require more energy to compensate for respiratory and cardiovascular adjustments. A low arteriovenous difference indicates that even at low levels of exercise, the anemic person is working close to the maximum threshold. The same maximum cardiac output can be reached in both anemic and nonanemic individuals (in the absence of long-term training); however, the level of physical exercise requiring maximum or near-maximum cardiac output would be significantly lower in the anemic subject. This clearly indicates that the threshold of maximum physical work is higher in nonanemic than in anemic individuals.

4.2. Human Studies

Cardiovascular adjustments in response to exercise on an upright bicycle ergometer were studied in anemic east African industrial workers before and after treatment with oral iron tablets (200 mg $FeSO_4$/day for three months). Significantly decreased heart rate (lower by 23 beats/min) and increased VO_2 max (higher by 530 ml/min), comparable to those of normal controls, were reported after iron treatment (Davies and Van Haaren, 1973). In another study of Tanzanian industrial workers using a stationary bicycle ergometer, Davies et al. (1973) showed that anemic subjects worked with higher heart rates and increased cardiac output. Severely anemic subjects (hemoglobin below 6.7 g/dl) and moderately anemic subjects (hemoglobin 6.8–9.2 g/dl) worked with 170 and 160 beats/min respectively, compared with control subjects (hemoglobin 9.3–14.5 g/dl) who had 127 beats/min; moreover, they also had significantly less predicted maximum aerobic power (VO_2 max): 1.90 liters/min and 2.20 liters/min respectively compared with 2.88 liters/min in controls. Gardner et al. (1977) studied physical work capacity and work tolerance in seven groups of females with hemoglobin levels ranging from 6 to 13 g/100 ml, using an 18-min multistage treadmill test. They reported an increase of 4.7% in heart rate with every g/dl decrease in hemoglobin level below 13 g/dl at moderate workload. Moreover, the percentage of subjects reaching the highest level of workload was shown to be low in groups with low hemoglobin levels. In fact, of the group of subjects with hemoglobin above 13 g/dl, all reached the highest workload; in the group with 6 g/dl hemoglobin, none reached the peak. Viteri and Torun (1974), using the Harvard step test, have shown physical work capacity to be proportional to the hemoglobin concentration of the subject. Edgerton et al. (1979) showed the work performance of tea pickers to be parallel to the hemoglobin content of their blood. Measured in quantity of tea leaves picked, work output in subjects with 9.0 g/dl of hemoglobin was 15.6 kg/day. Iron treatment for one month raised their hemoglobin to 11.5 g/dl, and the quantity of tea leaves picked rose to 17.5 kg/day. Iron treatment for one month resulted in a 12% increase in the work output, which amounts to an increase of 0.75 kg of tea leaves picked/day per g/dl increase of hemoglobin. In a similar study carried out in Indonesia on rubber plantation workers, it was shown that anemia even at the high cutoff level of 13.0 g/dl affected the workers' ability to perform on the Harvard step test (Basta et al. 1979). Anemic workers excavated approximately 20% less earth per day. Income from rubber tapping was directly proportional to the hemoglobin concentration. Treatment with ferrous iron and a small incentive

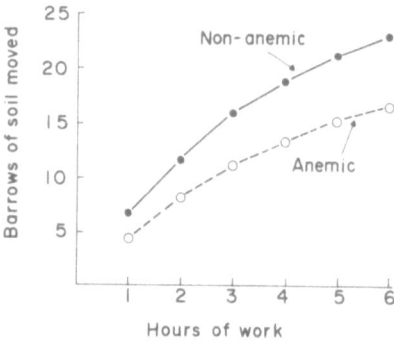

Figure 6. Physical work productivity in road workers related to duration of daily work. The iron-deficient anemic group is at a progressively greater disadvantage as the duration of work increases.

payment resulted in improved work output and hence productivity. Our data corroborate such findings relating anemia to physical work capacity (Figure 6). Furthermore, we differentiated the ability to perform short bursts of activity from endurance; the latter was affected much more in iron deficiency (Figure 7; Chandra, 1983b). In addition to increase in hemoglobin Ohira *et al.* (1979) noted increase in maximum work time and decrease in heart rate, in an iron-deficient anemic subject performing treadmill exercise after four days of iron treatment. They suggested that iron might be being incorporated into tissue, which in some way proves functionally beneficial in improving work tolerance.

4.3. Animal Studies

Animal experiments support the observations made in human studies of decreased physical work capacity in iron-deficiency anemia. The advantages of animal studies are many: namely, it is possible to monitor (increase or decrease)

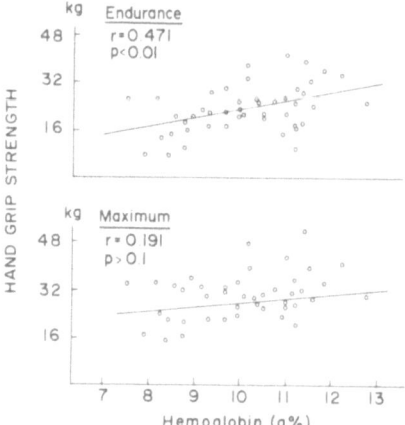

Figure 7. Hand-grip strength related to hemoglobin concentration. The maximum effort in a short burst of 10 sec was not affected by anemia, whereas endurance over a period of 1 min was significantly diminished in the anemic subjects and correlated with hemoglobin concentration.

hemoglobin level for a required length of time either by transfusion or bleeding, maximum threshold of exercise can be reached, effects of deprivation during development can be studied by selecting weanling animals, and biochemical effects can be studied by analyzing muscle for myoglobin and cytochrome content or for various enzymes of aerobic and glycolytic pathways. The most important is the delineation of the effect of anemia from iron deficiency *per se* by monitoring the hemoglobin levels of animals on deficient and sufficient diet.

Developing animals showed a differential response to iron-deficiency anemia compared with the adults. Developing rats on an iron-deficient diet had an impaired age-associated increase in myoglobin concentration of muscle (Dallman and Schwartz, 1965). Edgerton *et al.* (1972) reported a differential response of slow and fast muscle in 18-day-old male rats after 52 days of iron-deficient diet. The myoglobin concentration of the soleus muscle was lowered, while that of the gastrocnemius muscle was unaffected. In addition, they also reported a decrease in the cytochrome content of skeletal muscle but not in that of cardiac muscle. Work tolerance in forced exercise performance, studied by a running test on a motor-driven treadmill, also showed a significant decrease in anemia; normal levels were restored after iron repletion. Moreover, iron-deficient anemic rats were shown to be less active even in voluntary activity than the controls. Finch *et al.* (1976) have also shown poor running ability in iron-deficient rats. In two sets of experiments, they have studied the effect of iron deficiency with and without anemia. In the first set of experiments, all the animals had a hemoglobin level of 10 g/dl, adjusted by exchange transfusion. Different groups of animals were given iron-deficient, normal, and iron-supplemented diets for 4 weeks. Though the hemoglobin levels of all the animals was 10 g/dl, the animals on the iron-deficient diet ran for only 4 min, while those on iron-supplemented and normal diets ran for 16 to 20 min. Moreover, by supplementing iron to iron-deficient rats, running time was increased from 4 to 10 min in just 1 day and to 15 min in 2 days; after 3 days of iron treatment, it was comparable to normal. The decreased running time of iron-deficient rats was not attributed to hemoglobin levels, as all the animals were kept at a constant hemoglobin level of 10 g/dl; thus the difference is due to iron deficiency itself, which was confirmed further by a significant increase in the running time of iron-deficient animals after iron treatment for just for 1 day. In another set of experiments, it was shown that even after 9 days of increase in hemoglobin levels by transfusion, iron-deficient animals showed no increment in running time. On the other hand, the animals given iron supplements reached the maximum running time after only 4 days. These experiments clearly indicate that the debilitating effect of iron deficiency on exercise is independent of anemia. Muscles of iron-deficient rats, in addition to low levels of myoglobin and cytochrome content, showed lower rates of pyruvate–malate, succinate, and α-glycerophosphate-mediated phosphorylation. After iron supplementation, increased running time was parallel to increase in α-glycerophosphate while myoglobin and cytochrome content and phosphorylation with other substrates were still at a lower level. A biochemical lesion in skeletal muscle that impairs work performance in iron deficiency is thought to reside in the activity of α-glycerophosphate shuttle.

In adult rats, moderate anemia even of prolonged duration (hemoglobin 7.2 g/dl) and severe anemia of 30 days (hemoglobin 4.4 g/dl) had no effect on the myoglobin concentration and phosphofructokinase activity of the white vastus lateralis, red vastus lateralis, and soleus muscles (Koziol *et al.,* 1982). Cytochrome oxidase activity was decreased only in severe anemia and not in moderate anemia. However, the work performance was shown to be 33% and 59% less than control values in moderate and severe anemia respectively. Moreover iron-deficient rats had elevated heart rates and cardiomegaly.

4.4. Additional Comments

The differences in physical work tolerance of anemic and nonanemic individuals should hamper the work output only if the work involves tasks that are highly demanding physically. However, at low or moderate levels of physical tasks, both anemic and nonanemic subjects should be able to put in the same amount of work, though the energy cost would be greater in the anemic. Practically, almost none of the physical workers put in work at maximum threshold level except when there is a strong motivation and competition at personal level. In spite of this, the work outputs shown in various studies are much greater in the nonanemic than the anemic. The impaired work capacity of anemic subjects would seriously affect their productivity and is of greater importance in developing countries, where productivity depends upon the manual physical work output of laborers. Moreover, tiredness, weakness, and irregularity in performing work is also usually observed in anemic workers. All these, in turn, reflect on the workers in reducing their incomes. This limits their buying power and can therefore lead to undernutrition, thus adding to and aggravating the problem. The overall result would be ruined health and low income at a personal level and low productivity and hampered growth at the national level, which can be countered by inexpensive iron treatment.

5. COGNITION AND BEHAVIOR

The results of many recent studies on iron status and behavioral performance suggests that iron is a critical element for the normal functioning of the central nervous system. This may be due to the requirements for iron in many enzyme systems. The nonheme iron content of the extrapyramidal system of the human brain is 21 mg/100 ml, which is equivalent to that of the liver, the major storehouse of iron. Remaining parts of the brain contain about 2 to 5 mg iron/100 ml. The total amount of iron in brain tissue is much higher than the expected value obtained by the sum total of iron-containing enzymes and cofactors (Hallgren and Sourander, 1958). In addition to the observed fetal resorption and decreased body size and weight, deprivation of iron in the developing rat has been shown to reduce the nonheme iron content of the brain and is found to be more or less irreversible even after long-term iron treatment (Dallman *et al.*, 1975). Decreased monoamine oxidase activity has been observed in the liver and platelets of iron-deficient animals, while monoamine oxidase activity, cytochrome content, rate of phosphorylation, and catalase activity in the brain were unaffected (Mackler *et al.*, 1978). However, decreased specific activity of aldehyde oxidase and a concomitant increase in the accumulation of serotonin, 5-hydroxyindolacetaldehyde and 5-hydroxyindolacetic acid were reported in the brain of the iron-deficient rat. These putative neurotransmitters are known to induce drowsiness and decreased attentiveness as well as decreased ability to learn. Treatment of iron-deficient rats with 5 mg of iron dextran intraperitoneally restored the activity of aldehyde oxidase and also the levels of 5-hydroxyindole compounds to normal in one week. Voorhess *et al.* (1975) have observed increased urinary norepinephrine excretion in iron-deficient children, which returned to normal within 3–4 days of iron treatment. These biochemical alterations causing deranged catecholamine metabolism during deficiency and its normalization after iron treatment form the basis for a possible involvement of iron in cognitive function and behavior.

Clinical observations indicate that iron-deficient infants are usually irritable and listless (Mauer, 1969). There are several reports documenting impaired mental functions in iron-deprived animals and human subjects (Pollitt and Leibel, 1976; Vyas and Chandra, 1983). Massaro and Wildmayer (1981) have shown that iron-deficiency anemia in rats adversely affects some aspects of associative learning. There are controversial reports showing deficient and unaffected maze performance in iron-deficient rats (Bernhardt, 1936; Scarpelli, 1959). Howell (1971) reported that 3- to 5-year-old iron-deficient children with hemoglobin below 10 g/dl showed decreased attentiveness, short attention span, and perceptual restriction. Sulzer *et al.* (1973) have shown that 4- to 5-year-old anemic children with hemoglobin below 10 g/dl did poorly in a vocabulary test, had lower IQ scores, and showed impaired performance in measures of the latency and associative reactions. Iron deficiency has adverse effects on attention and memory control processes, which return to normal after iron treatment. Iron-deficient young adolescent subjects of the Philadelphia Junior High School were also shown to score comparatively lower on tests of academic performance, which included vocabulary, reading knowledge, comprehension, spelling, capitalization, punctuation and usage, map–graph–table reading, use of reference material, arithmetic concepts and problem solving. Moreover, they were found to be more disruptive, irritable, and restless in the classroom (Webb and Oski, 1973). In upstate New York, Oski and Honig (1978) studied infants 9–26 months of age. Those with hemoglobin levels below 10.5 g/dl were treated for 6–8 days. As a result, their performance on mental and developmental indices improved from an initial level of 96.25 points to 109.83 points. The increase in these scores after iron treatment was inversely related to the pretreatment hemoglobin levels. Behavioral performance (reactivity) also improved. In addition, iron treatment resulted in improved gross and fine motor coordination. Others have not found any relationship between IQ measures and degree of anemia among children (Chodorkoff and Whitten, 1963), although the type of anemia investigated was the hemolytic variety characteristic of sickle cell disease, in which iron deficiency is generally not seen.

A recent report by Lozoff et al. (1982) concluded that developmental deficits assessed by the Bayley method are more frequent in anemic children than nonanemic controls and that there was no improvement either in mental development index or psychomotor development index after short-term oral iron therapy. The lack of improvement may be due to the need for long-term therapy, as seen also in experimental animals, or perhaps the cause of lower developmental scores in anemic children may be an intervening variable closely linked to iron deficiency; lead toxicity could be considered one such factor.

In another study, Walter et al. (1983) have demonstrated the effect of mild iron deficiency on infant behavior, this was rapidly reversible with iron supplements. On the Bayley scales of infant development, iron-deficient anemic patients achieved a lower index of mental development. Improvement in the index following iron therapy was associated with an increase in attention span and cooperativeness.

Iron-deficiency anemia in infancy has been shown to have long-lasting effects. Infants, whose anemia was corrected at 6 to 18 months showed soft neurologic signs like clumsiness in balancing on one foot, tandem walking, and repetitive limb movements as well as low attentiveness and more hyperactivity even at 6 to 7 years of age—that is, 5 to 6 years after the correction of their anemia (Cantwell, 1974).

The contributory role of general nutritional inadequacy, and other social and genetic factors (in addition to iron deficiency and anemia) in the development of poor performance, perceptual disturbance, and conduct problems is not clearly dissected out in the majority of the studies. Many methodologic problems plague studies on this topic, however; not the least of which being those that involve the reliability of the testing procedures for young children, cross-cultural transfer of techniques, retrospective analyses, the adequacy of controls, and the definition of iron deficiency. Several investigations in progress are attempting to use improved assessment methods and should provide much-needed answers to the question of iron, cognitive ability, and behavior.

Iron deficiency may occasionally be associated with behavioral disorders such as pica, pagophagia, breath-holding spells, and temper tantrums (Coltman, 1969; Chandra, 1965). Abnormal eating behavior may be both the cause and the effect of iron deficiency. Iron therapy has been observed to accelerate the cessation of these generally self-limited aberrations of behavior.

REFERENCES

Andelman, M. B., and Sered, B. R., 1966, Utilization of dietary iron by term infants, *Am. J. Dis. Child.* 111:45–55.

Antia, A. U., McFarlane, H., and Soothill, J. F., 1968, Serum siderophilia in kwashiorkor, *Arch. Dis. Child.* 43:459–462.

Baliga, B. S., Kuvibidila, S., and Suskind, R. M., 1982, Effect of iron deficiency on the cell mediated immune response, *Ind. J. Pediatr.* 49:431–445.

Baltimore, R. S., Shedd, D. G., and Pearson, H. A., 1982, Effect of iron saturation on the bacteriostasis of human serum: In vivo does not correlate with in vitro saturation, *J. Pediatr.* 101:519–523.

Barry, D. M. J., and Reeve, A. W., 1977, Increased incidence of gram-negative neonatal sepsis with intramuscular iron administration, *Pediatrics* 60:908.

Basta, S. S., Soekirman, Karyadi, D., and Scrimshaw, N. S., 1979, Iron deficiency anemia and the productivity of adult males in Indonesia, *Am. J. Clin. Nutr.* 32:916–925.

Bernhardt, K. S., 1936, Phosphorus and iron deficiencies and learning in the rat, *J. Comp. Psychol.* 22:273.

Bhaskaram, C., and Reddy, V., 1975, Cell mediated immunity in iron and vitamin-deficient children, *Br. Med. J.* 3:522.

Buckley, R. H., 1975, Iron deficiency anemia: its relationship to infections susceptibility and host defense, *J. Pediatr.* 86:993–995.

Bünger, U., Pongé, J., and Schmoldt, P., 1982, Zur oralen und intramuskulären Ferri dextran intervention bei männlichen Aufzuchtkalbern. 2. Morbiditätstrten und Beh and lung shäufigkeiten an Pneumonie und/oder Durchfall, *Arch. Tierernährung* 32:673–684.

Burman, D., 1972, Hemoglobin levels in normal infants aged 3 to 24 months and the effect of iron, *Arch. Dis. Child.* 48:863–866.

Cantwell, R. J., 1974, The long-term neurological sequelae of anemia in infancy, *Pediatr. Res.* 3:342.

Chandra, R. K., 1965, Association of breath-holding attacks with anemia and their treatment, *Indian Pediatr.* 2:411–416.

Chandra, R. K., 1973, Reduced bactericidal capacity of polymorphs in iron deficiency, *Arch. Dis. Child.* 48:864–866.

Chandra, R. K., 1976a, Immune response in iron-deficient children, *J. Pediatr.* 88:698–699.

Chandra, R. K., 1976b, Iron and immunocompetence, *Nutr. Rev.* 34:129–132.

Chandra, R. K., 1977, Lymphocyte subpopulations in human malnutrition: Cytotoxic and suppressor cells, *Pediatrics* 59:423–427.

Chandra, R. K., 1980, *Immunology of Nutritional Disorders*, Arnold, London.

Chandra, R. K., 1981, Immunocompetence in nutritional assessment, in: *Nutritional Assessment— Present Status, Future Directions and Prospects*, (S. M. Levenson, ed.), Ross Laboratories, Columbus, Ohio, pp. 111–113.

Chandra, R. K., 1983a, Mucosal immunity in nutritional deficiency, in: *Secretory Immune System in*

Health and Disease (J. R. McGhee and J. Mestecky, eds.), pp. 345–352, New York Academy of Sciences, New York.

Chandra, R. K., 1983b, Unpublished data.

Chandra, R. K., and Saraya, A. K., 1975, Impaired immunocompetence associated with iron deficiency, *J. Pediatr.* 86:899–902.

Chandra, R. K., Au, B., Woodford, G., and Hyam, P., 1977, Iron status, immune response and susceptibility to infection, in: *Ciba Foundation Symposium on Iron Metabolism* Elsevier Excerpta Medica North-Holland, Amsterdam, pp. 249–261.

Chodorkoff, J., and Whitten, C. F., 1963, The intellectual status of children with sickle cell anemia, *J. Pediatr.* 63:29.

Coltman, C. A., Jr., 1969, Pogophagia and iron lack, *J.A.M.A.* 207:513–516.

Dallman, P., and Schwartz, H. C., 1965, Myoglobin and cytochrome response during repair of iron deficiency in the rat, *J. Clin. Invest.* 44:1631.

Dallman, P., Siimes, M. A., and Manies, E. C., 1975, Brain iron: Persistent deficiency following short term iron deprivation in the young rat, *Br. J. Haematol.* 31:209.

Davies, C. T. M., and VanHaaren, J. P. M., 1973, Effect of treatment on physiological responses to exercise in East African industrial workers with iron deficiency anemia, *Br. J. Indust. Med.* 30:335–340.

Davies, C. T. M., Chukweumeka, A. C., and Van Haaren, J. P. M., 1973, Iron-deficiency anemia: Its effect on maximum aerobic power and responses to exercise in African males aged 17–40 years, *Clin. Sci.* 44:555–562.

Dillman, E., Gale, C., Green, W., Johnson, D. G., Mackler, B., and Finch, C., 1980, Hypothermia in iron deficiency due to altered triiodothyronine metabolism, *Am. J. Physiol.* 238:R377–R381.

Editorial, 1974, Iron and resistance to infection, *Lancet* 2:325–326.

Edgerton, V. R., Bryant, S. L., Gillespie, C. A., and Gardner, G. W., 1972, Iron deficiency anemia and physical performance and activity of rats, *J. Nutr.* 102:381–400.

Edgerton, V. R., Gardner, G. W., Ohira, Y., Barnard, R. J., and Senewiratne, B., 1979, Iron deficiency anemia and its effect on worker productivity and activity patterns, *Br. Med. J.* 2:1546.

Finch, C. A., Miller, L. R., Inamdar, A. R., 1976, Iron deficiency in the rat: Physiological and biochemical studies of muscle dysfunction, *J. Clin. Invest.* 58:447.

Fletcher, J., Mather, J., Lewis, M. J., and Whiting, G., 1975, Mouth lesions in iron-deficient anemia: Relationship to *Candida albicans* in saliva and to impairment of lymphocyte transformation, *J. Infect. Dis.* 131:44–50.

Gardner, G. W., Edgerton, V. R., Senewiratne, B., Barnard, R. J., and Ohira, Y., 1977, Physical work capacity and metabolic stress in subjects with iron deficiency anemia, *Am. J. Clin. Nutr.* 30:910–917.

Gross, R., and Newberne, P. M., 1980, Role of nutrition in immunologic function, *Physiol. Rev.* 60:188–302.

Gross, R. L., Reid, J. V. O., Newberne, P. M., Burgess, B., Marston, R., and Hift, W., 1975, Depressed cell-mediated immunity in megaloblastic anemia due to folic acid deficiency, *Am. J. Clin. Nutr.* 28:225–232.

Guha, D. K., Walia, B. N. S., Tandon, B. N., Deo, M. G., and Ghai, O. P., 1968, Small bowel changes in iron deficiency anaemia of childhood, *Arch. Dis. Child.* 43:239–244.

Hallgren, B., and Sourander, P.,1958, The effect of age on the nonhaemin iron in the human brain, *J. Neurochem.* 3:41.

Hegenauer, J., and Saltman, P., 1975, Iron and susceptibility to infectious disease, *Science* 188:1038–1039.

Hershko, C. H., Karsai, A., Eylon, L., and Izak, G., 1970, The effect of chronic iron deficiency on some biochemical functions of the human hemopoietic tissue, *Blood* 36:321–329.

Hesse, H. deV., 1981, Iron status in South African mothers and infants: Perceptions, random thoughts and studies, in: *Iron Nutrition Revisited: Infancy, Childhood and Adolescence* (F. A. Oski and H. A. Pearson, eds.), Ross Laboratories, Columbus, Ohio, p. 15.

Higashi, O., Sato, Y., Takamatsu, H., and Oyama, M., 1967, Mean cellular peroxidase (MCP) of leukocytes in iron deficiency anemia, *Tohoku J. Exp. Med.* 93:105–113.

Higgs, J. M., and Wells, R. S., 1973, Chronic mucocutaneous candidiasis: Associated abnormalities of iron metabolism, *Br. J. Dermatol.* 86(Suppl. 8):88–97.

Hoffbrand, A. V., and Broitman, S. A., 1969, Effect of chronic nutritional iron deficiency on the small intestinal disaccharidase activities of growing dogs, *Proc. Soc. Exp. Biol. Med.* 130:595–602.

Howell, D., 1971, *Significance of Iron Deficiencies. Consequences of Mild Deficiency in Children. Extent and Meaning of Iron Deficiency in the United States,* National Academy of Sciences, Washington, D.C.

Jacobs, A., 1982, Non-haematological effects of iron deficiency, *Clin. Haematol.* 11:353–364.

James, J. A., Combes, M., 1960, Iron deficiency in the premature infant: Significance and prevention by the intramuscular administration of iron-dextran, *Pediatrics* 26:368–374.

Joynson, D. H. M., Jacobs, A., Walker, D. M., and Dolby, A. E., 1972, Defect of cell-mediated immunity in patients with iron-deficiency anaemia, *Lancet* 2: 1058–1059.

Koziol, B. J., Ohira, Y., Edgerton, V. R., and Simpson, D. R., 1982, Changes in work tolerance associated with metabolic and physiological adjustment to moderate and severe iron deficiency anemia, *Am. J. Clin. Nutr.* 36:830–839.

Kulapongs, P., Vithayasai, V., Suskind, R., and Olson, R., 1974, Cell-mediated immunity and phagocytosis-killing function in children with severe iron deficiency anaemia, *Lancet* 2:689–691.

Kuvibidila, S., Baliga, S. B., and Suskind, R. M., 1981, Effects of iron-deficiency anemia on delayed cutaneous hypersensitivity in mice, *Am. J. Clin. Nutr.* 34:2635–2640.

Kuvibidila, S., Nauss, K. M., Baliga, B. S. and Suskind, R. S., 1983, Impairment of blastogenic response of splenic lymphocytes from iron-deficient mice: in vivo repletion, *Am. J. Clin. Nutr.* 37:15–25.

Likhite, V., Rodvien, R., and Crosby, W. H., 1976, Depressed phagocytic function exhibited by polymorphonuclear leucocytes from chronically iron-deficient rabbits, *Br. J. Haematol.* 34:251–255.

Lozoff, B., Brittenham, G. M., Viteri, F. E., Wolf, A. W., and Urrutia, J. J., 1982, The effects of short-term oral iron therapy on developmental deficit in iron-deficient anemic infants, *J. Pediatr.* 100:351–357.

Lukens, J. N., 1975, Iron deficiency and infection: Fact or fable? *Am. J. Dis. Child.* 129:160–162.

MacDougall, L. G., Anderson, R., McNab, G. M., and Katz, J., 1975, The immune response in iron-deficient children: Impaired cellular defense mechanisms with altered humoral components, *J. Pediatr.* 86:833–843.

Mackay, H. M., 1928, Anaemia in infancy: its prevalence and prevention, *Arch. Dis. Child.* 3:117–147.

Mackler, B., Person, R., Miller, L. R., Inamdar, A. R., and Finch, C. A., 1978, Iron deficiency in the rat: Biochemical studies of brain metabolism, *Pediatr. Res.* 12:217–220.

Masawe, A. E. J., Muindi, J. M., and Swai, G. B. R., 1974, Infections in iron deficiency and other types of anaemia in the tropics, *Lancet* 2:314–317.

Massaro, T. F., and Wildmayer, P., 1981, The effect of iron deficiency on cognitive performance in the rat, *Am. J. Clin. Nutr.* 34:864–870.

Mauer, A. M., 1969, *Pediatric Hematology,* McGraw-Hill, New York.

Murray, M. J., Murray, A. B., Murray, M. B., and Murray, C. J., 1978, The adverse effect of iron repletion on the course of certain infections, *Br. Med. J.* 2:1113–1115.

Naiman, J. L., Oski, F. A., Diamond, L. K., Vawter, G. F., and Schwachman, H., 1964, The gastrointestinal effects of iron-deficiency anemia, *Pediatrics* 33:83–90.

Nalder, B. N., Mahoney, A. W., Ramakrishnan, R., and Hendricks, G. D., 1972, Sensitivity of the immunological response to the nutritional status of rats, *J. Nutr.* 102:535–542.

Nutrition Canada, 1973, *Nutrition: A National Priority,* Information Canada, Ottawa, Canada, pp. 45–123.

Ohira, Y., Edgerton, V. R., Gardner, G. W., Barnard, R. J., and Senewiratne, B., 1979, Work capacity heart rate and blood lactate responses to iron treatment, *Br. J. Haematol.* 41:365.

Oski, F. A., and Honig, A. S., 1978, The effects of therapy on the developmental scores of iron-deficient infants, *J. Pediatr.* 92:21–25.

Pollitt, E., and Leibel, R. L., 1976, Iron deficiency and behavior, *J. Pediatr.* 88:372–381.

Prasad, J. S., 1979, Leucocyte function in iron-deficiency anemia, *Am. J. Clin. Nutr.* 32:550–532.

Scarpelli, E. M., 1959, Maternal nutritional deficiency and intelligence of the offspring (thiamine and iron), *J. Comp. Physiol. Psychol.* 52:536.

Soyano, A., Candellet, D., and Layrisse, M., 1982, Effect of iron deficiency on the mitogen-induced proliferative response of rat lymphocytes, *Int. Arch. Allergy Appl. Immun.* 69:353–357.

Srikantia, S. G., Bhaskaram, C., Prasad, J. S., and Krishnamachari, K. A. V. R., 1976, Anemia and immune response, *Lancet* 1:1307–1309.

Sriratanaban, S., and Thayer, W. R., 1971, Small intestinal disaccharidase activities in experimental iron and protein deficiency, *Am. J. Clin. Nutr.* 24:411–415.

Stekel, A., and Heresi, G., 1982, Personal communication.

Sulzer, J. L., Wesley, H. H., and Leonig, F., 1973, Nutrition and behavior in head start children: Results from the Tulane study, in: *Nutrition Development and Social Behavior* (D. J. Kallen, ed.), DHEW Publication NIH-73-242, Washington, D.C.

Van Heerden, C., Oosthuizen, R., Van Wyk, H., Prinsloo, P., and Anderson, R., 1981, Evaluation of neutrophil and lymphocyte function in subjects with iron deficiency, *S. Afr. Med. J.* 59:111–113.

Viteri, F., and Torun, B., 1974, Anaemia and physical work capacity, *Clin. Haematol.* 3:609–626.

Voorhess, M. L., Stuart, M. J., Stockman, J. A., and Oski, F. A., 1975, Iron deficiency anemia and increased urinary norepinephrine excretion, *J. Pediatr.* 86:542–548.

Vyas, D., and Chandra, R. K., 1983a, Small intestinal structure and function in nutritional deficiency, in: *Disorders of Small Intestine* (C. C. Booth, ed.), Blackwell, London.

Vyas, D., and Chandra, R. K., 1983b, Functional implications of iron deficiency, in: *Iron Deficiency in Infants and Children* (A. Stekel, ed.), Raven Press, New York.

Walter, T., Kovalskys, J., and Stekel, A., 1983, Effect of mild iron deficiency on infant mental development scores, *J. Pediatr.* 102:519–522.

Webb, T. E., and Oski, F. A., 1973, Iron deficiency anemia and scholastic achievement in young adolescents, *J. Pediatr.* 82:827–830.

Weinberg, E. D., 1974, Iron and susceptibility to disease, *Science* 184:952–956.

WHO Expert Group, 1968, Control of nutritional anemia with special reference to iron deficiency, *W.H.O. Tech. Rep. Ser.* 580.

Wrigglesworth, J. M., and Baum, H., 1980, The biochemical functions of iron, in: *Iron in Biochemistry and Medicine* (A. Jacobs and M. Worwood, eds.) Academic Press, London.

5

Hypolactasia
Geographical Distribution, Diagnosis, and Practical Significance

G. C. Cook

Recent advances in our knowledge of primary and secondary hypolactasia have recently been reviewed (Flatz and Rotthauwe, 1977; Cook, 1978a, 1980; Ferguson, 1981). This chapter is a supplement to those works.

Hypolactasia and lactose intolerance are not synonymous terms (Johnson *et al.*, 1981); the former refers to the lactase concentration in the enterocyte brush border, whereas the latter indicates the presence of symptoms following lactose ingestion. Thus by no means all hypolactasic individuals are lactose-intolerant; this is to some extent influenced by dietary practices (see below). Persistence of lactase (PL) after infancy and childhood is an unusual event among mammals and is confined to a minority of mankind.

1. GEOGRAPHICAL DISTRIBUTION OF PRIMARY (GENETICALLY DETERMINED) HYPOLACTASIA AND PERSISTENCE OF LACTASE (PL)

The first detailed report of a striking ethnic variation in jejunal lactase concentrations in adult life was presented by Cuatrecasas *et al.* (1965); these authors, however, considered that enzyme concentrations were substrate-dependent (i.e., regulated by milk consumption). Clear evidence that intestinal lactase

G. C. Cook • Department of Clinical Tropical Medicine, London School of Hygiene and Tropical Medicine, London WC1H 7HT, England.

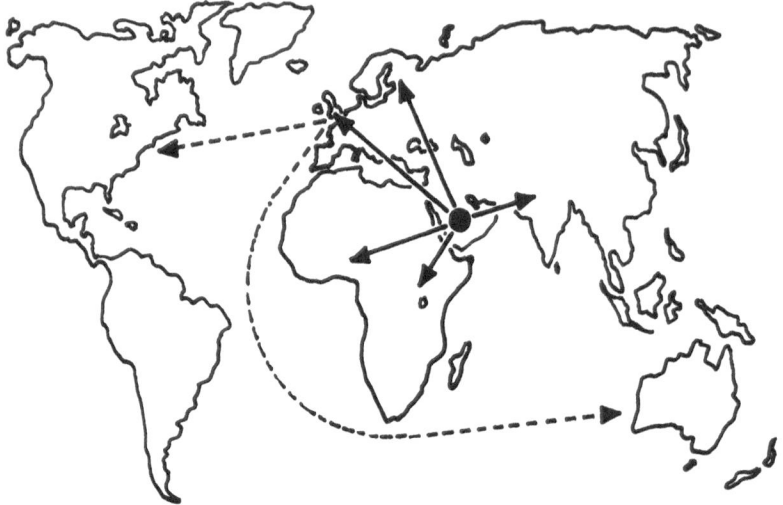

Figure 1. Probable routes of genetic drift of the gene for persistence of lactase (PL) into adult life, assuming that there was a single original focus. Solid lines indicate the ancient routes; interrupted lines indicate migration of northern European stock over the last two centuries.

concentration in adult life has a *genetic* basis was first produced by Cook and Kajubi (1966) working in Uganda. In a study involving African adults, a significant difference in incidence of PL was demonstrated between Bantu-speaking (low incidence) and Hamitic (high incidence) groups. Shortly after that, comparable evidence was produced from the United States in American whites (high incidence) and blacks (low incidence) (Bayless and Rosensweig, 1966). These early observations gave rise to an enormous number of studies in many different ethnic groups in numerous geographical locations (Cook, 1980; Simoons, 1981). Now it is entirely clear that hypolactasia is the normal state for adult *Homo sapiens,* including children over 10 years of age. In some populations in developing Third World countries, however, it includes those aged 5 and above.

Figure 1 summarizes current knowledge on the distribution of the gene for PL in a world context. The most important recent advances have been centered on the Indian subcontinent and northern Africa.

1.1. Distribution of PL in the Indian Subcontinent

In India, major differences in the incidence of PL have been recorded; these results have been summarized by Simoons (1982). Lactase status has been documented in a multicenter study (Tandon *et al.,* 1981). At a northern center (Delhi), 73% had PL, whereas at two southern centers (Trivandrum, in Kerala state, and Pondicherry) the incidence was only 33%. These results supplement data previously reported from India. Using a similar technique in New Delhi, 116 of

134 (87%) Punjabis were shown to have PL, in contrast to 32 of 46 (69%) non-Punjabis (Tandon *et al.*, 1977). Desai *et al.*, (1970) reported a 36% incidence of PL at Bombay (in the west); blood glucose response was recorded after 139 mmol lactose in 100 subjects. In Hyderabad (in the south) an incidence rate of 39% was recorded by Reddy *et al.* (1972); in that study, however, tests were performed in only 18 adults. In south India, Swaminathan *et al.* (1970) had previously shown a zero incidence of PL in 38 local Indians. These data are consistent with a genetic drift from Arabia involving the Aryan people, who invaded that country from the Middle East (Mourant *et al.*, 1976). The southern Indian population is largely derived from the Dravidians, who were the original inhabitants of India (they kept domestic animals but apparently never milked them).

In Pakistan, Rab and Baseer (1976) reported a 95% incidence of PL in 55 Punjabis, Sindhis, Baluchis, Pathans, and Mohajirs. That incidence rate contrasts strikingly with data from a large study in Afghanistan (Rahimi *et al.*, 1976); only 17% of 270 Tajik, Pashtun, Pasha-i, Uzbek, Hazara, and mixed urban people tested had PL. That percentage is perhaps lower than would be anticipated if the high incidence in Pakistan and north India resulted simply from a genetic drift from the Aryan populations of the Arabian peninsula.

1.2. Distribution of PL in Northern Africa

Several studies have indicated that the Hamitic populations of Africa (Mourant *et al.*, 1976) have a high incidence of PL (Cook and Kajubi, 1966; Cook, 1980), while the Bantu-speaking peoples usually have adult hypolactasia.

In Egypt, an overall PL incidence of 27% has been recorded in a study involving 570 apparently healthy people (Hussein *et al.*, 1982); the hydrogen breath test was used. A significant difference was documented between populations in the northern (15% PL) and southern (40% PL) sections of the Nile valley ($p < .001$). Milk has apparently been consumed there since the days of ancient Egypt.

In the Sudan, Bayoumi *et al.*, (1981, 1982) have studied two large groups of adults: (1) a northern group, traditional nomadic desert pastoralists (the Beja), at Port Sudan, and (2) a southern group, Nilotic people (mostly Dinka), at Bor. Of the former group, 83% had PL, compared with 25% of the latter. An important aspect of that study is that both groups drank considerable quantities of milk; the Nilotes, however, were not dependent on it nutritionally and seemed to adapt to small amounts throughout the day. This adaptation occurred after the first week or two of the dry season, when they became milk consumers of necessity. In Senegal, also, a significant difference in lactase status between African and Hamitic populations has recently been documented (Arnold *et al.*, 1980). The ethnic distribution of lactase demonstrated in those studies is consistent with that reported from Uganda, Rwanda, and Burundi (Cook, 1980). Only 22% of the black South African population has PL (Segal *et al.*, 1983).

New data on the distribution of PL in both northern Africa (Sudan) and the Indian subcontinent are thus of interest in relation to the previous demonstration of a high frequency of the gene in Saudi Arabia and the Yemen (Cook and Al-Torki, 1975). Furthermore, the suggestion of a genetic drift of PL from a focus in the Arabian peninsula (Cook, 1978a) receives further support.

1.3. Distribution of PL in Europe

Further studies in southern Europe have confirmed that hypolactasia is common in Italy (Porro *et al.*, 1981) and Greece (Vlachos *et al.*, 1976; Zuccato *et al.*, 1983). Using the breath-hydrogen technique (after 139 mmol oral lactose), 150 of 200 Greek adults (75%) had evidence of hypolactasia (Ladas, Papanikos, and Arapakis, 1982); that is, only 25% had PL. In those with slow small-intestinal transit, symptoms were less of a problem than in those with rapid transit. Rapid small-intestinal transit was considered to be a very important cause of symptoms in those with hypolactasia. There are marked individual differences in intestinal transit rate; enteroglucagon concentrations might be important (Cook, 1980). To date there are no comparisons of plasma enteroglucagon concentrations in relation to lactose ingestion in subjects with hypolactasia and those with PL.

Ninety-five percent of 150 white British adults in Scotland had PL (Ferguson *et al.*, 1984). In the U.S.S.R., an 85% incidence rate of PL has been reported at Leningrad (Isokoski *et al.*, 1981). In a study in Ireland, only 2 (4%) of 50 healthy volunteers of 16–68 years (both parents and at least three grandparents were Irish; the fourth grandparent, if not Irish, originated in England, Scotland, or Wales) had hypolactasia measured by jejunal lactase activity (Fielding *et al.*, 1981). These findings are in line with results from most northern European countries.

The likely direction of dispersal of the PL gene, assuming a single original focus existed in the Arabian peninsula, is shown in Figure 1 (see above).

1.4. Incidence of PL in Southeast Asia, the Pacific, and Australia

In areas with a very high incidence of hypolactasia, further reports have also appeared. In Indonesia, 90% of 53 healthy adults were shown to have hypolactasia (Surjono *et al.*, 1973). More important are four reports from Papua New Guinea (PNG), a country in which lactase status had not previously been adequately documented. Working at Port Moresby, Cook (1979) demonstrated a 2% incidence of PL in a study involving 50 Papua New Guineans from many parts of the country (Booth *et al.*, 1981); blood glucose response to 139 mmol oral lactose was studied. In a study at Goodenough Island (Gibney *et al.*, 1981), 35

Austronesian-speaking Papua New Guineans were similarly studied (venous instead of capillary blood was unfortunately used); milk is not consumed by that population. In 4 (14%) of 29, PL was considered to be present. The possibility of a recent founder effect was not excluded. Of 29 children, 5 (all above age 9) in the Milne Bay province of PNG were also shown to have PL. Furthermore, 3 (10%) of 30 adults at Tari (in the southern highlands) were also considered to have that condition (Jenkins *et al.*, 1981); these people are also not traditional milk drinkers. Five subjects with PL at Agaun were probably descended from a common ancestor (who could have been an immigrant) five generations ago. Using the hydrogen breath test, Arnhold *et al.*, (1981) studied 35 adults in northwest PNG and similarly produced evidence that a minority had PL.

It is noteworthy that occasional cases of PL have been reported in other studies in southeast Asia (Cook, 1978a; 1980; Surjono *et al.*, 1973); a zero incidence for that gene has not always been recorded.

Sixteen percent of 45 healthy aborigines in western Australia were also shown to have PL, using the breath hydrogen technique (Brand *et al.*, 1983).

1.5. Incidence of PL in Children in Population Groups with a High Incidence of Adult Hypolactasia

Further reports of lactase status in children in several ethnic groups in different geographical areas have appeared.

A high incidence of hypolactasia in 186 healthy children of approximately 1 year of age has been reported in Arabs in Jordan (Hijazi *et al.*, 1981); over the age of 3 years, more than 50% were lactose malabsorbers. In that study, the high incidence of hypolactasia in children less than 1 year old is likely to have some significance. In Greece, a 30% incidence of lactose intolerance was recorded in a 6-month to 3-year-old group (Vlachos *et al.*, 1976). In an investigation in Iran, 101 children ranging from ages 7–12 were studied (Sadre and Ghassemi, 1981); rates of lactose malabsorption of 64% and 100% were recorded in the 7–10 and 11–12 age groups respectively.

However, in the United States, lactose intolerance does not seem to be common until after age 5 (Shwachman and Lebenthal, 1975). A minority of American black children between 1 and 4 years of age does, however, have lactose intolerance (Bayless *et al*, 1975a); the significance of this is not clear. In Manitoba Indian schoolchildren (in whom there is a high incidence of lactose malabsorption in adult life), milk intolerance is not a major practical problem (Ellestad-Sayed *et al.*, 1980).

There seems, therefore, to be a significant difference between the rate of decline in lactase concentration in Western and Third World countries (Cook, 1967; Bayless *et al*, 1975a). The timing of the switch, which could have a resemblance to that governing fetal hemoglobin production (Orkin, 1983), might have a genetic basis, although hormonal factors have not been excluded; the timing of sexual development, for example, varies in different ethnic groups. In the rat, thyroxine has been shown to inhibit lactase activity, which seems to be under hormonal control (Raul *et al.*, 1983); during weaning blood thyroxine is increased.

2. EXPLANATIONS FOR THE SURVIVAL OF PL

It is possible, from the geographical evidence presented above, to account for the vast majority of cases of PL by *genetic drift* from an original focus (or foci). That focus seems most likely to have existed in a population in Arabia; radiation of the drift from there to northern African (Hamitic) and northern Indian (Aryan) populations is not difficult to envisage. Whether the high incidence of PL in northern Europeans and their descendants also arose from that or from another focus is impossible to determine. The presence of population groups in middle Europe (e.g., Lapps and Estonians) with intermediate incidence rates (44–77%) for PL (Isokoski *et al.*, 1981) is consistent with such an hypothesis.

Several hypotheses have been advanced to account for the survival advantage of PL (Cook and Nurse, 1980; Isokoski *et al.*, 1981). It has been estimated that a 1% increase in the survival rate resulting from the presence of PL over 400 generations is adequate to explain the changes in PL gene frequency from an original 0.05 to 0.60 (Isokoski *et al.*, 1981). Seeley (1982) has suggested incidentally that persistence of PL probably originated multicentrically and that if it resulted from a single mutation, it must have been at the level of Adam or Eve.

2.1. The Culture-Historical Hypothesis

This hypothesis (Simoons, 1970, 1978) is based on a possible Darwinian advantage of the PL gene in herders, in whom other sources of food are sparse for at least part of the year. That hypothesis is founded on the presence of a high frequency of PL in parts of the world where most people drink fresh, untreated milk.

Incidentally, the Sahara Desert was once, apparently, a green and pleasant land (Williams, 1981). In the Lake Turkana region of Kenya, there is evidence that in the later Holocene period a transition from a fishing-based economy to pastoralism took place (Owen *et al.*, 1982).

2.2. The Calcium-Absorption Hypothesis

This hypothesis (Flatz and Rotthauwe, 1973) is based on the fact that calcium absorption is known to be enhanced following lactose hydrolysis. There is good evidence that the effect of lactose on calcium absorption is dependent on lactase activity (Cochet *et al.*, 1983). Ability to absorb calcium in areas where adults are subjected to a dietary deficiency or to a marginally adequate intake of vitamin D would thus constitute a selective advantage. This would *not*, however, apply to three of the major areas where PL is common (i.e., the Arabian peninsula, northern Africa and northern India); there, sunlight is plentiful and vitamin D deficiency is not a problem.

2.3. The Water-Absorption Hypothesis

This hypothesis (Cook and Al-Torki, 1975) suggests that the survival advantage of PL is related to fluid rather than calorie intake. In areas where camel's milk has been widely consumed (as a source of energy and also water) over several millenia, the ability to hydrolyse lactose and to absorb its constituent monosaccharides would be followed by water transfer from the intestinal lumen and the consequent avoidance of severe dehydration. This could certainly have been very important in Arabia, northern Africa, and northern India, where there are not only high ambient temperatures during much of the year but also many dehydrating diseases (such as cholera) that have for long been exceedingly common.

2.4. The Weaning-Time Hypothesis

This view (Leiberman and Leiberman, 1978) presupposes that PL delays weaning because the infant continues to tolerate and thrive on maternal milk; this could be an advantage in an environment where other sources of infant food are inadequate. King (1972) has reported that in Zambia (where almost 100% of adults have hypolactasia) weaning time might be largely dependent on the rate of fall of lactase to the low adult concentration; cessation of breast-feeding there is followed by a cure of lactose-induced diarrhea. Continuation of breast-feeding would, however, depress maternal fertility over a prolonged period, and this would presumably act *against* the trait.

2.5. The Linkage-Disequilibrium Hypothesis

This hypothesis (Nurse, 1977) suggests that sporadic mutations *before* humans took to domestic milk consumption led to foci of such an adequate gene frequency of PL that milk as a major food source, and subsequently dairying, proved successful. The selective advantage might not, of course, have operated on the locus for intestinal lactase but on another locus in linkage disequilibrium with it.

2.6. The Rotavirus Receptor and Uncoating Hypothesis

This view (Holmes *et al.*, 1976) is based on the supposition that brush-border lactase provides a receptor site for the rotavirus. This infection is an important cause of infantile enteritis and hence infant mortality, especially in the Third World. However, the hypothesis has the disadvantage that it implies selection *against* PL.

2.7. Protection against Colonic Infections

In rats, an acid cecal pH encourages the growth of *Entamoeba histolytica* (Prasad and Bansal, 1983). In subjects with PL who consume milk, colonic pH is likely to be less acid because there is little or no substrate for colonic bacterial activity.

2.8. Resistance to Systemic Infections

The possibility that PL exerts a protective effect against some systemic infections (including parasites) has not been investigated adequately (Cook, 1980). Some evidence suggests that iron deficiency exerts a protective effect against certain infections, including malaria, tuberculosis, and brucellosis (Murray *et al.*, 1978a,b).

Milk has a low iron concentration; if it is used as a major calorie source, chronic iron deficiency results. This would place subjects with PL at an advantage.

2.9. Synthesis of the Various Hypotheses

As previously stated, a considerable bulk of evidence favors an original focus for PL in the Arabian peninsula; radiation would most likely have taken place in the directions shown in Figure 1 (see above).

The occurrence of small numbers of cases of PL in population groups who have not traditionally consumed milk, such as those of PNG (see above), is not, presumably, a result of genetic drift. They have most likely resulted from local mutations; in some areas a polymorphism exists. It is noteworthy that the brush-border concentration of lactase as evidenced by blood glucose responses to oral lactose (in those individuals who do have adequate lactase for some hydrolysis) seems to be lower than that in the very large numbers of cases of PL reported in the literature and which seem to have resulted from major genetic drifts (Cook and Nurse, 1980); it does not exclude the possibility of mild enzyme induction. Studies of jejunal lactase *concentrations* are urgently required in such individuals.

There is a tendency for genetic loci that interact by reinforcing each other to be present on the same chromosome. Thus a water-sparing locus would perhaps be in close linkage with the lactase locus and an allele for water conservation at one site would come selectively into linkage disequilibrium with one promoting water absorption at the other (Cook and Nurse, 1980). Linkage disequilibrium could presumably occur relatively rapidly once lactose became a regular dietary constituent.

3. GENETICS AND POSSIBLE UNDESIRABLE EFFECTS OF PL

Previous work has clearly demonstrated that PL has been transmitted by an autosomal dominant gene (Ransome-Kuti *et al.*, 1975; Cook, 1980). There is no point in continuing to regard hypolactasia as being inherited by an autosomal recessive gene; that situation is now known to be the normal state for adult *Homo sapiens* (Cook, 1973).

Studies in Greenlandic and Danish subjects with and without PL (using crossed immunoelectrophoresis) confirm that low enzymatic activity in adults with hypolactasia is caused by a low lactase concentration in the enterocyte and not by a modified inactive enzyme (Skovbjerg *et al.*, 1980a).

3.1. Atherosclerosis

It has been suggested that presence of the PL gene might be positively correlated with an increased atherosclerosis rate (Cook, 1980; Seeley, 1982). There is also some evidence that serum triglyceride concentrations are higher in subjects with PL than those without; this might render individuals with PL at greater risk for arterial disease. Seeley (1981a,b) has produced evidence for an association between the presence of atherosclerosis and the ingestion of unfermented milk protein.

Firm evidence that milk intake significantly influences total, low-, or high-density plasma lipoprotein cholesterol is, however, lacking (Thompson *et al.*, 1982).

3.2. Cataract Formation

Simoons (1982) has suggested that populations with PL have a higher incidence of cataracts than those without. Repeated galactose challenges result in an accumulation of galactitol, which cannot be readily metabolized; this results in senile cataract formation. Galactokinase is always present at a high concentration in infants; it falls in adults regardless of whether they have PL or hypolactasia.

4. SECONDARY (ACQUIRED) HYPOLACTASIA

Despite some impressions to the contrary (Griffin and Pasternak, 1982), it is likely that, in a world context, secondary hypolactasia in adult life is numerically less common than the primary form; in childhood that situation is probably reversed.

It is, incidentally, very important not to confuse symptoms resulting from cow's milk intolerance with those related to hypolactasia, especially in childhood (Kosnai *et al.*, 1980; Firer *et al.*, 1981).

4.1. Small-Intestinal Infections and Malignancy

Acute diarrheal attacks in children in tropical countries are frequently associated with *secondary* hypolactasia. Thus in Bangladesh, using the breath-hydrogen technique, 29, 35, 36, and 50% of 83 children between 1 and 36 months of age with rotavirus, enterotoxigenic *Escherichia coli*, non-cholera *Vibrio* and *Shigella* infections, respectively, had evidence of lactose malabsorption (Brown *et al.*, 1980). In another study also, a high incidence of secondary lactose malabsorption has been reported in young children with rotavirus infections (Hyams *et al.*, 1981). This organism represents the leading cause of acute non-bacterial gastroenteritis in some Third World countries. If overt malabsorption is also present, hypolactasia, as anticipated, is a common finding; in Mexico, 77% of such affected infants had evidence of hypolactasia (Lifshitz *et al.*, 1971). These studies are in line with several previous ones. However, in Birmingham, England, using a breath-hydrogen technique, hypolactasia was shown to be uncommon in association with acute infantile gastroenteritis (Gardiner *et al.*, 1981). Similarly, in lambs suffering from rotavirus diarrhea, lactose intolerance has been shown not to be a major problem (Ferguson *et al.*, 1981). Hypolactasia also occurs in postinfective tropical malabsorption and giardiasis (Cook, 1978b).

Similarly in small-intestinal malignancies, including the "Mediterranean lymphoma," secondary hypolactasia is very common (Nasrallah, 1979).

4.2. Malnutrition

In severe kwashiorkor, the pathogenesis of which is still not clearly understood (Coward and Lunn, 1981; Hendrickse, *et al.*, 1982), secondary hypolactasia is occasionally present.

In an attempt to ascertain whether hypolactasia associated with malnutrition is a direct result of the nutritional deficit or of the very commonly associated gastroenteritis, Jambunathan *et al.* (1981) carried out investigations on infant rats. Specific activity of intestinal disaccharidases was not significantly affected by poor nutritional status *per se;* there was some reduction in concentrations associated with mucosal atrophy. It seems overall, that hypolactasia in malnourished infants is more likely to be a result of a viral, bacterial, or parasitic enteritis than is the primary undernutrition.

Decreased concentrations of intestinal disaccharidases, and subsequent impairment of lactose absorption, has been demonstrated in preschool children with iron-deficiency anemia (*Nutr. Rev.*, 1982a); this is reversible after iron supplementation. Thus pastoralists living on milk are apt to get very low serum iron concentrations because bovine milk is a notoriously poor source of iron. This secondary hypolactasia might be important in certain groups in a Third World context.

4.3. Dietary Depression of Lactase Concentration

In the rat, dietary fiber in the presence of a high-fat diet has a significant effect on jejunal disaccharidase concentrations (Thomsen and Tasman-Jones, 1982). In that investigation, while galactomannan and tannin significantly lowered the lactase concentration, cellulose had no significant effect.

4.4. Miscellaneous Small-Intestinal Diseases

In childhood celiac disease it seems likely that secondary hypolactasia, and possibly interference with iron absorption also, precede the major mucosal changes (Egan-Mitchell *et al.*, 1981).

There does not seem to be an increased incidence of hypolactasia in the presence of inflammatory bowel disease unless there is extensive small bowel involvement in Crohn's disease (Kirschner *et al.*, 1981).

Although present in a minority of patients with the irritable bowel syndrome, lactose intolerance is not usually a major problem; however, in adults who have genetically determined hypolactasia together with that syndrome, withdrawal of dietary milk is well worth a clinical trial (Ferguson, 1981). Working in India (Meerut, Uttar Pradesh), Mittal *et al.*, (1981) found an incidence of 47% lactose malabsorption in 45 cases of irritable bowel syndrome compared with 28% in 25 healthy controls; the clinical significance of this is not clear.

Concentrations of lactase and other disaccharidases have been assayed after jejunoileal bypass operations for morbid obesity (Skovbjerg *et al.*, 1980b). Although there was a reduction in lactase (and other enzyme) concentrations in the jejunal mucosa, an increase in relation to other enzymes was recorded in the ileum.

Secondary hypolactasia is sometimes a sequel to pelvic radiotherapy (Weiss and Stryker, 1982); this probably contributes to the nausea, vomiting, and diarrhea often experienced by such patients.

A clinical syndrome of lactose intolerance (presumably secondary), aural dermatitis, and eczema has been suggested on limited evidence (Kirschenbaum, 1981). Three patients, all young women, were recorded (nickel sensitivity was ruled out in all of them).

5. CLINICAL SIGNIFICANCE OF HYPOLACTASIA

5.1. Symptoms Attributable to Hypolactasia

Classical symptoms associated with hypolactasia are abdominal colic and diarrhea, with osmotic and irritative elements.

Lactose malabsorption seems to be of little importance in recurrent abdominal pain of childhood (Wald *et al.*, 1982); in the cited study, most sufferers were not lactose malabsorbers. In a further study, in England, hypolactasia did not seem to be a common cause of abdominal pain in childhood (Dearlove *et al.*, 1983). Recurrent abdominal pain in childhood does not, therefore, seem to have a significant relationship to hypolactasia (Blumenthal *et al.*, 1981; Lebenthal *et al.*, 1981). This symptom seems to be unrelated to lactose intolerance. However, there seems little doubt that in Italy, hypolactasia does account for some cases of recurrent undiagnosed abdominal pain (Porro *et al.*, 1981). People with genetically determined hypolactasia are apt to get more symptoms after gastrectomy (Gudmad-Høyer, 1969).

5.2. Effect on Other Nutrients

Lactose malabsorption does not seem to impair significantly the absorption of dietary fat or nitrogen. Thus, in children with kwashiorkor, fat absorption is unaffected and nitrogen absorption only mildly impaired (Bowie, 1975). In Bowie's (1975) study, nitrogen *retention* was overall unaffected. It also seems unlikely that unabsorbed lactose in otherwise healthy hypolactasic subjects is of significant nutritional consequence regarding the absorption of other nutrients (Leichter, 1981).

The clinical importance of lactose intolerance in adults with hypolactasia has also been studied (Bayless *et al.*, 1975). Of those with hypolactasia, 72% had previously associated milk consumption with gastrointestinal symptoms; 59% and 68% respectively had symptoms after ingesting 240 ml of low-fat milk or the equivalent amount of lactose. None with PL had symptoms after milk or lactose. In the groups with hypolactasia and PL, 31% and 13% respectively, refused to drink 240 ml of low-fat milk.

Therefore, although lactose intolerance is little more than an inconvenience in adults, it does mean that less milk is normally ingested (Bayless *et al.*, 1975; Fowkes and Ferguson, 1980). Also, skimmed milk that is given, often as part of aid programs to the Third World is often rejected by both adults and children with either primary or secondary hypolactasia (Simoons *et al.*, 1977).

Although breast milk is often infected in Third World countries, it has a significant antibacterial activity (*Lancet*, 1981); lactoferrin, which is a powerful iron-binding protein, is largely responsible for that. In addition, it contains secretory IgA antibodies.

5.3. Lactose and Milk Supplements in the Presence of Hypolactasia

Because lactase is a noninducible enzyme (Gilat *et al.*, 1972), the best treatment for hypolactasia is removal of lactose from the diet. Thus fresh milk, powdered milk, and milk puddings must be avoided. Small amounts of milk—in margarine, sausages, and in baking, for example—can usually be tolerated.

Social policy with regard to usage of milk and dairy products in food supplement programs should perhaps be guided by data concerning lactose tolerance and not the incidence of hypolactasia (Johnson *et al.*, 1981).

Brown (1981) has suggested that in tropical countries, milk should not be donated as a *single* energy source; it should be combined with traditional weaning foods to bolster the protein and energy density. Milk should be introduced slowly and in relatively low dosage into the diet; when so used, it can provide important nutritional supplements in areas where adult hypolactasia is very common.

Lactose-hydrolyzed milk certainly reduces symptoms in hypolactasic subjects. Thus, Pedersen *et al.* (1982) demonstrated a lower incidence of symptoms after low-lactose milk processed by Lactozym 3000 L® for 24 hr at 4°C. A suggestion has been made, however, that absorption of calcium and magnesium may be concurrently reduced (Kobayashi *et al.*, 1975). Various other commercial preparations are available for treatment. A lactase preparation that can be added to milk before consumption has been compared with a milk product containing lactose-hydrolyzing, nonpathogenic *Lactobacillus acidophilus* (Payne *et al.*, 1981). Using the breath-hydrogen technique, only the former regime reduced the hydrogen response and diminished the symptoms. This study suggests that *L. acidophilus*-treated milk does not help people with hypolactasia. Lactose-free formulas or the addition of commercially available yeast lactase (Lact Aid) to milk is also of value (Kirschner *et al.*, 1981). Holsinger (1981) has reviewed the possibilities for widespread production of lactose-modified dairy products in the light of commercially available sources of β-galactosidase. Such lactose-modified milk preparations can be used with confidence by hypolactic individuals. Because lactase is released by bacteria within it. Yogurt is tolerated by hypolactasic individuals (Kolars *et al.*, 1984).

In India, 112 children below age 2 with secondary disaccharidase deficiency associated with gastroenteritis were studied (Raghupathy *et al.*, 1981). A low-cost groundnut protein formula that simulated energy and protein content of cow's milk was very well tolerated. In Singapore, in children with gastroenteritis, oral milk and rice water have been compared with respect to ileal osmolality and volume (Ho *et al.*, 1982); volume was substantially lower with rice water and osmolality was also decreased.

Lactose-hydrolyzed human milk has been used successfully in congenital hypolactasia (Similä *et al.*, 1982).

5.4. Alleviation of Symptoms Associated with Hypolactasia

Alleviation of symptoms of lactose intolerance after the ingestion of acetylsalicylic acid has been reported; it probably results from the drug's inhibiting effect on prostaglandin synthesis (Lieb, 1980). The major effect is probably on colonic motility, permitting a higher concentration of colonic gas (including hydrogen) from unabsorbed carbohydrate to be absorbed; this is detected by a high-breath-hydrogen concentration (Flatz and Lie, 1982). In the cited study, acetylsalicylic acid had no effect on the symptoms of lactose intolerance or on the time of hydrogen excretion after an oral load of 139 mmol.

5.5. Management of Portal–Systemic Encephalopathy in Hypolactasia

A controlled crossover comparison has been made using 139 mmol lactose twice daily or 3 g neomycin daily with milk of magnesia; the subjects were 10 Mexican patients with hypolactasia, cirrhosis, and chronic portal–systemic encephalopathy (Uribe *et al.*, 1980). Mild diarrhea and bloating were the only significant side effects. No patient became deeply comatose while on either regime; indeed, significant impairment in mental state, asterixis, number of connection tests, and electroencephalograms was observed during lactose treatment. The value of lactose in the management of portal–systemic encephalopathy in population groups with hypolactasia is thus confirmed.

5.6. Advantage of Hypolactasia in Reducing Intestinal Lead Absorption

Lactose seems to have a specific effect in enhancing lead absorption from the small intestine of rats (*Nutr. Rev.*, 1982b); the mechanism might be similar to that which increases calcium absorption.

5.7. Importance of Falling Lactase Concentration in Infant Malnutrition

There seems no doubt that faltering growth curves in infancy in developing countries (Waterlow *et al.*, 1980; Dobbing, 1981) are to some extent a result of hypolactasia that occurs before weaning takes place (see above). Other factors, however, are also important. The importance of breast-feeding in developing Third World countries (Villar and Belizan, 1981) has been strongly emphasized—to such an extent, in fact, that the possibility that continued milk ingestion could possibly have deleterious effects is never considered.

6. ADAPTATION TO HYPOLACTASIA

6.1. Upper Gastrointestinal Factors in Adaptation

Tolerance to milk in hypolactasic subjects can be increased by giving it in divided doses throughout the day. Decreasing the gastric emptying rate after milk ingestion is also of value. Some dietary fibers (cellulose and psyllium) delay gastric emptying in lactose malabsorbers, although others (pectin) have no effect (Nguyen *et al.*, 1982). Small intestinal transit is clearly important (see above); when that is increased (e.g., in the presence of small intestinal infections), symptoms related to hypolactasia are exacerbated. When relative slowing of transit occurs—for example, in severe postinfective tropical malabsorption—symptoms are reduced in intensity.

In 70% of people with hypolactasia, 139 mmol lactose produce symptoms of lactose intolerance, whereas 28 to 42 mmol lactose (i.e., the equivalent of 0.5 pint milk) produce symptoms in 30–60% (Bedine and Bayless, 1973; Bayless *et al.*, 1975b; Jones *et al.*, 1976). Those considerable differences in the incidence of symptoms in people with an intact colon are not easily explained (Caspary *et al.*, 1981).

6.2. Colonic Adaptation

Lactose intolerance may be considered to be *basically* a colonic problem—that is, either a failure of colonic salvage or a failure of the colonic flora to hydrolyze lactose (Szatlóczky, 1982); the coronary dilator prenylamin, which has an antibacterial effect, releases β-galactosidase by increasing bacterial cell-wall permeability and reduces symptoms of lactose intolerance.

Colonic adaptation (Read, 1982) is clearly of importance (Levitt and Bond, 1981). The normal human colon is able to absorb 4–7 liters of water/24 hr. Thus, in the event of a failure of colonic salvage in the presence of a diseased colon, diarrhea results (Read, 1982). Colonic mucosal damage is marked in shigellosis, amebic colitis, *Campylobacter* infections, and so on; it would be expected, therefore, that subjects with those diseases and also with hypolactasia would have increased diarrhea after milk intake. Abnormality in colonic function has also been demonstrated in "tropical sprue," where the brunt of the injury involves the enterocyte (Ramakrishna and Mathan, 1982). Abnormalities in colonic water and electrolyte absorption might be a result of impaired fatty acid absorption (Tiruppathi *et al.*, 1983); unsaturated fatty acids inhibit Na,K–ATPase and Mg–ATPase in the basolateral membranes not only of enterocytes but also of colonocytes. Therefore in that condition also, diarrhea will be exacerbated if milk or lactose is ingested, because secondary hypolactasia is common (Cook, 1978b). The following mechanisms for impaired colonic function in tropical sprue might thus be important: (1) colonocyte damage (as occurs in the enterocyte), (2) enterotoxin production by colonic bacteria, (3) action of bile acids unabsorbed by the small intestine, and (4) effect of free fatty acids on the enterocyte. Bile acids can be converted by colonic bacteria to deconjugated, dihydroxy bile acids, which impair the colonic salvage of water and salt by stimulating colonic secretion and propulsion (Binder, 1980; Snape *et al.*, 1980). In a similar way, unabsorbed long-chain fatty acids are converted by colonic bacteria to hydroxy fatty acids, which stimulate colonic secretion (Binder, 1980), modify colonic motility (Christensen and Freeman, 1972), and cause copious diarrhea.

Similar observations apply to electrolyte absorption from the colon (Phillips and Giller, 1973; Emonts *et al.*, 1979; Edmonds, 1981; Palma *et al.*, 1981).

The normal colon is able to absorb 100 to 160 mmol carbohydrate (from ileal effluent) every 24 hr as volatile fatty acids, before carbohydrate appears in the stool, with resulting diarrhea (Saunders and Wiggins, 1981). While that observation probably explains why many subjects with hypolactasia do not get diarrhea after drinking milk or lactose, it presumably also explains why diarrhea after milk or lactose is potentially severe in the hypolactasic subject with colonic disease.

An increase in colonic propulsive movements has been demonstrated in ulcerative colitis (Spriggs *et al.*, 1951); it is likely that this also occurs in some tropical colonic diseases. Increased propulsion would also reduce the pool of colonic bacterial flora, with the result that conversion of carbohydrate to volatile fatty acids is slowed and fluid absorption subsequently impaired (Read, 1982).

These observations might also be relevant to the survival of PL in nomadic desert populations (see above); colonic disease is prevalent in them and milk the major source of calories.

7. DIAGNOSIS OF LACTASE STATUS

Diagnosis of lactase status is usually by an oral lactose tolerance test (Cook, 1973), assay of lactase concentration in a jejunal biopsy specimen, or the breath-hydrogen test (Barr, 1981; Solomons, 1981).

Serum galactose concentrations after glucose and galactose have been shown to be not significantly different in subjects with hypolactasia and PL (Williams and MacDonald, 1982).

The hydrogen-breath test is reproducible and has proved of value in delineating the incidence of hypolactasia in basically fit population groups (Welsh *et al.*, 1981). However, in the presence of acute diarrhea, deceptively low levels of hydrogen production have been demonstrated (Solomons *et al.*, 1979). This results from quantitative or qualitative changes in colonic flora (with reduction in the concentration of fermentive bacteria) or increased colonic motility with an increased loss of hydrogen per rectum. Concurrent administration of antibiotics may also decrease hydrogen production. Colonic pH is another factor known to have a significant effect on the H_2 breath test (*Nutr. Rev.*, 1982c). An acidic environment in lactose-fed adults attenuated the breath-H_2 response to nonabsorbed carbohydrate; this was less marked, however, in preterm infants.

Further evaluation is still necessary (Sheps, 1982); in gastroenteritis in children, false-negative results have been recorded (Robb and Davidson, 1982). These are usually a consequence of antimicrobial therapy or a mechanical failure in the breath test.

In another study in children, an increase of breath hydrogen above 10 ppm by 120 min after lactose administration gave complete reliability as a diagnostic test for primary hypolactasia when compared with jejunal lactase measurements (Barr *et al.*, 1981). An increase in hydrogen after 120 min was less discriminatory and was often associated with secondary hypolactasia.

A recent modification that is a simple and more sensitive method for detecting hydrogen uses an electrochemical detector rather than the conventional gas chromatographic system (Corbett *et al.*, 1981).

In epidemiological studies, a simple urinary test in which galactose is measured by a strip test after a lactose and ethanol load has given encouraging results (Arola *et al.*, 1982); it is of value in mass screening.

REFERENCES

Arnhold, R. G., Perman, J. A., and Nurse, G. T., 1981, Persistent high intestinal lactase activity in Papua New Guinea: The breath hydrogen test in a Sepik population, *Ann. Hum. Biol.* 8:481–484.

Arnold, J., Diop, M., Kodjovi, M., and Rozier, J., 1980, L'intolérance au lactose chez l'adulte au Sénégal, *C. R. Soc. Biol.* 174:983–992.

Arola, H., Koivula, T., Jokela, H., and Isokoski, M., 1982, Simple urinary test for lactose malabsorption, *Lancet* 2:524–525.

Barr, R. G., 1981, Limitations of the hydrogen breath test and other techniques for predicting incomplete lactose absorption, in: *Lactose Digestion: Clinical and Nutritional Implications* (D. M. Paige and T. M. Bayless, eds.), Johns Hopkins University Press, Baltimore, pp. 110–114.

Barr, R. G., Watkins, J. B., and Perman, J. A., 1981, Mucosal function and breath hydrogen excretion: Comparative studies in the clinical evaluation of children with nonspecific abdominal complaints, *Pediatrics* 68:526–533.

Bayless, T. M., and Rosensweig, N. S., 1966, A racial difference in incidence of lactase deficiency: A survey of milk intolerance and lactase deficiency in healthy adult males, *J.A.M.A.* 197:968–972.

Bayless, T. M., Paige, D. M., Rothfeld, B., and Huang, S.-S., 1975a, Lactose tolerance in children, *N. Engl. J. Med.* 293:306.

Bayless, T. M., Rothfeld, B., Massa, C., Wise, L., Paige, D., and Bedine, M. S., 1975b, Lactose and milk intolerance: Clinical implications, *N. Engl. J. Med.* 292:1156–1159.

Bayoumi, R. A. L., Saha, N., Salih, A. S., Bakkar, A. E., and Flatz, G., 1981, Distribution of the lactase phenotypes in the population of the Democratic Republic of the Sudan, *Hum. Genet.* 57:279–281.

Bayoumi, R. A. L., Flatz, S. D., Kühnau, W., and Faltz, G., 1982, Beja and nilotes: Nomadic pastoralist groups in the Sudan with opposite distributions of the adult lactase phenotypes, *Am. J. Phys. Anthrop.* 58:173–178.

Bedine, M. S., and Bayless, T. M., 1973, Intolerance of small amounts of lactose by individuals with low lactase levels, *Gastroenterology* 65:735–743.

Binder, H. J., 1980, Pathophysiology of bile acid and fatty acid induced diarrhea, in: *Secretory Diarrhea* (M. Field, J. S. Fordtran, and S. G. Schultz, eds.), American Physiological Society, pp. 157–178.

Blumenthal, I., Kelleher, J., and Littlewood, J. M., 1981, Recurrent abdominal pain and lactose intolerance in childhood, *Br. Med. J.* 282:2013–2014.

Booth, P. B., Mourant, A. E., Tills, D., Kopéc, A. C., Warlow, A., Teesdale, P., Hornabrook, R. W., Crane, G. G., and Saave, J. J., 1981, Genetic surveys from the Central, Morobe and Northern districts, Papua New Guinea. *Ann. Hum. Biol.* 8:435–445.

Bowie, M. D., 1975, Effect of lactose-induced diarrhoea on absorption of nitrogen and fat, *Arch. Dis. Child.* 50:363–366.

Brand, J. C., Gracey, M. S., Spargo, R. M., and Dutton, S. P., 1983, Lactose malabsorption in Australian aborigines, *Am. J. Clin. Nutr.*, 37:449–452.

Brown, K. H., 1981. Milk supplementation for children in the tropics, in: *Lactose Digestion: Clinical and Nutritional Implications* (D. M. Paige and T. M. Bayless, eds.), Johns Hopkins University Press, Baltimore, pp. 194–202.

Brown, K. H., Black, R. E., and Parry, L., 1980, The effect of diarrhea on incidence of lactose malabsorption among Bangladeshi children, *Am. J. Clin. Nutr.* 33:2226–2227.

Caspary, W. F., Lembcke, B., and Elsenhans, B., 1981, Bacterial fermentation of carbohydrates within the gastrointestinal tract, *Clin. Res. Rev.* 1 (Suppl. 1):107–117.

Christensen, J., and Freeman, B. W., 1972, Circular muscle electromyogram in the cat colon: Local effect of sodium ricinoleate, *Gastroenterology* 63:1011–1015.

Cochet, B., Jung, A., Griessen, M., Bartholdi, P., Schaller, P., and Donath, A., 1983, Effects of lactose in intestinal calcium absorption in normal and lactase-deficient subjects, *Gastroenterology* 84:935–940.

Cook, G. C., 1967, Lactase activity in newborn and infant Baganda, *Br. Med. J.* 1:527–530.

Cook, G. C., 1973, Incidence and clinical features of specific hypolactasia in adult man, in: *Proceedings of the Eleventh Symposium of the Swedish Nutrition Foundation, Stockholm: Intestinal Enzyme Deficiencies and Their Nutritional Implications,* (B. Borgström, A. Dahlqvist, and L. Hambraeus, eds.), Almqvist & Wiksell, Uppsala, pp. 52–73.

Cook, G. C., 1978a, Did persistence of intestinal lactase into adult life originate on the Arabian peninsula? *Man* 13:418–427.

Cook, G. C., 1978b, Breath hydrogen concentrations after oral lactose and lactulose in tropical malabsorption and adult hypolactasia, *Trans. R. Soc. Trop. Med. Hyg.* 72:277–281.

Cook, G. C., 1979, Intestinal lactase status of adults in Papua New Guinea. *Ann. Hum. Biol.* 6:55–58.

Cook, G. C., 1980, *Tropical Gastroenterology,* Oxford University Press, New York, pp. 325–339.

Cook, G. C., and Al-Torki, M. T., 1975, High intestinal lactase concentrations in adult Arabs in Saudi Arabia, *Br. Med. J.* 3:135–136.

Cook, G. C., and Kajubi, S. K., 1966, Tribal incidence of lactase deficiency in Uganda, *Lancet* 1:725–730.

Cook, G. C., and Nurse, G. T., 1980, The intestinal lactase polymorphism in Papua New Guinea, *Papua New Guinea Med. J.* 23:141–145.

Corbett, C. L., Thomas, S., Read, N. W., Hobson, N. Bergman, I., and Holdsworth, C. D., 1981, Electrochemical detector for breath hydrogen determination: Measurement of small bowel transit time in normal subjects and patients with the irritable bowel syndrome, *Gut* 22:836–840.

Coward, W. A., and Lunn, P. G., 1981, The biochemistry and physiology of kwashiorkor and marasmus, *Br. Med. Bull.* 37:19–24.

Cuatrecasas, P., Lockwood, D. H., and Caldwell, J. R. 1965, Lactase deficiency in the adult: A common occurrence, *Lancet* 1:14–18.

Dearlove, J., Dearlove, B., Pearl, K., and Primavesi, R., 1983, Dietary lactose and the child with abdominal pain, *Br. Med. J.* 286:1936.

Desai, H. G., Gupte, U. V., Pradhan, A. G., Thakkar, K. D., and Antia, F. P., 1970, Incidence of lactase deficiency in control subjects from India: Role of hereditary factors, *Indian J. Med. Sci.* 24:729–736.

Dobbing, J., 1981, Faltering growth and human milk, *Lancet* 1:386.

Edmonds, C. J., 1981, Water and ionic transfer pathways of mammalian large intestine, *Clin. Sci.* 61:257–263.

Egan-Mitchell, B., Fottrell, P. F., and McNicholl, B., 1981, Early or pre-coeliac mucosa: Development of gluten enteropathy, *Gut* 22:65–69.

Ellestad-Sayed, J. J., Levitt, M. D., and Bond, J. H., 1980, Milk intolerance in Manitoba Indian school children, *Am. J. Clin. Nutr.* 33:2198–2201.

Emonts, P., Vidon, N., Bernier, J.-J., and Rambaud, J.-C., 1979, Étude sur 24 heures des flux liquidiens intestinaux chez l'homme normal par la techniques de la perfusion lente d'un marqueur non absorbable, *Gastroenterol. Clin. Biol.* 3:139–146.

Ferguson, A., 1981, Diagnosis and treatment of lactose intolerance, *Br. Med. J.* 283: 1423–1424.

Ferguson, A., MacDonald, D. M., and Brydon, W. G., 1984, Prevalence of lactase deficiency in British adults, *Gut* 25:163–167.

Ferguson, A., Paul, G., and Snodgrass, D. R., 1981, Lactose intolerance in lambs with rotavirus diarrhoea, *Gut* 22:114–119.

Fielding, J. F., Harrington, M. G., and Fottrell, P. F., 1981, The incidence of primary hypolactasia amongst native Irish, *Irish J. Med. Sci.* 150:276–277.

Firer, M. A., Hosking, C. S., and Hill, D. J., 1981, Effect of antigen load on development of milk antibodies in infants allergic to milk, *Br. Med. J.* 283:693–696.

Flatz, G., and Lie, G.-H., 1982, Effect of acetylsalicylic acid on symptoms and hydrogen excretion in the disaccharide tolerance test with lactose or lactulose, *Am. J. Clin. Nutr.* 35:273–276.

Flatz, G., and Rotthauwe, H. W., 1973, Lactose nutrition and natural selection, *Lancet* 2:76–77.

Flatz, G., and Rotthauwe, H. W., 1977, The human lactase polymorphism; Physiology and genetics of lactose absorption and malabsorption, in: *Progress in Medical Genetics* (A. G. Steinberg, A. G. Beam, A. G. Motulsky, and B. Childs, eds.), Saunders, Philadelphia, pp. 205–249.

Fowkes, F. G. R., and Ferguson, A., 1980, Prevalence of self-diagnosed irritable bowel syndrome and cows' milk intolerance in white and non-white doctors, *Scot. Med. J.* 26:41–44.

Gardiner, A. J., Tarlow, M. J., Sutherland, I. T., and Sammons, H. G., 1981, Lactose malabsorption during gastroenteritis, assessed by the hydrogen breath test, *Archs Dis. Child.* 56:364–367.

Gibney, S. F. A., Munroe, V., Nurse, G. T., and Schofield, E. C., 1981, Lactose absorption in a Western Massim population, *Ann. Hum. Biol.* 8:477–480.

Gilat, T., Russo, S., Gelman-Malachi, E., and Aldor, T. A. M., 1972, Lactase in man: A nonadaptable enzyme, *Gastroenterology* 62:1125–1127.

Griffin, G. E., and Pasternak, C. A., 1982, The cell surface and disease, *Clin. Sci.* 63:1–9.

Gudmand-Høyer, E., 1969, Lactose malabsorption in patients operated upon for peptic ulcer, *Scand. J. Gastroenterol.* 4:705–711.

Hendrickse, R. G., Coulter, J. B. S., Lamplugh, S. M., MacFarlane, S. B. J., Williams, T. E., Omer, M. I. A., and Suliman, G. I., 1982, Aflatoxins and kwashiorkor: A study in Sudanese children, *Br. Med. J.* 285:843–846.

Hijazi, S., El-Khateeb, M., and Abdulatif, D., 1981, Lactose malabsorption in Jordanian infants and young children, *Acta Paediatr. Scand.* 70:759–760.

Ho, T. F., Yip, W. C. L., Tay, J. S. H., and Vellayappan, K., 1982, Rice water and milk: Effect on ileal fluid osmolality and volume, *Lancet* 1:169.

Holmes, I. H., Rodger, S. M., Schnagl, R. D., Ruck, B. J., Gust, I. D., Bishop, R. F., and Barnes, G. L., 1976, Is lactase the receptor and uncoating enzyme for infantile enteritis (rota) viruses? *Lancet* 1:1387–1389.

Holsinger, V. H., 1981, Potential applications for lactose-hydrolysed milk and whey fractions in dairy foods, in: *Lactose Digestion: Clinical and Nutritional Implications* (D. M. Paige and T. M. Bayless, eds.), Johns Hopkins University Press, Baltimore, pp. 231–246.

Hussein, L., Flatz, S. D., Kühnau, W., and Flatz G., 1982, Distribution of human adult lactase phenotypes in Egypt, *Hum. Hered.* 32:94–99.

Hyams, J. S., Krause, P. J., and Gleason, P. A., 1981, Lactose malabsorption following rotavirus infection in young children, *J. Pediatr.* 99:916–918.

Isokoski, M., Sahi, T., Villako, K., and Tamm, A., 1981, Epidemiology and genetics of lactose malabsorption, *Ann. Clin. Res.* 13:164–168.

Jambunathan, L. R., Neuhoff, D., and Younoszai, M. K., 1981, Intestinal disaccharidases in malnourished infant rats, *Am. J. Clin. Nutr.* 34:1879–1884.

Jenkins, T., Gibney, S. F. A., Nurse, G. T., and Penketh, R. J. A., 1981, Persistent high intestinal lactase activity in Papua New Guinea: Lactose absorption curves in two populations, *Ann. Hum. Biol.* 8:447–451.

Johnson, R. C., Cole, R. E., and Ahem, F. M. 1981, Genetic interpretation of racial/ethnic differences in lactose absorption and tolerance: A review, *Hum. Biol.* 53:1–13.

Jones, D. V., Latham, M. C., Kosikowski, F. V., and Woodward, G. 1976, Symptom response to lactose-reduced milk in lactose-intolerant adults, *Am. J. Clin. Nutr.* 29:633–638.

King, F., 1972, Intolerance to lactose in mother's milk? *Lancet* 2:335.

Kirschenbaum, M. B., 1981, Ear dermatitis, lactose intolerance, and eczema, *Arch. Dermatol.* 117:523.

Kirschner, B. S., De Favaro, M. V., and Jensen, W., 1981, Lactose malabsorption in children and adolescents with inflammatory bowel disease, *Gastroenterology* 81:829–832.

Kobayashi, A., Kawai, S., Ohbe, Y., and Nagashima, Y., 1975, Effect of dietary lactose and a lactase preparation on the intestinal absorption of calcium and magnesium in normal infants. *Am. J. Clin. Nutr.* 28:681–683.

Kolars, J. C., Levitt, M. D., Aouji, M., and Savaiano, D. A. 1984, Yogurt: An autodigesting source of lactose, *N. Engl. J. Med.,* 310:1–3.

Kosnai, I., Kuitunen, P., Savilahti, E., Rapola, J., and Köhegyi, J., 1980, Cell kinetics in the jejunal crypt epithelium in malabsorption syndrome with cows' milk protein intolerance and in coeliac disease of childhood, *Gut* 21:1041–1046.

Ladas, S., Papanikos, J., and Arapakis, G., 1982, Lactose malabsorption in Greek adults: Correlation of small bowel transit time with the severity of lactose intolerance, *Gut* 23:968–973.

Lancet, 1981, The how of breast milk and infection, *Lancet* 1:1192–1193.

Lebenthal, E., Rossi, T. M., Nord, K. S., and Branski, D., 1981, Recurrent abdominal pain and lactose absorption in children, *Pediatrics* 67:828–832.

Lieb, J., 1980, Lactose intolerance, *N. Engl. J. Med.* 302:178.

Leiberman, M., and Leiberman, D., 1978, Lactase deficiency: A genetic mechanism which regulates the time of weaning, *Am. Nat.* 112:625–627.

Leichter, J., 1981, Effects of lactose on the absorption of other nutrients: Implications in lactose-intolerant adults, in: *Lactose Digestion: Clinical and Nutritional Implications* (D. M. Paige and T. M. Bayless, eds.), Johns Hopkins University Press, Baltimore, pp. 142–147.

Levitt, M. D., and Bond, J. H., 1981, Quantitative measurement of lactose malabsorption and colonic salvage of nonabsorbed lactose: Direct and indirect methods, in: *Lactose Digestion: Clinical and Nutritional Implications* (D. M. Paige and T. M. Bayless, eds.), Johns Hopkins University Press, Baltimore, pp. 80–87.

Lifshitz, F., Coello-Ramirez, P., Gutierrez-Topete, G., and Cornado-Cornet, M. C., 1971, Carbo-hydrate intolerance in infants with diarrhoea, *J. Pediatr.* 79:760–767.

Mittal, S. K., Mital, H. S., Dwivedi, K. K., Mehrotra, T. N., Kumar, M., Elhence, G. P., Singh, V. S., and Pratap, V. K., 1981, Lactose malabsorption in irritable colon syndrome, *J. Assoc. Phys. India* 29:751–756.

Mourant, A. E., Kopéc, A. C., and Domaniewska-Sobczak, K., 1976, *The Distribution of the Human Blood Groups and Other Polymorphisms,* 2nd ed., Oxford University Press, New York.

Murray, M. J., Murray A. B., Murray, M. B., and Murray, C. J., 1978a, The adverse effect of iron repletion on the course of certain infections, *Br. Med. J.* 2:1113–1115.

Murray, M. J., Murray, A. B., Murray, N. J., and Murray, M. B., 1978b, Diet and cerebral malaria: The effect of famine and refeeding, *Am. J. Clin. Nutr.* 31:57–61.

Nasrallah, S. M., 1979, Lactose intolerance in the Lebanese population and in Mediterranean lymphoma, *Am. J. Clin. Nutr.* 32:1994–1996.

Nguyen, K. N., Welsh, J. D., Manion, C. V., and Ficken, V. J., 1982, Effect of fiber on breath hydrogen response and symptoms after oral lactose in lactose malabsorbers, *Am. J. Clin. Nutr.* 35:1347–1531.

Nurse, G. T., 1977, The importance of intestinal lactase and milk tolerance in Southern Africa, *Leech Johannesb.* 47:8–10.

Nutr. Rev., 1982a, Iron deficiency and intestinal absorption of sugars, *Nutr. Rev.* 40:205–207.

Nutr. Rev., 1982b, Effect of lactose on intestinal absorption of lead, *Nutr. Rev.* 40:116–117.

Nutr. Rev., 1982c, The influence of colonic pH on the hydrogen breath-analysis test, *Nutr. Rev.* 40:172–175.

Orkin, S. H., 1983, Controlling the fetal globin switch in man, *Nature (Lond.)* 301:108–109.

Owen, R. B., Barthelme, J. W., Renaut, R. W., and Vincens, A., 1982, Palaeolimnology and archeology of Holocene deposits north-east of Lake Turkana, Kenya, *Nature [London]* 298:523–529.

Palma, R., Vidon, N., and Bernier, J. J., 1981, Maximal capacity for fluid absorption in human bowel, *Dig. Dis. Sci.* 26:929–934.

Payne, D. L., Welsh, J. D., Manion, C. V., Tsegaye, A., and Herd, L. D., 1981, Effectiveness of milk products in dietary management of lactose malabsorption, *Am. J. Clin. Nutr.* 34:2711–2715.

Pedersen, E. R., Jensen, B. H., Jensen, H. J., Keldsbo, I. L., Hylander Møller, E., and Nørby Rasmussen, S., 1982, Lactose malabsorption and tolerance of lactose-hydrolysed milk: A double-blind controlled crossover study, *Scand. J. Gastroenterol.* 17:861–864.

Phillips, S. F., and Giller, J., 1973, The contribution of the colon to electrolyte and water conserva-tion in man, *J. Lab. Clin. Med.* 81:733–746.

Porro, G. B., Petrillo, M., Parente, F., Sangaletti, O., and Vedova, G. D., Recurrent abdominal pain and lactose intolerance, *Br. Med. J.* 283:501.

Prasad, B. N. K., and Bansal, I., 1983, Inter-relationship between faecal pH and susceptibility to *Entamoeba histolytica* infection in rats, *Trans. R. Soc. Trop. Med. Hyg.* 77:271–273.

Rab, S. M., and Baseer, A., 1976, High intestinal lactase concentration in adult Pakistanis, *Br. Med. J.* 1:436.

Raghupathy, P., Pereira, S. M., and Sarala, T. C., 1981, A comparison between children with and without secondary disaccharide intolerance and management with a low-cost lactose-free formula, *Ann. Trop. Med. Parasitol.* 75:211-216.

Rahimi, A. G., Delbruck, H., Haeckel, R., Goedde, H. W., and Flatz, G., 1976, Persistence of high intestinal lactase activity (lactose tolerance) in Afghanistan, *Hum. Genet.* 34:57-62.

Ramakrishna, B. S., and Mathan, V. I., 1982, Water and electrolyte absorption by the colon in tropical sprue, *Gut* 23:843-846.

Ransome-Kuti, O., Kretchmer, N., Johnson, J. D., and Gribble, J. T., 1975, A genetic study of lactose digestion in Nigerian families, *Gastroenterology* 68:431-436.

Raul, F., Noriega, R., Nsi-Emvo, E., Doffoel, M., and Grenier, J. F., 1983, Lactase activity is under hormonal control in the intestine of adult rat, *Gut* 24:648-652.

Read, N. W., 1982, Diarrhoea: The failure of colonic salvage, *Lancet* 2:481-483.

Reddy, V., and Pershad, J., 1972, Lactase deficiency in Indians, *Am. J. Clin. Nutr.* 25:114-119.

Robb, T. A., and Davidson, G. P., 1982, Hydrogen breath test in gastroenteritis, *Arch. Dis. Child.* 57:561-562.

Sadre, M, and Ghassemi, H. 1981, Milk intolerance among Iranian school children, *J. Trop Pediatr.* 27:312-314.

Saunders, D. R., and Wiggins, H. S., 1981, Conservation of mannitol, lactulose and raffinose by the human colon, *Am. J. Physiol.* 241:G397-G402.

Seeley, S., 1981a, Diet and coronary heart disease: A survey of mortality rates and food consumption statistics of 24 countries, *Med. Hypotheses* 7:907-918.

Seeley, S., 1981b, Diet and coronary heart disease: A survey of female mortality rates and food consumption statistics of 21 countries, *Med. Hypotheses* 7:1133-1137.

Seeley, S., 1982, Diagnosis and treatment of lactose intolerance, *Br. Med. J.* 284:598.

Segal, I., Gagjee, P. P., Essop, A. R., and Noormohamed, A. M., 1983, Lactase deficiency in the South African black population, *Am. J. Clin. Nutr.* 38:901-905.

Sheps, S., 1982, Lactose breath hydrogen test, *Pediatrics* 69:827-828.

Shwachman, H., and Lebenthal, E., 1975, Lactose tolerance in children, *N. Engl. J. Med.* 293:305.

Similä, S., Kokkonen, J., and Kouvalainen, K., 1982, Use of lactose-hydrolysed human milk in congenital lactase deficiency, *J. Pediatr.* 101:584-585.

Simoons, F. J., 1970, Primary lactose intolerance and the milking habit: A problem in biological and cultural interrelations. II. A culture historical hypothesis, *Am. J. Dig. Dis.* 15:695-710.

Simoons, F. J., 1978, The geographic hypothesis and lactose malabsorption: A weighing of the evidence, *Am. J. Dig. Dis.* 23:963-980.

Simoons, F. J., 1981, Geographic patterns of primary adult lactose malabsorption: A further interpretation of evidence for the old world, in: *Lactose Digestion: Clinical and Nutritional Implications* (D. M. Paige and T. M. Bayless, eds.), Johns Hopkins University Press, Baltimore, pp. 23-48.

Simoons, F. J., 1982, A geographic approach to senile cataracts: Possible links with milk consumption, lactase activity and galactose metabolism, *Dig. Dis. Sci.* 27:257-264.

Simoons, F. J., Johnson, J. D., and Kretchmer, N., 1977, Perspective on milk-drinking and malabsorption of lactose, *Pediatrics* 59:98-109.

Skovbjerg, H., Gudmand-Høyer, E., and Fenger, H. J., 1980a, Immunoelectrophoretic studies on human small intestinal brush border proteins—amount of lactase protein in adult-type hypolactasia, *Gut* 21:360-364.

Skovbjerg, H., Gudmand-Høyer, E., Norén, O., and Sjöström, H., 1980b, Immunoelectrophoretic studies on human small intestinal brush border proteins: Cellular alterations in the levels of brush border enzymes after jejunoileal bypass operation, *Gut* 21:662-668.

Snape, W. J., Shiff, S., and Cohen, S., 1980, Effect of deoxycholic acid on colonic motility in the rabbit, *Am. J. Physiol.* 238:G321-G325.

Solomons, N. W., 1981, Diagnosis and screening techniques for lactose maldigestion: Advantages of the hydrogen breath test, in: *Lactose Digestion: Clinical and Nutritional Implications,* (D. M. Paige and T. M. Bayless, eds.), Johns Hopkins University Press, Baltimore, pp. 91–109.

Solomons, N. W., García, R., Schneider, R., Viteri, F. E., and von Kaenel, V. A., 1979, H_2 breath tests during diarrhea, *Acta Paediatr. Scand.* 68:171–172.

Spriggs, E. A., Code, C. F., Bargen, J. A., Curtis, R. K., and Hightower, N. C., 1951, Motility of the pelvic colon and rectum of normal persons and patients with ulcerative colitis, *Gastroenterology* 19:480–491.

Surjono, A., Sebodo, T., Sunarto, J., and Moenginah, P. A., 1973, Lactose intolerance among healthy adults, *Paediatr. Indonesiana* 13:49–54.

Swaminathan, N., Mathan, V. I., Baker, S. J., and Radhakrishnan, A. N., 1970, Disaccharidase levels in jejunal biopsy specimens from American and south Indian control subjects and patients with tropical sprue, *Clin. Chim. Acta* 30:707–712.

Szatlóczky, E., 1982, Cause, diagnosis and chemotherapy of lactose intolerance, *Br. Med. J.* 284:1405.

Tandon, R. K., Goel, U., Mukherjee, S. N., Pandey, S. C., and Lal, K., 1977, Lactose intolerance during pregnancy in different Indian communities, *Indian J. Med. Res.* 66:33–38.

Tandon, R. K., Joshi, Y. K., Singh, D. S., Narendranathan, M., Balakrishnan, V., and Lal, K., 1981, Lactose intolerance in north and south Indians, *Am. J. Clin. Nutr.* 34:943–946.

Thompson, L. U., Jenkins, D. J. A., Amer, V., Reichert, R., Jenkins, A., and Kumulsky, J., 1982, The effect of fermented and unfermented milks on serum cholesterol, *Am. J. Clin. Nutr.* 36: 1106–1111.

Thomsen, L. L., and Tasman-Jones, C., 1982, Disaccharidase levels of the rat jejunum are altered by dietary fibre, *Digestion* 23:253–258.

Tiruppathi, C., Balasubramanian, K. A., Hill, P. G., and Mathan, V. I., 1983, Faecal free fatty acids in tropical sprue and their possible role in the production of diarrhoea by inhibition of ATPases, *Gut* 24:300–305.

Uribe, M., Márquez, M. A., García-Ramos, G., Escobedo, V., Murillo, H., and Lisker, R., 1980, Treatment of chronic portal-systemic encephalopathy with lactose in lactase-deficient patients, *Dig. Dis. Sci.* 25:924–928.

Villar, J., and Belizan, J. M., 1981, Breastfeeding in developing countries, *Lancet* 2:621–623.

Vlachos, P., Liakakos, D., and Boviatsi, E., 1976, Childhood lactose intolerance, *N. Engl. J. Med.* 294:163.

Wald, A, Chandra, R., Fisher, S. E., Gartner, J. C., and Zitelli, B., 1982, Lactose malabsorption in recurrent abdominal pain of childhood, *J. Pediatr.* 100:65–68.

Waterlow, J. C., Ashworth, A., and Griffiths, M., 1980, Faltering in infant growth in less-developed countries, *Lancet* 2:1176–1178.

Weiss, R. G., and Stryker, J. A., 1982, ^{14}C-lactose breath tests during pelvic radiotherapy: The effect of the amount of small bowel irradiated, *Radiology* 142:507–510.

Welsh, J. D., Payne, D. L., Manion, C., Morrison, R. D., and Nichols, M. A., 1981, Interval sampling of breath hydrogen (H_2) as an index of lactose malabsorption in lactase-deficient subjects, *Dig. Dis. Sci.* 26:681–685.

Williams, C. A., and MacDonald, I., 1981, Serum galactose levels in lactose-intolerant persons receiving a galactose:glucose mixture, *Hum. Nutr. Clin. Nutr.* 36C:149–153.

Williams, M., 1981, Prehistoric Sahara of green and plenty, *Nature [London]* 292:277.

Zuccato, E., Andreoletti, M., Bozzani, A., Marcucci, F., Velio, P., Bianchi, P., and Mussini, E., 1983, Respiratory excretion of hydrogen and methane in Italian subjects after ingestion of lactose in milk, *Europ. J. Clin. Invest.* 13:261–266.

6

Immune Response to *Leishmania*

Reza Behin and Jacques Louis

1. *LEISHMANIA* AND LEISHMANIASIS

"Leishmaniasis" is a term applied to a variety of clinical conditions caused by flagellated protozoans belonging to the genus *Leishmania*. Prefixes indicating the tissues or organs involved—such as cutaneous, mucocutaneous, or visceral—are commonly used to provide a semieological basis for classifying the various manifestations of the disease. Geographical classifications, such as American mucocutaneous leishmaniasis or Indian kala-azar, are less and less used since—despite differences in the species of the parasite or the vector involved—the clinical manifestations of the disease does not basically differ in various regions of the world.

The public health significance of leishmanial diseases has been generally underestimated. It has been through the efforts of the WHO's Special Programme in Tropical Diseases that interest in leishmaniasis has remained alive and its importance as a health hazard more fully realized. Some 400,000 new cases have been estimated to occur annually, and outbreaks of cutaneous and visceral leishmaniasis have been registered in recent years in Asia and Africa. Effective vaccines are nonexistent, and chemotherapy is not always effective, particularly against more severe forms such as espundia, the mutilating mucocutaneous form, or diffuse cutaneous and post-kala-azar dermal leishmaniasis.

Household insecticide spraying carried out for malaria control has apparently reduced the incidence of leishmanial diseases in some areas. However,

Reza Behin and Jacques Louis • World Health Organization, Immunology Research and Training Center, Biochemistry Institute, University of Lausanne, 1066 Epalinges, Switzerland.

insecticide attacks on the sandfly vectors can be of value only in areas where the disease is of anthroponotic form. Almost all forms of leishmaniasis are zoonoses, with a large variety of wild animals harboring species of *Leishmania*. Possible exceptions are kala-azar in India and the urban cutaneous leishmaniasis seen in the Middle East and Russia, for which no reservoir hosts have so far been identified.

It is gratifying to see that the magnitude of the problem has been appreciated, and as the result of the Special Programme, a resurgence in research activity on various aspects of leishmaniases has taken place.

1.1. The Parasite

The genus *Leishmania* comprises flagellated protozoans that are obligate parasites of a large variety of vertebrates including lizards but not birds. No reference is made in this review to lizard *Leishmania* because detailed information concerning the immunopathological aspects of infected reptilian hosts is not available.

The mammalian leishmanias are digenetic parasites having two distinct phases in their life cycle. Each phase is characterized by a specific host, in which the parasite assumes a distinct morphology and location. In the tissue of mammalian hosts, leishmanias are found exclusively in the "amastigote" form within the phagosomal vacuoles of phagocytic cells of the macrophage–histiocyte series. The amastigotes are small oval bodies of 3–5 μm containing a relatively large nuclei and the basal apparatus of a flagellum. They are completely dependent on the host cells in which they repeatedly multiply, presumably causing their eventual rupture. The liberated parasites are then phagocytosed by neighboring macrophages. The cell-to-cell transfer of the parasite may also occur during cell division or giant cell formation. In the body of the insect vector, a species of phlebotomine sandfly, the ingested amastigote transforms itself into the motile extracellular "promastigote," a slender, long-bodied (10–15 μm) organism with a single anterior flagellum. Promastigotes multiply in the gut of the insect vector and are inoculated into a new host by the bite of the infected fly. They can easily be grown *in vitro* in a variety of culture media at ambient temperature. Extreme similarities among the species, particularly at their promastigote stages, preclude the use of morphology as a taxonomic tool in differenting them. Although morphometric studies (Gardener *et al.*, 1977) have demonstrated species-characteristic differences in certain ultrastructural features of leishmanial amastigotes, this difficult technique leads only to the grouping of species rather than species identification. The same objection holds for newer techniques such as the measurement of the buoyant densities of nuclear and kinetoplastic DNA or isoenzyme characterization of the parasites. The use of monoclonal antibodies seems to provide promising advances in the taxonomy of leishmanial parasites.

At least 12 species of leishmanial parasites have been shown to cause human diseases. There is no general agreement on the nomenclature of these parasites; despite considerable progress in recent years in biochemical and serological characterization, it is not yet possible to separate with any degree of certainty some closely related species and varieties. Discussion on this aspect of the parasite is outside the scope of this review. However, in the opinion of the authors, the trinomial nomenclature of Hoare (1965), despite its inconvenience, reduces confusion and provides a better reference to the etiological agents of human leishmaniasis. Using the trinomial system of nomenclature and clinicoepidemiological data, the following species complexes have been recognized (Lainson and Shaw, 1972; Lumsden, 1974).

The *Leishmania donovani* complex includes species causing visceral leishmaniasis (kala-azar) in various parts of the world. *L. d. donovani* of India is perhaps the only member of this complex for which no reservoir host has so far been identified (Zuckerman and Lainson, 1977). *L. d. infantum*, of Mediterranean regions, has a reservoir host in dogs and is known to affect mainly children (Lysenko, 1971). *L. d. archibaldi* is distributed in northeastern parts of Africa, where several species of carnivores and rodents harbor the parasite (Zuckerman and Lainson, 1977). *L. d. chagasi* is the causative agent of visceral leishmaniasis in Venezuela and other South American countries. Among many animal hosts incriminated as reservoirs, foxes and dogs are the most important (Lainson and Shaw, 1972, 1978). Like the rest of South American *Leishmania*, *L. d. chagasi* is transmitted by species of *Lutzomyia* (Lainson and Shaw, 1978).

Parasites of the *Leishmania tropica* complex are the cause of the classical as well as the aberrant forms of cutaneous leishmaniasis in the old world. The "dry sore" or urban cutaneous leishmaniasis is apparently an anthroponotic form with no reservoir host. It is caused by *L. t. tropica* (*L. t. minor*), with endemic foci in the middle Asia and Mediterranean regions (Lysenko, 1971).

L. t. major is the causative agent of the "moist sore" or rural cutaneous leishmaniasis (Figure 1), with widely distributed through Asia and the Mediterranean region. Species of gerbils and jirds act as the reservoir hosts of this parasite. *L. t. aethiopica* causes moist sores and is apparently limited to Ethiopia. The parasite is thought to cause occasionally diffuse cutaneous leishmaniasis (Figure 2). The rock hyrax is considered as the reservoir (Ashford, 1970; Bray, 1974).

The *Leishmania mexicana* complex includes several species causing mild dermal lesions as well as the more serious disseminated cutaneous infections in south Central America. Species of *Lutzomyia* are incriminated as the vectors, and a large variety of forest mammals host the parasites in nature. The following three species are known to infect man: *L. m. mexicana*, *L. m. amazonensis* and

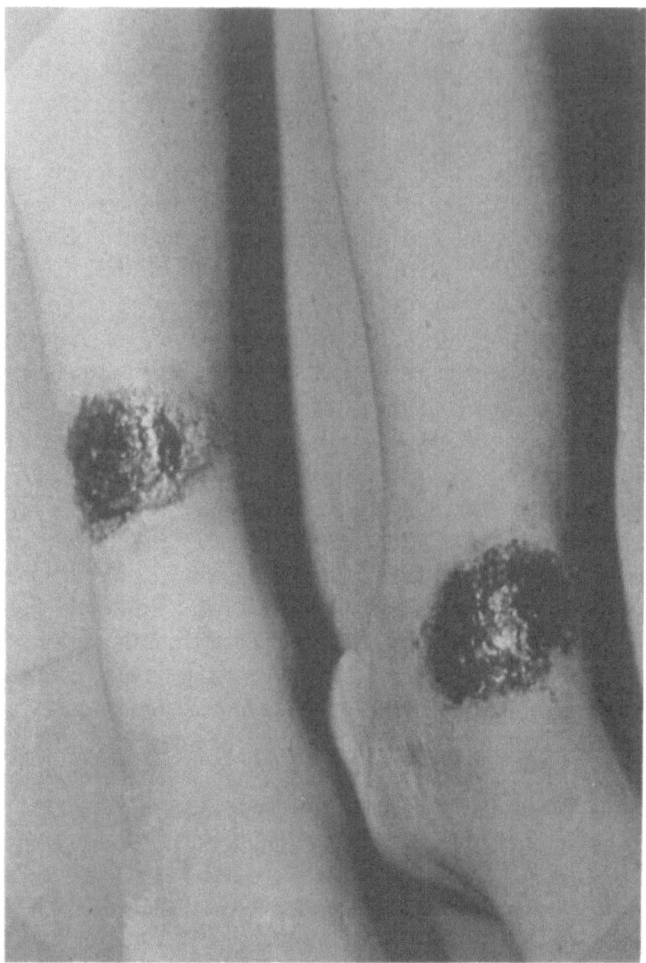

Figure 1.   Oriental sore, wet type (rural), due to *L. t. major*.

L. m. pifanoi. Diffuse cutaneous leishmaniasis of Latin America is attributed to the latter two species (Lainson and Shaw, 1978).

The *Leishmania braziliensis* complex comprises species of enzootic origin widely distributed among forest mammals including various rodents, carnivores, opposums, anteaters, sloths, small primates, and armadillos. The only exception is *L. b. peruviana* of the Peruvian Andes and Argentinean highlands, for which no reservoir other than the domestic dog has been so far identified (Lainson and Shaw, 1978). Species of *L. braziliensis* complex include *L. b. braziliensis*, the etiological agent of the mucocutaneous disease called espundia (Figure 3); *L. b.*

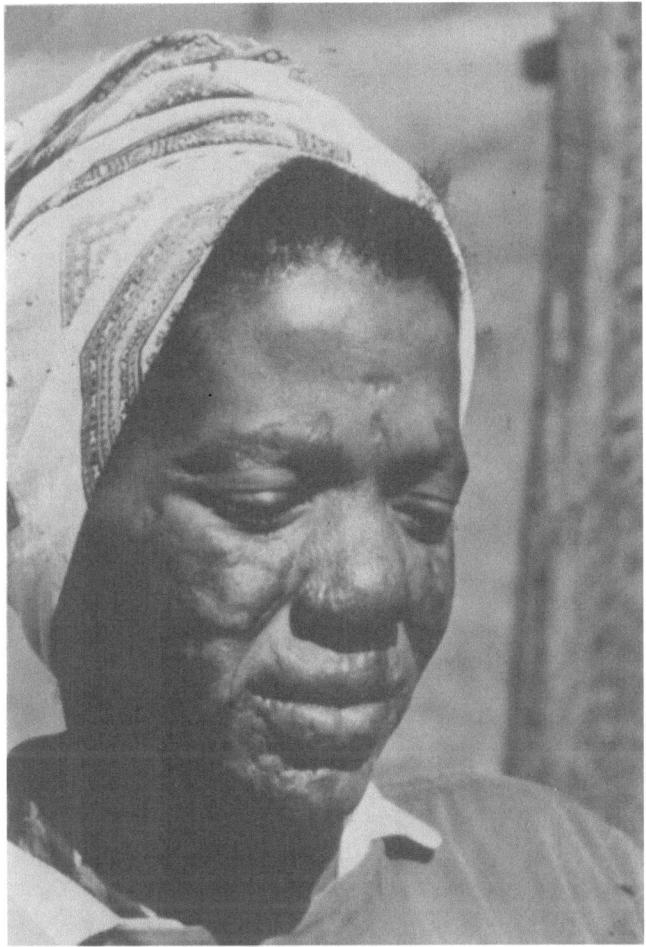

Figure 2. A case of diffuse cutaneous leishmaniasis from Ethiopia. (Courtesy of the late Dr. A. Belehu.)

guyanensis, the cause of forest yaws (Figure 4); and *L. b. panamenensis*, which causes cutaneous disease in Panama and neighboring countries (Lainson and Shaw, 1978).

1.2. The Clinical Forms

Human infections with species of leishmania can best be classified simply on the basis of the type of tissues involved. On this basis, and irrespective of geographical boundaries, three categories of infection can be identified. They

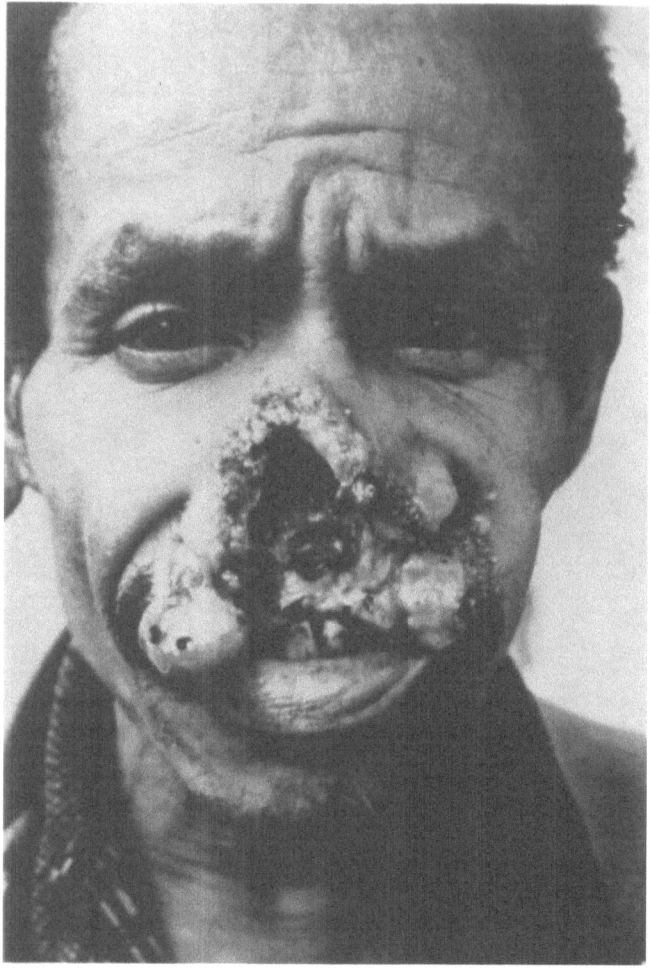

Figure 3.   A case of Espundia from Bolivia. (Courtesy of Dr. Elio-Calvo.)

include (1) the purely cutaneous forms, (2) the mucocutaneous forms, and (3) the systemic variety commonly known as kala-azar or visceral leishmaniasis. The etiological agents of these principal forms are rather well defined in each endemic zone, their histopathological changes are sufficiently characterized, and a set of immunological parameters are recognized as being typical of each type of the infection. These clinical entities are not immutable however; deviation from the general rules occasionally occurs, giving rise to clinical conditions that do not match the characteristics of the form involved either in terms of histology or immunology. Since the histopathological features of the basic forms as well as the aberrant infections are crucial to an understanding of the immune responses of infected host to parasite, a brief review of this subject seems essential.

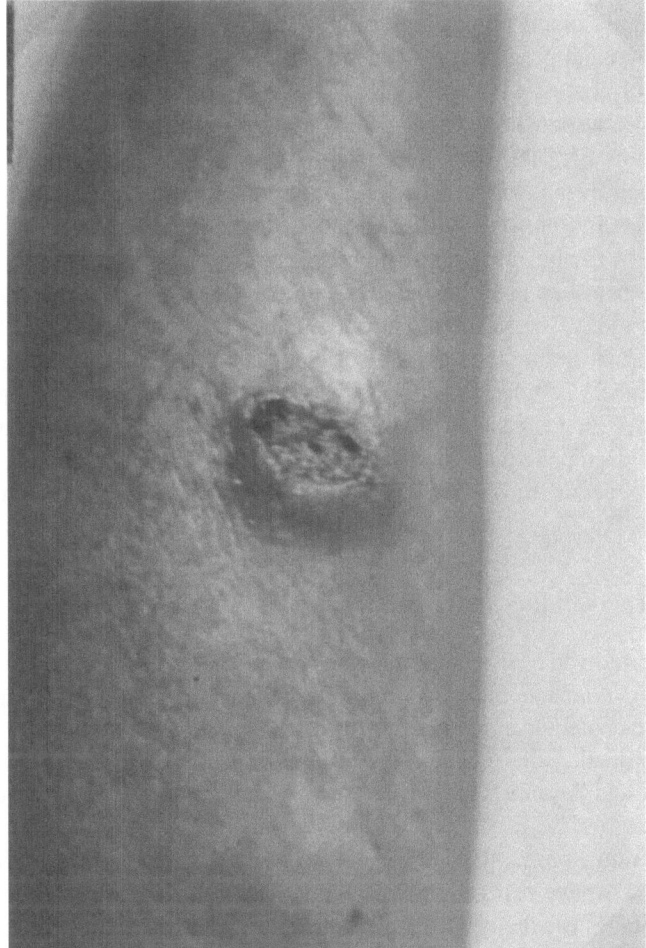

Figure 4.   A primary skin lesion due to *L. b. guyanensis*. (Courtesy of Dr. J. Shaw.)

1.2.1. Simple Cutaneous Leishmaniasis

The classical "oriental sore" in Asia, the "Chiclero's ulcer" in Mexico, the "uta" of Peru, and many vernacular equivalents in other endemic areas are benign cutaneous infections caused by species belonging to *L. tropica* and *L. mexicana* complexes of species. Parasites belonging to the *L. braziliensis* complex may also be involved in similar clinical conditions in Latin America. Although the epidemiological features and gross clinical manifestations of the disease may vary slightly from one place to another, the histopathology of the disease and the immunological responses of the host to the causative agents remain the same universally. The first manifestation of the cutaneous disease is the appearance of a firm, painless papule at the site of the insect bite. The papule grows slowly but progressively without forming the pinpoint white center characteristic of abscesses caused by pyogenic bacteria. Histologically, the papule consists of a histiocytoma accompanied by hypertrophy of the papilla and stratum corneum. Parasite-laden macrophages become more and more evident in the dermis; their eventual destruction, seemingly due to repeated multiplication of the parasite, is followed by disintegration of the papillae and necrosis of the epidermis. A sizable crust is formed on the skin, which soon becomes detached, leaving a crater-like ulcer behind. The edge of the wound thickens; limiting the size of the ulcer. The surface of the wound then takes a very red and "bumpy" appearance, indicating the formation of granulation tissue with many anastomosing capillaries. Cellular changes at this stage consist of a heavy lymphocytic infiltration with increasing number of plasma cells and multinucleated giant cells. The macrophages are less frequently seen, and the few remaining parasites are of degenerate forms. Spontaneous recovery without recourse to chemotherapy is the general rule in most cases.

1.2.2. Mucocutaneous Leishmaniasis

The prototype of this clinical form is the espundia of Brazil, which is a non-self-healing infection of the nasopharyngial mucosa following an apparently simple cutaneous ulceration caused by *L. b. braziliensis*. A primary mucosal infection affecting the mouth and nasal cavity has occasionally been reported from Asia and Africa (Naik *et al.*, 1978; Abdalla *et al.*, 1975). The causative agent of the disease in the latter two continents has not been determined.

In its initial phase, the mucocutaneous disease starts as a skin infection very similar to a simple self-healing cutaneous leishmaniasis. Metastatic spread to mucosal tissues usually occurs some years later, when the initial lesion has long been healed and forgotten. The parasite may, however, be present on the mucosal surface of the nose during the active phase of the initial lesion (Garnham, 1971). The secondary mucosal infection, whether concomitant with the skin lesion or latent, runs a slow but progressively necrotic course, resulting in irreversible damage to both the soft and cartilaginous tissues of the nasopharyngeal cavities.

The evolution of the disease is very complex; no single histological picture can be drawn to represent the whole range of changes that occur in an infected individual. In an extensive study involving 60 patients presenting various leishmanial dermatoses, Ridley *et al.*, (1980) described two groups that comprised most of the mucocutaneous cases. The histology of one group was indistiguishable from normal skin, differing only in having small patches of collagen degeneration, some fibrinoid necrosis, and a slight increase in fibroblasts. In this group inflammatory cells were absent and there was no sign of granuloma formation. The second group was characterized by a marked granulomatous reaction involving giant cells, numerous plasma cells, poor lymphocytic infiltrate, and no necrosis. A third group with a mixed histological character, considered as a transitional phase, was also described.

1.2.3. Visceral Leishmaniasis

The viscerotropic *Leishmania* species belonging to the *L. donovani* complex are the causes of the systemic reticuloendotheliosis best exemplified by the kala-azar of India. The disease is widely distributed around the world and often ends fatally. Although slight clinical and epidemiological differences exist among geographical variants of the disease, the principal clinical and histopathological features of the infection remain the same throughout the endemic areas. Briefly, they consist of a rather generalized hyperplasia of the reticuloendothelial cells in most internal organs, particularly of the spleen, liver, and—in certain forms—the lymph nodes. Other predominant features include anemia, leukopenia, hemorrhage, intestinal ulceration, myocardial damage, amyloidosis, and cloudy swelling of the liver and kidneys. Synthesis of plasma proteins is disturbed, leading to hypoproteinemia and hypergammaglobulinemia. Microscopically, two types of lesions may be observed in the liver: (1) a granulomatous reaction consisting of histiocytes and lymphogranulocytic cells or (2) more or less extensive areas of hemorrhagic necrosis, congestive changes, extravasation, reticular collapse, and eventually disappearance of hepatocytes (Pampiglione *et al.*, 1974). Histological changes of spleen and lymph nodes consists of a marked atrophy of the splenic white pulp and of the paracortical areas of lymph nodes. The depleted areas in both organs are compensated by accumulation of parasite-laden histiocytes and plasma cells (Veress *et al.*, 1977).

1.2.4. The Aberrant Clinical Forms

Two abnormal conditions are known to follow an apparently simple cutaneous leishmaniasis and a third to follow nonradically cured cases of kala-azar. The three aberrant conditions are chronic nonhealing skin manifestations of undetermined etiology. The first two include leishmaniasis recidivans (LR) and diffuse cutaneous leishmaniasis (DCL); the third is known as post-kala-azar dermal leishmaniasis (PKDL).

LR is the consequence of an earlier infection of the urban type of Oriental sore. The lesions often appear some years after an apparent cure of the initial cutaneous disease. They resemble a lupoid skin eruption near or at some distance from the scar of the initial ulcer. Histologically, the lesion is caused by an intense lymphocytic infiltration, numerous giant cells, some epitheloid cells and rare histiocytic elements. The parasites are scanty and often undetectable (Pettit, 1962, Ardehali *et al.*, 1980).

DCL, which is better known from Venezuela and Ethiopia, was first described and named by Convit (1958) as leishmaniasis tegumentaria diffusa. Although most cases in the New World have been recognized and described from Venezuela, the disease is certainly not confined to this country. Similar conditions have been reported from Brazil, Bolivia, and the Dominican Republic. The distribution of DCL in the Old World is much more limited: the majority of cases so far reported have been from Ethiopia. The condition involves the exposed parts of the skin, particularly the face and the extremities, on which numerous papular or nodular eruptions appear. The multiplicity of lesions is certainly due to metastic spread of the parasite from an initial single cutaneous lesion. Metastasis to the internal organs never occurs however, and the parasite remains confined to the skin. The lesions are painless, nonulcerating nodules consisting predominantly of parasite-laden macrophages. The remarkable histological feature of the disease is the scarcity of lymphocytic elements and, despite the chronicity of the condition, the absence of giant and epitheloid cells.

PKDL is a skin disease that follows an incompletely treated case of visceral leishmaniasis. The onset of the skin manifestation may vary from several months to many years after an apparent cure from the visceral infection. Intriguingly enough, the disease does not accompany an internal infection and, despite the presence of the parasite in dermal lesion sometimes in considerable number, no parasites are found in the viscera. The clinical picture consists of numerous nodular eruptions on various parts of the skin, particularly on the face, limbs, or trunk. The lesions may be depigmented or erythematous, but they are usually nonulcerative. The depigmented types are associated with granulomatous reactions, some vascular reactions, and few parasites. The erythematous types show a considerable edema, many newly formed blood vessels, a marked granulomatous infiltration, and numerous parasites (Sen Gupta and Bhattacharjee, 1953).

2. THE IMMUNE RESPONSE OF MAN IN VARIOUS LEISHMANIAL INFECTIONS

2.1. Immune Response in Cutaneous Leishmaniasis

The classical cutaneous leishmaniasis of the Old World as well as the Oriental sore and its many equivalents in the New World are characterized by three immunological parameters: (1) the development of marked cell-mediated reactions detectable by both *in vivo* and *in vitro* techniques, (2) a low level of circulating antibody, and (3) the development of long-lasting immunity following spontaneous cure.

It has long been known that inoculation of the parasite extract (Wagener, 1923) or a phenolized suspension of leishmanial promastigotes "leishmanin" into the skin of an individual infected or recovered from cutaneous leishmaniasis evokes a delayed skin reaction of tuberculin type within 12–24 hr (Montenegro 1926). The diagnostic value of the test was confirmed by Buss (1929), Pessôa and Pestona (1940) for *L. braziliensis,* and Dostrovsky and Sagher (1946) for *L. tropica.* The test, often referred to as the "Montenegro reaction," has been used widely in all endemic areas as a diagnostic tool and for epidemiological studies. The diagnostic value of the test is questionable, since exposure to various *Leishmania* species (including lizard and rodent *Leishmania*) may result in the development of a positive skin reaction (Mayrink *et al.,* 1979; Manson-Bahr, 1961, 1963).

Depending on the species of the parasite involved, a positive delayed skin reaction may be obtained as soon as a week or many months after the onset of the infection. Once positive, the reaction is said to remain so for decades (Guirges, 1971). It must be mentioned however, that loss of skin reactivity in 52% of treated cases of American cutaneous leishmaniasis has been reported (Mayrink *et al.,* 1976). It is interesting to note that despite the parallelism that often is believed to exist between the development of a positive delayed hypersensitivity reaction and a functional cell-mediated immune response in leishmanial infection, the cutaneous disease runs its normal course long after the onset of skin positivity. The appearance of a delayed skin reaction does not correspond to the time of healing, nor does it constitute an indication of resistance against the parasite. Individuals bearing an active sore and presenting positive skin reactions are shown to be susceptible to reinoculation with the same parasite. An ulcer rapidly grows at the site of the reinoculation, becoming isophasic with the initial lesion and healing at the same time (Dostrovsky *et al.,* 1952a). Attempts in transfer of delayed skin reaction from positive to negative subjects by leukocytes have so far been equivocal (Adler and Nelken, 1965; Bray and Lainson, 1965; Mendes, 1979). Demonstration of cellular immune responses in human cutaneous leishmaniasis by *in vitro* techniques have not been numerous. A few available reports (Tremonti and Walton, 1970; Witztum *et al.,* 1978; Neva *et al.,* 1979) indicate that peripheral blood lymphocytes from individuals bearing a leishmanial lesion or recovered from the disease undergo blast transformation in the presence of leishmanial antigen. The significance of these observations in relation to a protective immune response against the parasite remains to be elucidated.

Earlier attempts to demonstrate circulating antibodies in cutaneous leishmaniasis have generally been unsuccessful. Equivocal results were reported by indirect hemoagglutination, which was later shown to be poorly suited for this purpose (Bray and Lainson, 1967; Mannweiler *et al.*, 1978; Menzel and Bienzle, 1978). By the use of more sensitive techniques such as indirect immunofluorescence and enzyme-linked immunosorbent assay circulating antibodies have repeatedly been shown to be present in this disease (Behforouz *et al.*, 1976; Menzel and Bienzle, 1978; Roffi *et al*, 1980; Anthony *et al.*, 1980). In a more recent study, Moriearty, *et al.* (1982) have demonstrated, by immunofluorescence, the presence of plasma cells in all the biopsies taken from all the 20 cases of human cutaneous leishmaniasis in Brazil. Although the IgG-producing plasma cells were detected in most cases, small numbers of IgM-producing cells were found in 17 cases and rare IgA-producing cells in only 9 of 18 cases examined. Antileishmanial antibodies of the IgG class were found in 15 patients; 2-mercaptoethanol-sensitive agglutinin for promastigotes were found in 19 cases. Total serum immunoglobulin levels were found normal or slightly raised, and no perceptible changes were detected in the level of complement components. The authors concluded that in cutaneous leishmaniasis, serum Ig or antipromastigote antibody levels are not indicative of the actual role of humoral factors in cutaneous leishmaniasis.

2.2. Immune Response in Mucocutaneous Leishmaniasis

As described earlier, mucocutaneous leishmaniasis may arise from an existing cutaneous lesion or appear, as is more frequently the case, some years after the primary skin lesion has healed, when it might be thought that the patient had acquired full immunity. Although nasal involvement occurs in 80% of infections with *L. b. braziliensis*, not more than 30% of cases develop mucocutaneous disease. The development of a mucosal lesion is therefore not an inescapable fatality following infection with this parasite; spontaneous recovery from the primary ulcer and the absence of relapse in many cases point to an effective protective mechanism that prevents reactivation of the parasite in the nasopharyngeal cavities. It is the breakdown of this protective mechanism in an apparently immunocompetent individual that is intriguing. Patients with mucocutaneous leishmaniasis respond normally in tests of immunological reactivity. Delayed skin reaction is positive in most cases, and the presence of antibodies has repeatedly been demonstrated (Convit and Pinardi, 1969; Walton *et al.*, 1972). A reverse correlation seems to be indicated between the level of antibody and the degree of mucosal involvement. The percent positivity for antibody response, determined by indirect immunofluorescence, was shown to be 56 and 83 for patients exhibiting 90% and 67% mucosal involvement respectively (Ridley 1980). Both groups were 100% positive on the delayed skin test. Circulating immune complexes and anti-IgG antibodies have also been demonstrated, particularly in cases exhibiting multiple mucosal lesions (Desjeux *et al.*, 1980).

2.3. Immune Response in Visceral Leishmaniasis

Two immunological phenomena—an exaggerated production of immunoglobulin and a negative delayed skin reaction to "leishmanin"—characterize an active human infection with species of *L. donovani*. The augmented level of immunoglobulin is mainly due to a remarkable increase in the levels of IgG and IgM (Irunberry *et al.*, 1968; Rezai *et al.*, 1977; Ghose *et al.*, 1980). Much of this increase appears to be nonspecific, and polyclonal B-cell activation has been suggested as its underlying mechanism (Ghose *et al.*, 1980). Specific antibodies at high titer can, however, be detected by a variety of serological tests, including complement fixation (Moses, 1919; Da Cunha and Dias, 1938; Sen Gupta, 1943; Alencar *et al.*, 1966, 1968); indirect and direct hemoagglutination (Cascio *et al.*, 1963; Bray and Lainson, 1967; Allain and Kagan, 1975); electrophoretic techniques (Ranque *et al.*, 1969; Ranque and Quilici, 1970; Rezai *et al.*, 1977; Aikat *et al.*, 1979b); immunofluorescence (Araujo and Mayrink, 1968; Camargo and Rebonato, 1969; Duxbury and Sadun, 1964; Quilici *et al.*, 1968); and finally, the enzyme-linked immunosorbent assay (Hommel, 1976; Hommel *et al.*, 1978; Edrissian and Darabian, 1979; Guimares *et al.*, 1981).

Soluble immune complexes have been detected and shown to contain IgM, IgG, C1q, C1r, C1s, C3c, and C3d; on dissociation at acid pH, the purified complex was found to contain anti-IgG and anti-*Leishmania* antibodies (Casali and Lambert, 1979). Red blood cells have also been found coated with C3d (Puguin and Miescher, 1979). No alteration in the complement system other than a significant decrease in the level of C3 (Ghose *et al.*, 1980) has been reported.

The hyperreactivity of humoral response in active kala-azar most often parallels a state of hyporeactivity in T-cell-mediated systems of the immune responses. The absence of low reactivity of the T-cell-dependent responses is best exemplified by the negative skin tests generally observed during the active phase of the disease in most endemic areas. The partially dermotropic *L. d. archibaldi* of East Africa often causes positive delayed skin reaction before visceralization (Manson-Bahr, 1961). The conversion from negative to positive skin test in India as well as in other endemic area does occur, however, once the cure is achieved by chemotherapy or spontaneously (Sen Gupta and Mukherjee 1962; Southgate and Manson-Bahr, 1967; Rezai *et al.*, 1978; Wyler *et al.*, 1979). The defective skin hypersensitivity has been shown to parallel poor lymphocytic response to specific parasite antigen *in vitro* (Wyler *et al.*, 1979). The lymphocytic response and the skin test became positive after a successful course of therapy. Similar results have been reported by Carvalho and co-workers

(1981) from Brazil. In their study, the impaired response of lymphocytes from untreated patients could not be attributed to either reduced numbers of circulating T cells or the inhibitory effect of monocytes or serum factors. In other reports, T cells in peripheral circulation were reported to be reduced in number (Rezai *et al.*, 1978) and were said to respond poorly to mitogens *in vitro* (Ghose *et al.*, 1979). Perturbation in cell-mediated responses and T-cell subpopulations associated with circulating immune complexes as well as an increase in T gamma cells, a population believed to contain suppressor T cells, have also been reported (Narayanan *et al.*, 1979). It is of interest to note that the reduced T-cell-mediated responses, particularly delayed skin reaction, turn slowly to normal levels when the disease is already eradicated by chemotherapy or spontaneously. This situation does not seem to support a T-cell-mediated protective mechanism, which is currently believed to have a prominent role against leishmanial diseases.

2.4. Immune Response in Aberrant Forms of Leishmaniasis

The lupoid or tuberculoid leishmaniasis of the skin (LR, or leishmaniasis recidivans) is, as described earlier, the result of reactivation of the parasite in the site or adjacent to the scar of a former Oriental sore. Patients with lesions of recidiva type display strong skin hypersensitivity to small doses of leishmanin (Sagher, 1947; Ardehali *et al.*, 1980). The tuberculoid histology of the lesion, the scarcity of the parasite, and strong delayed skin reaction have been interpreted as a state of exaggerated allergy to the parasite (Turk and Bryceson, 1971).

Little information is available concerning the nature and titer of antibodies, which are demonstrated by the Prausnitz-Küstner reaction (Dostrovsky and Sagher, 1946). In a more recent study, antibodies were shown to be present at variable titers among LR patients (Ardehali *et al.*, 1980).

The peculiarities of the host's immune response have been suggested to explain the persistence and reactivation of the parasite in hyperreactive LR patients. This opinion is mainly based on the observation that the injection of parasites from classical oriental sore into LR patients produced an LR-type lesions (Dostrovsky *et al.*, 1952). However, the possibility that a different species or variant of the parasite may be responsible for this form of the disease has been considered (Zuckerman 1975; Handman *et al.* 1981).

In contrast to leishmaniasis recidivans, discussed above, DCL is immunologically characterized by an absence of reactivity to *Leishmania* antigen as measured by delayed skin reaction and the presence of circulating antibodies with titers above those reported for the simple cutaneous leishmaniasis (Turk and Bryceson, 1971; Convit *et al.*, 1972; Bray and Lainson, 1965, 1966, 1967; Bittencourt and Guimares, 1968; Convit and Pinardi, 1969). The absence or low reactivity of the skin to leishmanin is shown to be specific, since the patients present no evidence of a generalized immunodepression and react normally to unrelated antigens such as lepromin or tuberculin (Turk and Bryceson, 1971). Recently (Petersen *et al.*, 1982), a new focus of diffuse cutaneous leishmaniasis was reported from Dominican Republic, where four cases of DCL have been examined immunologically. The tests performed included skin test with leishmanin and with nonleishmanial antigens (candidin and PPD); lymphocyte proliferation assay; lymphocyte response after passage over nylon wool columns, and proliferation after treatment of lymphocyte culture with indomethacin. The results obtained confirmed previous reports so far described. In brief, none of the patients responded to leishmanin although 18 close relatives did, suggesting that the latter had been exposed to leishmanial antigen. Two patients did not respond to *Candida* and PPD. The lymphocyte proliferation assays to *Leishmania* antigen were negative in all four patients. Passage of the lymphocytes over the nylon wool column, which removes the adherent cells, restored the lymphocyte response to the parasite antigen. Finally, the lymphocyte response was also restored after treatment with indomethacin. The rather fashionable conclusion was therefore drawn that an adherent suppressor cell population is responsible for the specific anergy in diffuse cutaneous leishmaniasis.

As in LR, the actual etiology of DCL remains unknown. Although geographical confinement of cases favors the belief that a particular variant of the *Leishmania* parasite may be responsible for this condition, inoculation of the parasite isolated from a DCL patient to a normal recipient was found to produce a skin ulcer typical of simple cutaneous leishmaniasis (Convit *et al.*, 1972).

PKDL, unlike LR or DCL, manifests itself in a variety of clinical and histological forms. Therefore, the immunological features of the syndrome have often been found variable from one case to another and difficult to categorize. The macular form shares certain features with LR, with the presence of chronic inflammatory cells and no or few parasites. The nodular form shows a histology reminiscent of DCL, with a histiocytoma and many parasites. The maculonodular form may show any combination of cells (Girgla *et al.*, 1977; Khan, 1977). Although it is generally agreed that most patients with PKDL respond negatively to the Montenegro test and that the circulating antibodies are often present, no attempt has so far been made to correlate the immunological features of cases under study with their histological pictures.

The humoral aspects of 20 cases of post-kala-azar dermal syndrome have recently been presented by Haldar and his co-workers (1981), who measured immunoglobulin levels and the third component of the complement and compared them with sera from normal controls and from kala-azar patients. The mean values of serum IgG and IgM of PKDL patients were found to be significantly above those of controls but substantially lower than those of kala-azar sera. No difference in the values of IgA and C3 was detected between PKDL and control sera. Specific anti-*Leishmania* antibodies, mostly IgG and to a lesser extent IgM, were also demonstrated. The cell-mediated responses of these patients were not studied.

2.5. The Spectral Concept in Leishmaniasis

It is evident from the foregoing that a wide range of clinical manifestations may consequently follow the entry of a given species of *Leishmania* parasite into an individual. The resulting infection may run its anticipated course, as is often the case, or take an abnormal path, giving rise to conditions such as diffuse cutaneous leishmaniasis, leishmaniasis recidivans, or post-kala-azar dermal leishmaniasis. The question of the etiology of these conditions has been difficult to answer and a consensus of opinions has yet to be reached. Certainly, possible contributing factors related to the parasite or to the host must always be considered. The parasite-related factors may include the species and the variant involved, its antigenicity and virulence, the initial number inoculated into the host, and perhaps the association of the parasite with a particular species of the reservoir animal or the insect vector transmitting it. The host-related factors involve genetic constitution, ethnic origin, and the level of the host's immune competence. Unfortunately, the close morphological similarity among members of the genus *Leishmania,* the absence of a precise taxonomic tool capable of differentiating closely related species and variants, and the difficulty of characterizing the relevant antigens leave the question of identities of the parasites unanswered. Information concerning the association of the parasite with various reservoir hosts and its insect vectors are lacking. Less adequate still is our knowledge concerning the impact of genetic and ethnic background of people at risk. However, despite the complexity of the situation, the spectral concept of leishmanial diseases, in analogy with leprosy, was adopted by Destombes (1960), who considered different *Leishmania*-related dermal manifestations to be the consequence of hosts's various levels of cell-mediated immune responses. A scale was therefore proposed on which various clinical forms of cutaneous leishmaniasis were ranked according to their histological pictures and levels of cell-mediated immunity (CMI), measured by skin tests. Thus, the allergic LR type, with predominance of lymphocyte and strongly positive delayed skin reaction, was placed at one pole of the scale, and the CDL form, with highly macrophagic histology and negative skin test, at the other pole. Bryceson elaborated the spectral concept of the disease still further by considering kala-azar as the visceral equivalent of the polar DCL form of leishmaniasis (Turk and Bryceson, 1971).

The polar or spectral concept clearly stresses the intimate association of the host's cell-mediated immune responses to various forms of leishmanial disease, but it disregards the humoral aspects of the immune response and completely ignores the parasite-related factors. Unlike leprosy, for which a universal causative agent (*Mycobacterium leprae*) is recognized, the leishmanial diseases are caused by several well-established, legitimate species that are responsible for various clinicoepidemiological manifestations of the disease. It must also be remembered that leishmanias are primarily parasites of lower mammals, with an expanding host range. The success of their existence is due to their highly specialized characteristics of being able to live and multiply inside the host macrophages—the cells that are responsible for nonspecific resistance and are considered to be the effector arm of the immune response.

It may be difficult or even impossible to differentiate a parasite causing a self-limiting cutaneous leishmaniasis from an isolate that has given rise to the chronic nonhealing DCL. However, the nonulcerative, nonfatal nature of DCL, which does not provoke the cell-mediated responses of an otherwise immunocompetent host, is indicative of something particular about the parasite as well as the host. Parasites isolated from a case of DCL were shown to produce classic self-healing cutaneous disease (Convit *et al.*, 1972), and patients with negative skin reactions to leishmanin were shown to respond normally to other antigens (Bryceson, 1970; Turk and Bryceson, 1971). The absence of reaction to leishmanin in DCL cases is generally considered as an indication of a state of defective cell-mediated immune response. The conversion to positive skin test occurs after a protracted course of therapy, when masses of parasites are eliminated by toxic drugs and not by the host's cellular defense mechanism. In the opinion of the authors, much of the existing confusion concerning the pathogenesis of the disease and the immune responses of the host stems from the overemphasis and often misinterpretation of the role and the mechanism of induction of cell-mediated immune response and its earmark, the delayed skin reaction, in leishmanial infections. An interesting view that has not yet been fully appreciated was constructed by Ridley (1979, 1980), after a detailed histological study of over 60 cases of cutaneous and mucocutaneous leishmaniasis from South America. In Ridley's opinion, the necrotic phase in cutaneous leishmaniasis represents an optimal antigenic load that sets in operation the necrotizing process. He considers this process to be more important for the elimination of parasites than delayed hypersensitivity. The granuloma formation was also found to be a postnecrotic phenomenon. It is interesting to recall the nonulcerative nature of the lesions and the absence of lymphocytic granuloma in DCL patients. Considering the enormous load of parasites in DCL cases, it is not surprising that intradermal injection of leishmanin fails to elicit a skin reaction. The conversion of negative to positive skin hypersensitivity after prolonged treatment, when the load of the parasite has considerably been reduced, demonstrates that there is no inherent specific anergy or defective cell-mediated immune response.

3. THE EXPERIMENTAL MODELS OF LEISHMANIASIS AND THEIR RELEVANCE TO THE DISEASE IN MAN

There is an ever-increasing list of animal species found naturally infected with species of leishmanial parasites. In a majority of cases, these infections are detected by meticulous inspection of wild-caught animals on which no appreciable superficial lesions may be noticed. Most dermal ulcerations, if present, are inflicted on the animals by trapping or due to animal's struggle to escape from its caging. Although nothing is known of the nature of the host–parasite relationship in the reservoir host of leishmanial infections, the dissimilarity between cryptic infections in animal reservoirs of leishmanial diseases on the one hand and those of man on the other renders the use of such animal models obsolete.

Existing knowledge concerning the immunology of experimental leishmaniasis has largely been derived from laboratory models that have been presumed to mimic certain forms of leishmaniasis in man. It is evident that results from animal experimentation do not necessarily provide a direct insight into a specific human disease. The question remains, therefore, as to what extent laboratory models of the infections represent or simulate human leishmanial diseases. A general consensus of opinion has yet to be reached as to the choice of the host–parasite combinations that are reasonably analogous to various forms of the disease in man. Even with the most analogous experimental host–parasite combination involving laboratory animals, it has to be assumed that similar immunological mechanisms operate in man. With this notion in mind, it will not be difficult to find experimental models for simpler forms of the disease, such as cutaneous leishmaniasis. For more complicated clinical conditions, reliance on immunomodulatory methods is required. Three general approaches have been taken to simulate the more severe forms of the disease in man:

1. Immunosuppression by physical or chemical methods such as removal of certain organs, irradiation, or treatment with immunosuppressive drugs.
2. Administration of very large doses of parasites or their inoculation into surgically altered sites.
3. The utilization of genetically manipulated strains of animals.

Obviously, such artificial models can hardly be considered to mimic any form of disease that occurs spontaneously in man. However, in the absence of other means and better models for study, reliance has to be placed—obviously with all necessary precautions—on experimental animal systems.

3.1. Genetics of Resistance and Susceptibility in Animal Models

The present state of knowledge concerning the genetic aspect of leishmanial infections has been derived exclusively from experimental infections of inbred mice with *L. donovani*, *L. t. major*, and to some extent *L. m. mexicana*. The resistant or susceptible phenotypic reactions of various mouse strains to *Leishmania* parasites and the availability of mouse populations of altered genetic makeup have particularly helped genetic study of leishmanial infections in the mouse. A detailed discussion of the subject is beyond the scope of this review; interested readers are referred to excellent articles by Gorczynski (1982), Bradley (1982), Blackwell (1982), and Howard *et al.* (1982). The available information may be summarized in the following terms:

1. A single major gene or tight linkage group named Lsh controls initial susceptibility of mice to *L. donovani* infection. The Lsh is located on chromosome 1 of the mouse.
2. The same regulatory genes seem to be involved in the control of phylogenetically distant pathogens.
3. The immune expressions of inbred mice to *L. donovani* infection is controlled by at least three genes—H-2 linked, H-11 linked, and Ir-2 linked.
4. There is no parallelism between susceptibilities of various mouse strains to *L. donovani* and *L. t. major*.
5. The pattern of disease by *L. t. major* in highly susceptible Balb/c mice segregates according to a single autosomal non-H-2-linked gene prediction in progeny of a cross with a resistant strain. This gene is unlikely to be identified with Lsh.

The dogmatic situation concerning the nonidentity of genetic regulation of infections due to *L. donovani* and *L. tropica* (mentioned in point 4) is further accentuated by our observation that a mouse strain exhibiting susceptibility to *L. donovani* of Indian origin may be categorized as resistant to *L. donovani* of Mediterranean origin. However, despite the great deal of interesting information that has been gathered on genetic aspects of leishmanial infections in mice, their relevance to human leishmaniasis is yet to be shown.

3.2. Cutaneous Leishmaniasis

3.2.1. The Guinea-Pig Model

Ever since the discovery of *Leishmania enriettii* in an spontaneous infection of the guinea pig in Brazil (Muniz and Meding, 1948), this host–parasite combination has been a favored model for cutaneous leishmaniasis in most laboratories engaged in studying various aspects of the disease.

Subcutaneous injection of the parasite in the hairless areas of the guinea pig's skin, the tip of the nose, the feet, or the skin of the ears results in the development of a cutaneous ulcer resembling the Oriental sore. Depending on the numbers of parasites injected, a nodule appears within one to several weeks. This ulcerates and then heals, leaving the animal permanently immune against reinfection. Metastatic lesions may occasionally appear in a small proportion of infected animals or after the injection of a large dose of the parasite (Bryceson *et al.*, 1974).

Histology of the lesion shows an early infiltration of the dermis by macrophages harboring in their cytoplasm an increasing number of the parasites. Multinucleated giant cells with masses of parasites become progressively abundant and the lymphoplasmocytic elements, which are present practically throughout the evolution of the lesion, eventually dominate the scene (Rezai *et al.*, 1972a, Radwanski *et al.*, 1974; Sordat and Behin, 1977). Destruction of the parasite, at least in part, seems to take place inside giant cells and is concomitant with the transfer of electron-dense material from cytoplasmic vesicles to the parasitophorous vacuoles, indicating fusion of the lysosomes with phagosomes (Sordat and Behin, 1977). Recovery occurs within 12–16 weeks, leaving a permanent scar at the site of the lesion. The frequency of metastatic spread and reappearance of the lesion seems to be dependent on the origin and strain of the animal.

3.2.2. The Mouse Model

Inoculation of *L. t. major* into the shaven skin of mice produces an ulcer of variable outcome depending on the strain of the mouse used (Behin *et al.*, 1979). Although the initial ulcerative phase of the infection appears to be the same in all mouse strains so far tested, the regressive and healing phase is largely dependent on the genetic background of the animal. The superficial skin ulcer of CBA or C_3H mice heals within a few months, while similarly induced lesions on mice of DBA/2 or Balb/c origin fail to heal and remain on the skin as long the animals live. Thus, the designation of healer and nonhealer strains refers to mouse strains that are capable of recovery from *L. tropica* infection as opposed to those that remain infected throughout their lives. Complete agreement on the designation of healer and nonhealer characteristics does not exist among various laboratories. This stems mainly from the lack of standards as to the source, maintenance, and methods of manipulating the parasite as well as the host animal.

Cutaneous infection of healer mice with *L. t. major* does not, as a rule, give rise to systemic infection, although the infected animals exhibit a moderate splenomegaly during the course of the infection. The nonhealer mice, in contrast, produce in the later phase of the infection a marked hepatosplenomegaly from which the parasite can be isolated. Infection of Balb/c has generally been found to be dramatic, involving most regional lymph nodes; the spleen, and the liver (Weintraub and Weinbaum, 1977; Nasseri and Modabber, 1979; Packchanian, 1979). Systemic infection with *L. t. major* has also been reported from healer mice such as CBA (Leclerc *et al.*, 1981).

Infection of mice with *L. m. mexicana* follows a similar pattern, depending on the strain of animal used. The infection may produce a self-resolving ulcer, a nonhealing, nonulcerating nodule, or a progressive lesion with metastases to the extremities and varying degrees of visceral involvement (Alexander and Phillips, 1978; Párez *et al.*, 1979b; Grimaldi *et al.*, 1980a).

3.3. Visceral Leishmaniasis

3.3.1. The Hamster Model

The hamster has been shown to be susceptible to several species of *Leishmania*, including several South American species (Wilson *et al.*, 1979). Even *L. enriettii*, which is one of the most host-specific parasites, can produce a transient lesion in the animal (Belehu and Turk 1976). Earlier studies employed the hamster as the host of *L. donovani*, which produces a fulminating, eventually fatal infection. However, from an immunological point of view, the usefulness of the hamster as a model of visceral infection by *L. donovani* has proved to be disappointing, because the animal seems unable to mount an immune response even with the help of chemotherapy (Stauber 1963).

More recent studies indicate that the route of infection may be crucial in the outcome of the disease and immune reactions of the host. Whereas intracardial injection of the hamster with *L. donovani* produces masses of the parasites in the liver and spleen and terminates fatally, subcutaneous injection of the parasite was found to induce protection against visceral disease in a proportion of infected animals.

The hamster is used in many laboratories for the mass production of amastigotes used in various experiments and to safeguard the virulence of *L. donovani*.

3.3.2. The Mouse Model

The outbred Swiss Webster mice have generally been used in earlier studies of infection by *L. donovani*. In one study, Smrkovski *et al.* (1974) reported that 70% of infected animals died within 58–200 days, with pathological manifestations including hepatosplenomegaly and thymic involution. The use of inbred strains of mice, however, indicates that the level of susceptibility to infection by *L. donovani* varies considerably according to the genetic background of the animal. Monitoring the parasite burden in liver imprints taken at 15-day intervals from 25 strains of inbred mice infected with an Ethiopian strain of *L. donovani*, Bradley (1974, 1977) recognized one group of mice that was acutely susceptible to the infection and another that was acutely resistant. A third type comprised one strain that behaved as susceptible initially but then exhibited a marked resistance, as evidenced by a rapid fall in parasite number present in the liver imprint. Pathology included hepatosplenomegaly and granuloma formation, which was more dramatic in resistant mouse strains. Similar results have been obtained in our center with three geographically distinct isolates of *L. donovani*.

3.3.3. Other Models

Since the pioneering studies of Stauber on animal models of leishmanial infections, little experimental work has been carried out with *Leishmania* parasites using animal models other than inbred mice. Although interesting information may be obtained from experimental work on potential reservoir hosts of the disease, the logistic difficulties and the inherent artificiality of experimental systems in simulating natural infection in wild-caught animals have probably been the most deterrent factors in such investigations.

The available information concerning experimental leishmanial infection in nonconventional host animals comes from Stauber and his co-workers. Having established a standard system for measuring the growth pattern of *L. donovani* in hamsters, Stauber (1955, 1958, 1962, 1964) and Stauber and colleagues (1966) employed the system in a comparative study of susceptibility to *L. donovani* of various animal species. The standard system consisted of inoculation by cardiac route of leishmanial amastigotes (200,000–500,000/g body weight) and estimation of parasite load in the spleen and liver of test animals eight days after infection. Animal species tested included the gerbil (*Meriones unguiculatus*), guinea pig, Nile grass rat (*Arvichanthis n. niloticus*), white rat (Wistar), rabbit, chinchilla (*Chinchilla lanigera*), and cotton rat (*Sigmodon h. hispidus*).

The results of this comparative study clearly demonstrated a range of host responses to *L. donovani* infection in the animal species tested. Whereas the infection readily killed chinchilla, animals such as the white rat, rabbit, gerbil, and guinea pig were found very resistant to the parasite. More interesting still was the infection of the cotton rat, which, despite a continuous rise in its parasite population, did not succumb and showed no external sign of infection.

4. IMMUNE RESPONSE IN EXPERIMENTAL MODELS OF INFECTION

4.1. Immune Response of the Guinea Pig

In vivo studies on guinea pigs infected with *L. enriettii* are unanimous in the conclusion that inoculation of a standard infective dose of 1 million parasites into the skin of the animal elicits a strong immune response, demonstrable by the delayed skin reaction within a week or two. Exaggerated doses of the parasite result in a diminished but transient skin reactivity, which return to normal as the infection regresses. Lowered skin hypersensitivity also coincides with the appearance of metastatic lesions and incapacity of the animal to eliminate the parasite (Bryceson *et al.*, 1974; Preston and Dumonde, 1976). It is worthy of notice that despite the presence of a positive skin reaction in the early phase of the infection, the disease runs its course, becomes a florid ulcer, and then heals.

The presence of antibodies has been demonstrated by immunofluorescence, with an increasing level from day 10 postinfection until convalescence, when the titer declines (Bryceson *et al.*, 1972, 1974; Radwansky *et al.*, 1974; Poulter, 1980a).

Spontaneous recovery is the rule in uncomplicated infections of guinea pigs with *L. enriettii*. Recovery accompanies strong resistance to challenge infection. Injection of the parasite elicit a transient inflammatory reaction in an immune animal but no disease. Histology of the injection site shows rapid disappearance of the parasite within eight days (Rezai *et al.*, 1972). Resistance to challenge infection has been shown to develop even before recovery from the initial lesion is accomplished (Poulter, 1979).

A peculiar feature of the protective mechanism in the guinea pig is its local aspect; that is, the mechanism seems to exercise its effect in one site and not in another. Animals developing metastatic lesions carry scars of healed primary lesions and strongly resist a challenged infection (Bryceson *et al.*, 1974; Poulter 1979). An interesting personal observation is that many months after an apparent cure, a guinea pig with a fibrous scar may develop on a paw a hypertrophic condition that does not ulcerate and contains an enormous load of the parasite. The lesion may involve one paw or all four, with a characteristic heavy keratinization of the footpads. It is interesting to speculate that if such animal were hairless, it might have developed a condition reminiscent of DCL in man.

Induction of metastatic leishmanial lesions in the guinea pig has been achieved by a variety of methods, including an elevated dose of parasites (Bryceson *et al.*, 1974), injection of the parasite into skin flaps with reduced lymphatic drainage (Kadivar and Soulsby 1975), immunosuppressive regimens such as whole body x-irradiation, the use of antilymphocytic serum and cyclophosphamide (Turk and Bryceson, 1971; Lemma and Yau, 1973; Belehu *et al.*, 1976), and the induction of tolerance through injection of a soluble parasite antigen into the fetus at 3–4 weeks of age (Bryceson *et al.*, 1972). Injection of the parasite or parasitized macrophages by intracardial or intravascular routes has also resulted in the development of metastatic lesions in the recipient animals (Kanan, 1975; Poulter, 1980b). As interesting as these observations may be, no definite conclusions can be drawn concerning the underlying mechanism responsible for the aberrant leishmanial disease observed in man or in guinea pigs bearing the scar of leishmanial lesions and a parasite-loaded metastatic nodule at the same time.

Earlier studies on *in vitro* correlates of cell-mediated immune responses in

L. enriettii-infected guinea pigs have demonstrated the presence in infected animals of lymphocytes capable of responding to parasite antigen by transforming to blast cells or by inhibiting the migration of macrophages (Bryceson *et al.*, 1970; Blewett *et al.*, 1971; Walton, 1970). In an extensive study, Bryceson and his co-workers (1970) reported that sensitized lymphocytes from draining lymph nodes of convalescent animals could destroy *L. enriettii*-infected peritoneal macrophages and the parasites contained in them within 24–48 hr of contact in culture at 37°C. Control cultures containing nonparasitized macrophages were reported unaffected. A specific recognition by sensitized lymphocytes of macrophages, presumably bearing parasite antigens on their surface, was proposed to explain the phenomenon. However, the specificity of this recognition was not absolute, since lymphocytes from animals immunized against Freund's complete adjuvant displayed similar cytotoxicity. Although these interesting observations have not been confirmed by other workers, particularly in our center (Mauel *et al.*, 1975), the cytotoxic effect of sensitized lymphocytes for parasitized macrophages is certainly far from being completely excluded as a mechanism of host defense in this infection.

The role of macrophages in the protective mechanism against leishmanial infections has been the focus of interest in many laboratories, including our own. Unfortunately, the results of most investigations *in vitro* involving guinea pig macrophages are disappointing because their fragility and rather short life span do not permit extended observation of their behaviour in culture. A previous report on light and electron microscopy of infected guinea pig tissue indicated that in the resolving ulcer, parasites seemed to be destroyed inside multinucleated giant cells (Sordat and Behin, 1977). This information led to a series of experiments in order to define more precisely whether macrophages have the capacity to destroy the ingested parasites. Peritoneal macrophages explanted from a normal or convalescent guinea pig did not differ in their capcity to ingest the amastigotes of *L. enriettii,* and they did not exhibit any measurable hostile effect on the survival of the phagocytosed parasites (Mauel *et al.*, 1975). In fact, the phagocytic capacity of macrophages from the ''immune'' guinea pig seemed to be higher than that of the normal animal.

In a long series of experiments, the effect of macrophage activation on intracellular survival of *L. enriettii* in the peritoneal macrophages of the guinea pig was studied (Mauel *et al.*, 1975; Behin *et al.*, 1975). Activation, based on the method described by Simon and Scheagran (1971) as well as by the aid of BCG or *Toxoplasma gondii*, failed to induce in macrophages the capacity to destroy the ingested parasites. The state of activation was demonstrated by the capacity of macrophages in parallel culture to eliminate within 4 hr 95% of ingested *Listeria monocytogenes* (Mauel *et al.*, 1975). Strong activation was also achieved after ingestion of *L. enriettii* amastigotes by macrophages obtained from peritoneal cavities of *Leishmania*-immune animals. While a considerable degree of microbicidal capacity was manifested by such activated cells, the number and viability of the parasites inside similarly treated macrophages did not change after 72 hr of incubation (Behin *et al.*, 1975).

The induction of a long-lasting, local delayed hypersensitivity in the guinea pig was shown to render the animal refractory to the development of a leishmanial lesion provided that the infecting dose of the parasite was inoculated at an existing site of delayed skin reaction. Inoculation of 10^6 *L. enriettii* in the ear skin of guinea pigs previously sensitized to dinitrochlorobenzene (DNCB) was found not to cause an ulcerating lesion if the state of skin hypersensitivity was continuously maintained by regular application of DNCB on the ear. The development of a leishmanial lesion was also strongly inhibited if a mixture of *L. enriettii* and BCG was inoculated into the ear skin of a BCG-immunized guinea pig. Inoculation of the same mixture into a nonimmunized animal resulted in the development of a typical leishmanial ulcer at the injected site (Behin *et al.*, 1977a).

The acquired capacity of DNCB or BCG-sensitized guinea pigs to inhibit the development of leishmanial infection was shown to be a localized phenomenon, since the absence of the lesion on the ear receiving regular application of DNCB did not prevent the development of a typical lesion on the opposite ear if the same number of parasites was injected but DNCB was not applied. The absence of a leishmanial ulcer following injection of BCG–parasite mixture in the ear of a BCG-immune animal was also found to have no effect on the development of a typical lesion on the opposite ear receiving an inoculum of the parasite without BCG. A possible candidate mechanism for the observed inhibition of lesion development in animals inoculated with viable parasites was sought in local activation of macrophages. However, the necessity for continuous presence of local delayed hypersensitivity to achieve this inhibition was taken to suggest that the absence of parasiticidal activity of guinea pig macrophages *in vitro* might be due to failure to cause activation of sufficient duration under culture conditions. Therefore, the behavior of guinea pig macrophages in culture may not reflect their actual potentialities *in vivo*.

4.2. Immune Responses of the Mouse

4.2.1. Infection by *L. t. major*

As discussed earlier, the outcome of a skin infection by *L. t. major* of inbred mice depends on the genetic background of the animals used. The designation of ''healer'' and ''nonhealer'' signifies the mouse strains that are capable of resolving the infections spontaneously within several weeks as opposed to those that remain infected for the rest of their lives. The persistence of the skin lesions in nonhealer animals usually accompanies the involvement of regional lymph nodes, the spleen, and the liver, from which the parasite can be isolated. Report of parasite isolation from the liver and spleen of healer mice long after recovery from a skin ulcer (Leclerec *et al.*, 1981) is not in conformity with our own experience. It indicates, however, a need for standardization of techniques and more precise characterization of the parasite under investigation.

The humoral responses of various mouse strains to infection with *L. t. major* have largely been neglected. In a pilot study (Behin, unpublished), levels of immunoglobulins of the IgG and IgM classes were found to increase in the healer CBA mice in a relatively rapid manner during the evolution of the lesion, followed by an immediate fall when regression of the lesion was well under way. The levels of these immunoglobulins in nonhealer DBA/2 mice were found to be lower in the early phase of the infection but increased progressively, with no tendency to fall off. These results are consistent with a possible polyclonal B-cell activation by the parasite or its metabolic by-products (Djoko-Tamnou *et al.*, 1981). Histopathology of the spleen and liver of healer and nonhealer mice revealed extensive amyloidosis of these organs in nonhealer animals. The amyloid nature of the deposits was established by their birefringence after specific staining and by demonstration of their antiparallel protein chain organization as revealed by electron microscopy. The amyloid deposits stained intensely with fluoresceinated anti-mouse IgG and IgM. Amyloid degeneration was never observed in tissues of healer animals and fluorescent staining showed only a very delicate fluorescence on the membrane of hepatocytes (Behin, unpublished).

The cellular aspects of the immune responses of inbred mice following infection with *L. t. major* have received more attention and a considerable amount of information, although not necessarily elucidating, has become available. Thus, the percentage of splenic T and B cells were found decreased and the spleen and lymph nodes were shown repopulated with large Ig^-, $Thy\text{-}1.2^-$ "null" cells (Djoko-Tamnou *et al.*, 1981). The immune response of nonhealer mice to sheep erythrocytes and to various mitogens was shown, both *in vivo* and *in vitro*, to be enhanced in the early phase of *L. tropica* infection but markedly depressed at the later stages (Leclerc *et al.*, 1982). In the healer mice, the regional lymph nodes were shown to undergo hyperplastic changes in the follicular and paracortical regions and to gain weight within the first 8–10 weeks of infection (Preston *et al.*, 1972).

The delayed-type hypersensitivity reaction was shown to peak within the first 10 days of the infection in the healer animals and to be insignificant in the nonhealer counterparts (Preston and Dumonde, 1976a; Nasseri and Moddaber, 1979). No absolute correlation was found to exist between the process of healing and the development of delayed hypersensitivity, as progressive lesions were found, in certain cases, to coexist with a positive skin test (Preston *et al.*, 1978; Moddaber *et al.*, 1980; Grimaldi *et al.*, 1980b; Hale and Howard, 1981).

The healer animals have been shown to be resistant to challenge with homologous and certain heterologous species of parasite. Thus recovery from *L. t. major* infection protects against the same parasite as well as against *L. m. mexicana* (Alexander and Phillips, 1978; Pérez *et al.*, 1979a). Resistance to a challenge inoculum is shown to develop before healing of the primary lesion. Finally, delayed skin reaction and partial protection may be transferred by lymphoid cells to intact syngeneic recipients. Simultaneous transfer of immune cells and serum is shown to be more effective in the passive transfer of resistance (Preston and Dumonde, 1976b).

Alteration of the immune system of the healer or nonhealer mice by physical or chemical means, before or after the infection with *L. t. major,* has produced inconclusive results. Inoculation of a large dose (10^8) of *L. t. major* in healer CBA mice was shown to produce nonhealing ulcers concomitant with a depressed skin reaction as well as an inability to reject allogeneic skin grafts and to produce antibody to foreign antigens (Preston *et al.*, 1978). Similar alterations in the immune responses of CBA mice infected with 10^6 parasites have been reported following thymectomy, irradiation, and bone-marrow reconstitution (Preston *et al.*, 1972). Conversely, thymectomy of nonhealer Balb/c mice prior to infection with *L. t. major* was shown to induce in the animal a reversion to positive skin reactivity but no healing (Howard *et al.*, 1980). Contrasting effects have also been observed following treatment of healer and nonhealer mice with cyclophosphamide, while nonhealer Balb/c mice reacted positively to skin test after cyclophosphamide treatment (Howard *et al.*, 1980). The same treatment has been reported to augment the skin reaction of healer CBA mice but prolong recovery from the infection (Preston *et al.*, 1978). Recovery of nonhealer mice from infection with *L. t. major* has been reported following treatment with BCG or sublethal x-irradiation (Weintraub and Weinbaum, 1977; Howard *et al.*, 1981). In our center, treatment of nonhealer mice with a similar dose of radiation caused death in a proportion of experimental animals and a certain degree of shrinkage and scabbing of the lesions of surviving animals, whose health was severely impaired (Behin, unpublished).

4.2.2. Infection by *L. mexicana mexicana*

The outcome of the infection with *L. m. mexicana* in inbred mice, as in the case *L. t. major,* depends largely on the strain of the animal used. Certain strains recover spontaneously from the infection while others remain infected throughout life, with a stagnant ulcer or a metastatic lesion involving internal organs (Pérez *et al.*, 1981, 1979b; Alexander and Phillips, 1978; Grimaldi *et al.*, 1980a).

Animals of resistant strains are shown to develop humoral as well as cell-mediated responses, demonstrable by agglutinating antibodies and delayed skin reaction (Pérez *et al.*, 1979b). The susceptible strains, in contrast, fail to exhibit skin hypersensitivity and show impaired production of antibodies. The nonhealer mice, however, may show a transitory blastogenic response to mitogens and an increase in IgM producing cells following immunization against sheep red blood cells. These responses occur only in the early phase of the infection; a drastic decrease in these responses was found to develop as the infection aged. Treatment with BCG or levamisole of C_3H mice, which normally develop nonhealing, nonulcerating lesions upon infection with *L. m. mexicana,* is shown to induce positive skin reaction and humoral responses in the face of a persistent, nonresolving ulcer (Grimaldi *et al.,* 1980b).

4.2.3. Infection by *L. donovani*

Infection of mice of susceptible or resistant phenotype with *L. donovani* results in the early development of a moderate hepatosplenomegaly accompanied by an increase of the parasite loads in these organs. In acutely susceptible animals, the infection takes an inexorably progressive course; in the resistant mice, the infection is contained and the spleen and liver eventually revert to their normal sizes. Histologically, all mouse strains develop a scattered histiocytoma consisting of parasitized and unparasitized macrophages throughout the liver. In acutely susceptible animals, the situation becomes more and more aggravated without an appreciable change in the cellular composition of the lesions. In the resistant mice, in contrast, the histiocytomas develop to granulomatous reactions, with the appearance of numerous lymphocytes and plasma cells. Areas of necrosis become apparent and macrophages no longer contain parasites (Bradley and Kirkley, 1977; Blackwell, 1982). These dramatic histological changes are manifestations of the host's immune response in its effort to eliminate the parasite. The residual survival of the parasite in most resistant mice indicates, however, that the defense machinery of the host is not always successful in terminating the infection.

Experimental evidence suggest that an intact, functional T-cell compartment is essential for the expression of an immune response and most probably for the development of an effective reaction against the parasite. Congenitally athymic mice are shown to display less resistance and lowered delayed skin hypersensitivity than control animals with normal thymus (Smrkovski *et al.,* 1979). Chronic infection has been produced in healer animals after immunosuppressive manipulation such as thymectomy, irradiation, and reconstitution with antiteta-serum-treated bone-marrow cells (Skov and Twohy, 1974a). Resistance of such animals was shown to be restored following transfer of normal lymph node or thymic cells but not with cell populations depleted of T lymphocytes (Skov and Twohy, 1974b; Rezai *et al.,* 1980). Conversely, however, neonatal thymectomy was not found to affect the acute resistance of healer animals (Bradley 1980), suggesting that the underlying mechanism of resistance may be independent of cell-mediated immune reaction. This notion is gaining ground increasingly.

Treatment with cyclophosphamide prior to infection is shown to significantly decrease the parasite loads of the spleen and liver (Herman and Farrell, 1977). Postinfection treatment of mice with cyclophosphamide was found to have an inverse effect.

Administration of BCG in presensitized Balb/c mice infected with *L. donovani* has also been shown to cause a considerable reduction in splenic parasite. This phenomenon is attributed tentatively to macrophage activation (Smrkovski and Larson, 1977a, 1977b).

4.3. Miscellaneous

More recent studies include observations on cross-immunity in monkeys and man infected with various South American species of *Leishmania* (Lainson and Shaw, 1977); the detection of antibody response to *L. mexicana* in African white-tailed rats (Sayles *et al.*, 1981); the study of immune response to *L. tropica* in *Maccaca mulata* (Wolf, 1976); and the investigation of the susceptibility of *Aotus trivirgatus* to *L. braziliensis* and *L. mexicana* (Christensen and de Vasquez, 1981).

4.4. Assessment of the Role of Suppressor T Cells in the Outcome of the Disease

Several recent reports indicate that the severity of diseases induced by *Leishmania* species could be related to a decreased antiparasite T-cell responsiveness resulting from a generalized nonspecific impairment of the immune response or from only an antigen-specific hyporesponsiveness. Recent reports pertaining to the state of generalized or antigen-specific immunosuppression that has been associated with nonhealing leishmanial infections in some strains of mice will be briefly summarized.

Using a murine model of visceral leishmaniasis, it has been observed that there is a close correlation between the capacity of the host to generate macrophage-activating lymphokines and its susceptibility to infection (Murray *et al.*, 1982). It was found that macrophages from the peritoneal cavity of mice genetically susceptible (Balb/c) or resistant (DBA/2) to *L. donovani* infection were both fully capable of destroying amastigotes once activated *in vitro* by a proper lymphokine preparation. Interestingly, this observation was made with peritoneal macrophages obtained from infected mice of both strains, irrespective of the duration of the *L. donovani* infection (Balb/c mice were susceptible to *L. donovani* infection, since rapid proliferation of amastigotes was observed in liver and spleen). Although normal spleen lymphocytes from both DBA/2 and Balb/c generated, after stimulation with Con A, lymphokines capable of activating peritoneal macrophages to kill intracellular parasites, mitogen stimulation of 4-weeks-infected Balb/c was not capable of generating these lymphokines. Similarly, the antigen-specific lymphokine response of spleen cells from infected Balb/c mice was suppressed 4 weeks after infection. This suppression of lymphokines production by Balb/c-infected spleen cells after stimulation with either *L. donovani*-specific antigens or nonspecific mitogen (Con A) was paralleled by a suppression of the lymphocyte proliferative response induced by these two stimuli. Furthermore, spleen cells from 4-weeks-infected Balb/c mice were able to suppress the proliferative capacity and the lymphokine-generating activities of either normal Balb/c spleen cells after stimulation by Con A or immune Balb/c spleen cells after stimulation by parasite antigens. Attempts to characterize the types of suppressor cells involved indicated that they were plastic adherent, comprised less than 4% of the total spleen cell population, and did not secrete inhibitory factors in response to mitogen or antigen (Murray *et al.*, 1982). Observations showing that the simultaneous infection of Balb/c mice with *L. donovani* and *T. gondii* did not suppress the lymphokine production of their spleen cells upon stimulation with the latter protozoan parasite are puzzling. As postulated by the investigators, it could be that, in the spleen of four-weeks-infected Balb/c mice, there is a selective defect in the secretion of lymphokines capable of activating macrophages to kill ingested *L. donovani* amastigotes.

Other reports document a state of nonspecific immunosuppression in the spleens of susceptible mice (Balb/c) after infection with *L. tropica* (Scott and Farrel, 1981). The lymphocytes' transformation response to various mitogens such as PHA and Con A (T-cell mitogens) and LPS (B-cell mitogen) was markedly suppressed. This suppression appears to be the result of the activity of a cell population having the characteristics of macrophages. Interestingly, indomethacin could reverse the depressed responses to T-cell mitogens, suggesting that prostaglandin E released by the suppressor macrophage-like cell population was responsible for mediating suppression, perhaps through the action of another cell type. Observations showing that these suppressor cells were not formed in C57 Bl/6 mice (a strain of mice resistant to *L. tropica*) indicate a role for these cells in suppressing an antileishmanial effector cell response. Similar to the situation observed in this experimental model of infection, suppressor adherent cells have been shown in patients suffering from diffuse cutaneous leishmaniasis; this suppressive activity was also abolished in the presence of indomethacin.

Taken together, these results suggest that adherent cells (presumably macrophages) can be responsible for the nonspecific suppression seen in certain forms of leishmaniasis and that this suppression may account for the clinical course of the disease. However, the possibility still exists that the suppression observed was mediated by an adherent T-cell population with low amounts of T-cell markers on its surface.

It has recently been shown that most antigen- or mitogen-activated T cells express a receptor for interleukin 2 (IL-2; a T-cell growth factor necessary for T-cell proliferation). One could postulate that in mice susceptible to *Leishmania*, the infection is accompanied by a nonspecific T-cell activation that induces the expression of receptor for IL-2 at the surface of activated T cells. Since IL-2 appears to provide one of the signals necessary for T-cell triggering by specific antigens, it is therefore possible that, during infection with *Leishmania*, the IL-2 produced as a result of antigenic stimulation of specific T cells is absorbed by nonspecifically activated T blasts resulting from polyclonal T-cell activation.

A role for T cells in the development of an *L. tropica*-specific suppression in susceptible Balb/c mice has been demonstrated by the group of Howard. They clearly demonstrated that the lack of resistance to *L. tropica* infection exhibited by Balb/c mice was correlated with the establishment of a specific suppression of delayed-type hypersensitivity (DTH) reaction to the parasite (Howard *et al.*, 1980). This selective impairment of *L. tropica*-specific DTH response in Balb/c mice resulted from the activity of a suppressor T-cell population, as demonstrated in cell transfer experiments. The suppressive activity described by Howard *et al.* in Balb/c mice was limited to the induction phase of DTH to *L. tropica*, since no suppression of the effector arm of specific DTH reaction was observed. This conclusion was confirmed by our own observations, which showed that *in-vitro*-generated *Leishmania*-specific Balb/c T-cell populations and clones were able to transfer specific DTH responses in both normal and infected Balb/c recipients (Louis *et al.*, 1982a). The generation of suppressor T cells was impaired by sublethal irradiation (550 rads) prior to the infection (Howard *et al.*, 1981). Interestingly, this treatment resulted in the healing of the lesions in normally highly susceptible Balb/c mice. The surface phenotype of cells mediating suppression in Balb/c mice was found to be Lyt 1^+2^-, a phenotype identical to that of cells responsible for the transfer of acquired immunity in resistant mice (Liew *et al.*, 1982). Furthermore, suppression appeared to be restricted to DTH responses, a finding which could suggest that T cells mediating DTH responses are distinct from those implicated in antibody response. This observation is at the present time difficult to reconcile with recent studies demonstrating that *L. tropica*-specific Lyt 1^+2^- cell clones are capable of multiple functions: (1) helper activity for antibody responses *in vitro*, (2) transfer of antigen-specific DTH responses after local or systemic injection into normal mice, and (3) specific activation of parasitized macrophages (Louis *et al.*, 1982b).

The induction of suppressive T cells in susceptible mice (Balb/c) could be the result of a defect at the macrophage level. This hypothesis is supported by recent observations of Gorczynski, which showed that adherent skin macrophages from Balb/c mice, once infected by *L. tropica*, cannot induce (fail to induce) immune T cells. Interestingly, they were functionally equivalent to macrophages from resistant mice in the presentation of degraded parasite antigens (Gorczynski and MacRae, 1982; Gorczynski, 1982). As suggested by Gorczynski, the difference in the expression of antigen on parasitized resistant and susceptible macrophages could account for the differential triggering of T-cell subsets. Clearly, more work needs to be done in order to elucidate the possible defect of infected macrophages from susceptible mice in their antigen presenting function.

5. *IN VITRO* ANALYSIS OF CMI RESPONSES

5.1. The T Lymphocytes

Even though the exact mechanism by which the immune system plays a role in the destruction of *Leishmania* parasites is not yet known, the crucial role of T lymphocytes has been recognized. Observations showing that mice thymectomized, irradiated, and reconstituted with bone marrow cells are very susceptible to *L. t. major* infections support an essential role for T lymphocyte in the healing process (Preston *et al.*, 1972). This conclusion is supported by the recent finding that, in susceptible Balb/c mice, DTH reactions to *L. t. major* antigens are specifically suppressed (Howard *et al.*, 1980). The direct proof of a crucial role for T lymphocytes in immunity to *Leishmania* derives from experiments demonstrating that athymic *nu/nu* mice exhibit a generalized and fatal disease upon infection with *L. t. major* (Handman *et al.*, 1979) and that transfer of syngeneic T cells induces resistance in susceptible *nu/nu* mice (Mitchell *et al.*, 1980). The precise mechanisms by which T cells mediate this protective effect is not yet known.

In order to evaluate the role of T-cells in the healing process directly, we have generated *in vitro* homogenous populations and clones of T lymphocytes specific for *L. t. major* antigens and analyzed their functional activities (Louis *et al.*, 1982a). In the following sections we will summarize the main characterization of these T-cell populations and clones.

5.1.1. Generation *in Vitro* of Murine T Lymphocytes Specific for *Leishmania* Antigens

In order to evaluate the mechanisms of activation of T lymphocytes by *L. t. major*, a method has been devised for the measurement of *Leishmania*-induced proliferation of primed T cells (Louis *et al.*, 1979). Lymphocytes from draining lymph nodes of mice primed with *L. t. major* subcutaneously at the base of the tail (Corradin *et al.*, 1977) exhibited intense proliferative responses upon challenge *in vitro* with the parasite. This response was dependent upon specific T lymphocytes; furthermore, purified T cells responded as efficiently as unfractionated lymph node cells in the presence of additional macrophages. Homogeneous populations of *L. t. major*-specific T cells free of contaminating macrophages were obtained by maintaining blasts cells, harvested from cultures of primed lymph node lymphocytes responding to *L. t. major*, in medium conditioned with IL-2. In these antigen-free cultures, growth was observed for several days and 98% of lymphocytes expressed the Thy 1.2 and Lyt 1^+2^- surface phenotypes. These T lymphocytes, after removal from the IL-2 conditioned medium, could be restimulated to proliferate upon challenge with *L. t. major* provided that I-A identical irradiated spleen cells were added as a source of macrophage (Louis *et al.*, 1981). Therefore, these data extend to a protozoan parasite system observations that have shown a requirement for I-A compatible macrophages in the induction of proliferative responses by protein antigens (Schwartz *et al.*, 1978).

5.1.2. Functional Analysis of Murine T Lymphocytes Specific for *Leishmania* Antigens

The helper activity of *L. t. major*-specific T blasts was investigated in an *in vitro* antihapten antibody response (Zubler and Louis, 1981). B lymphocytes from mice immunized with TNP-KHL were mixed with various numbers of *L. tropica*-specific T blasts and the cultures challenged with TNP-*L. tropica*. After 5 days the number of plaque-forming cells specific for TNP were enumerated; it was found that TNP *L. t. major* induced high anti-TNP responses in those cultures, indicating that *L. t. major*-specific T cells display helper activity.

The presently described *L. t. major*-specific T blasts were also capable to transfer specific DTH reactions to naive recipient mice. Normal mice injected either locally into the footpad or intravenously with *L. t. major*-specific T blasts exhibited intense DTH responses after antigen exposure. Furthermore, a need for identity at the level of the MHC between parasite-specific T cells and recipient mice for transfer of specific DTH reactions was observed (Louis *et al.*, 1982a).

It is believed that destruction of intracellular leishmanial parasites by activated macrophages is a major mechanism by which these parasites are eliminated from infected hosts. The possibility that *L. t. major*-specific T blasts, after activation by specific antigens, release lymphokines capable of activating *Leishmania*-infected macrophages resulting in the destruction of intracellular organisms was examined. Incubation of macrophages parasitized with *L. enriettii*- and *L. tropica*-specific T blasts resulted in the killing of *L. enriettii* by activated macrophages. Specific recognition of *L. enriettii* antigens by *L. tropica*-specific T blasts is not surprising in view of the extensive antigenic cross-reactivity between these two parasites at the T-cell level.

Interestingly, those *L. tropica*-specific T blasts were not directly cytolytic for parasitized macrophages (Louis *et al.* 1982a).

5.1.3. Characteristics and Immunological Function of Cloned T-Cell Lines Specific for *Leishmania* Antigens

Results described above indicate that the *L. t. major*-specific T cells resulting from stimulation *in vitro* of primed lymph node cells with parasite antigens and subsequently maintained in IL-2 containing medium are able to perform various immunological functions such as (1) helper activity for antibody responses, (2) transfer of DTH reactions to unimmunized syngeneic mice, and (3) specific activation of *Leishmania*-infected macrophages. It was therefore of interest to know whether or not these different functional activities could be attributed to different T-cell populations. Attempts were made to derive clones of *L. t. major*-specific T cells and to analyze them functionally.

Limited numbers of T cells (0.5 cell per microtiter well) were cultured together with irradiated spleen cells (as a source of filler cells) *L. t. major* and IL-2. Microcultures in which growth was observed were subcultured 10 days later in a larger volume together with fresh filler spleen cells, parasite antigens, and IL-2. Clones were maintained by reculturing them approximately every 2 weeks. In other cloning experiments, individual T lymphocytes were micromanipulated into microtiter wells. Clones obtained by these two approaches could be maintained for up to 3 months in continuous culture.

Characterization of several cloned T-cell lines has revealed that (1) they all displayed the Thy 1.2, Lyt 1^+2^- phenotype; (2) after removal from IL-2-conditioned medium, they were capable of a specific proliferation upon challenge with the parasites *in vitro;* (3) they possessed helper activity as tested in a secondary antihapten antibody response *in vitro.* T-cell clones recognized parasite antigens in the context of H-2-identical macrophages and their helper activity was also restricted to B cells compatible at the I-A region of the MHC.

Approximately one-half of the total number of clones tested were also demonstrated to transfer specific DTH responses after transfer to unimmunized mice and to activate specifically *Leishmania*-infected macrophages. These results confirm in a parasite antigen system previous observations which demonstrated that a given T-cell clone can perform a variety of immunological functions (Bianchi *et al.*, 1981; Lin and Askonas, 1981).

We hope that the presently described homogenous populations and clones of *L. t. major*-specific T cells will permit a more definitive assessment of the role played by parasite-specific Lyt 1^+2^- cells in both the healing process and the development of protective immunity. The availability of parasite-specific cloned T-cell lines which, by definition, should be of restricted specificity also represents an important step in the identification of parasite antigens implicated in the activation of T-cell responses beneficial for the host.

5.2. The Killing of *Leishmania* by Macrophages

The mononuclear phagocytic cells of the reticuloendothelial system, collectively referred to as macrophages, are the only cells in which the *Leishmania* species of mammals can live and multiply. Although a rather strict tissue preference is exhibited by various *Leishmania* parasites, the underlying topical factors that render macrophages of a particular tissue more acceptable to a given *Leishmania* species remain to be discovered. For the time being, terms such as "cutaneous," "mucocutaneous," or "visceral" leishmaniasis are only references to tissues where macrophages are preferentially infected and more likely to be found. The dermotropic parasites cause formation of a histiocytoma in the tegument and the viscerotropic species induce a systemic accumulation and hyperplasia of histiocytes and other macrophages. The ensuing pathological changes that occur in various clinical forms of the disease are the consequences of degenerative processes that occur in infected macrophages. The necrosis of the epithelium in cutaneous and mucocutaneous disease and pathological changes of liver and spleen in kala-azar are secondary to the presence and multiplication of the parasite in the macrophage—the very host cell that is the prime element of nonspecific resistance against various intruders and is considered an effective arm of the host's immune response. The inability of macrophages to eliminate the ingested parasites in the first place and the residual survival of *Leishmania,* as occurs in chronic forms of the disease, in the second are not compatible with anticipated role of the mononuclear phagocytes as we know them today. However, indications from studies *in vivo* and direct evidence from experiments *in vitro* suggest that under optimal experimental conditions, macrophages can be induced to kill and digest phagocytosed parasites.

A longitudinal study by light and election microscopy of evolving infection of guinea pigs by *L. enriettii* (Sordat and Behin, 1977) demonstrated an increasing giant cell formation and evidence of intracellular parasite destruction. In another study, the arrested development of a leishmanial lesion at the site of a delayed skin reaction in a DNCB- or BCG-sensitized guinea pig was interpreted as the result of a local macrophage activation in the inflamed tissues (Behin *et al.,* 1977a). Severity of infection with *L. tropica* (Weintraub and Weinbaum, 1977) and with *L. donovani* (Smrkovski and Larson, 1977a) of highly susceptible Balb/c mice is shown to be reduced by BCG treatment. This effect is attributed to activation of macrophages.

In vitro functional analysis of *Leishmania*-infected macrophages from healer or nonhealer mice has shown that intracellular multiplication of *L. tropica*

(Handman *et al.*, 1979) and of *L. donovani* (Bradley, 1979) is arrested in explanted macrophages of resistant phenotypes. Finally, peritoneal macrophages of
mice recovered from *L. tropica* or *L. donovani* infection have been shown to be
capable of killing or inhibiting multiplication of the relevant parasites (Miller and
Twohy, 1969; Handman and Spira, 1977). In our hands, no antiparasitic effect
could be demonstrated in guinea pig macrophages recovered from *L. enriettii*
infection (Behin *et al.*, 1975).

Infection of mouse macrophages *in vitro* with *L. enriettii*, to which mice are
totally refractory, has been particularly advantageous in the study of the mechanism of intracellular killing of leishmanial parasites by activated macrophages
(Büchmuller and Mauel, 1979, 1981). *L. enriettii* is readily phagocytosed and
survives well in peritoneal macrophages of the mouse. Activation of the latter
cells by a variety of methods results in total destruction of the ingested parasite
within 24–28 hr (Behin *et al.*, 1975, 1977b, 1979; Mauel *et al.*, 1975). Advantage was taken of this observation, and destruction of *L. enriettii* in activated
mouse macrophages was used as a positive index of activation to determine the
fate of ingested *L. t. major* in macrophages of healer and nonhealer mice (Behin
et al., 1979). It was found that activation of macrophages of healer mice (with
respect to *L. t. major* infection), through the mediation of concanavalin (Con-A)-
stimulated lymphocytes, destroyed both *L. enriettii* and *L. t. major*, while similarly treated cells from nonhealer animals destroyed only *L. enriettii* but not *L. t.
major*. The inability of nonhealer macrophages to eliminate the ingested *L. t.
major* was found to be of a quantitative rather than qualitative nature. *L. t.
major*-infected nonhealer macrophages could indeed be activated to kill the
parasite provided that a state of sustained activation was maintained for 72–96
hr. This was done by repeatedly pulsing infected macrophages with a lympho-
kine-rich medium prepared from Con-A-stimulated mouse splenic lymphocytes
(Behin *et al.*, 1979). The apparent inability of nonhealer mice to destroy *L. t.
major* was tentatively attributed to the higher threshold of activation required by
macrophages of nonhealer animals to eliminate the parasite.

The mechanism of intracellular destruction of leishmanial parasites by macrophages has been subject of several recent studies. It appears that toxic metabolites of oxygen, such as superoxide anion and particularly hydrogen peroxide, are
responsible for the parasiticidal capacity of macrophages (Murray 1981a, 1981b,
1982). Incubation of activated macrophages with exogenous peroxidase has been
shown to enhance destruction of *L. enriettii* by activated mouse macrophage—an
effect that is blocked by amiotriazole, an inhibitor of the enzyme (Buchmüller
and Mauel, 1981).

Although these observations suggest that the generation of the activated
state in host macrophages might result in the elimination of leishmanial parasites,
it is impossible, as yet, to explain why this does not happen early enough or at
all.

6. ANALYSIS OF HUMORAL RESPONSE TO *LEISHMANIA* PARASITE

Despite the general consensus that the mechanism of immune protection against leishmanial diseases is largely cell-mediated, the view is gaining ground that humoral response may be essential not only in recovery from the disease but also important in the pathogenesis of certain severe forms.

Antileishmanial antibodies are highly agglutinating and, in the presence of the complement, are very toxic to the parasite (Behin, unpublished observation). Thus, amastigotes liberated from ruptured macrophages may be eliminated by antibodies present in the immediate vicinity. Antibody may also opsonize the liberated parasites and render them more likely to invoke phagocytosis and activation of macrophages. Formation of immune complexes and release of the mediators of complement activation may induce necrotic processes; this is now believed to be an essential step in recovery from the disease. Conversely, antibodies in sufficient quantity may block parasite antigen, preventing the host from becoming sensitized and making it unable to mount an effective cell-mediated immune response; this enhancing effect might be exemplified in kala-azar. The following observations may support some of these views.

The presence of lytic and agglutinating factors in normal sera was demonstrated by Adler in 1940. These factors or so-called natural antibodies were later shown to occur in large variety of mammalian hosts including man (Ben Rashid, 1967; Ulrich *et al.*, 1968; Schmunis and Herman, 1970; Pearson and Steigbigel, 1980). The agglutinating factor of normal rabbit serum was identified with IgM fraction, which, with the addition of complement, was also lytic (Schmunis and Herman, 1970). The biological function of these natural antibodies, however, remains obscure; despite their universal presence in sera of most mammals, natural infections occur and the parasites readily bypass the antibodies lethal effects.

Artificially raised antibodies to *Leishmania* parasites have been shown to have lytic, agglutinating, and growth-inhibitory activities against the parasite (Rezai *et al.*, 1972b).

Antibodies in naturally occurring leishmanial infections have largely been known in association with kala-azar, of which hypergammaglobulinemia is the paramount feature. Other clinical forms were not generally known to induce detectable levels of circulating antibodies, although it was certainly known that healing coincides with large accumulations of plasma cells and that the parasites disappear in the vicinity of these antibody producing cells (Adler, 1964; Bryceson *et al.*, 1972; Rezai *et al.*, 1972a; Sordat and Behin, 1977). In a recent histological study of human cutaneous leishmaniasis (Moriearty *et al.*, 1982), the plasma cells were observed with reference to the class of globulins they produced and the possible relationship they may have had with circulating antibody to

Leishmania. Plasma cells comprised 10–50% of cells infiltrating lesions of the 20 patients examined. Antileishmanial antibodies were detected by indirect immunofluorescence in 15 patients and 2-mercapto-ethanol-sensitive agglutinins for promastigotes in 19 patients. No correlation was found between class and frequency of Ig-producing cells in the lesion and serum antibody and serum immunoglobulin levels. The authors concluded that in cutaneous leishmaniasis, serum immunoglobulins or anti-*Leishmania* antibody levels do not offer an accurate estimate of the possible role of antibody in protection.

Results of passive transfer experiment to demonstrate the protective value of antileishmanial antibodies are not convincing. In the guinea pig, transfer of serum from recovered animals to normal recipients failed to protect the animals from a challenge infective dose of the parasite (von Kretschmar 1965). Passive transfer of serum from immune CBA mice to intact recipients was found ineffective in conferring protection. However, good protection was achieved when a mixture of immune cells and serum was transferred to normal animals before challenge (Preston and Dumonde, 1976). The synergistic effect of immune cells and serum in passive protection experiments has also been documented in the guinea pig–*L. enriettii* model (Poulter 1980). Furthermore, the same report indicates that serum taken 24 hr after boosting an immune animal is alone capable of transferring protection to a normal guinea pig.

It is evident from the forgoing that no conclusive proof can as yet be found in favor of humoral response as the sole factor responsible for protection against leishmanial disease. Evidence suggests, however, that antibodies may have much to contribute in the pathogenesis as well as in the mechanism of recovery in leishmanial diseases.

7. CONCLUSION

It is the general consensus that the longer a host–parasite association has been in existence, in the evolutionary sense, the more likely it is to be a relationship unaccompanied by exaggerated reactions on either side. As Sprent (1963) expresses it in his book *Parasitism,* it may be wrong to consider that a nicely balanced host–parasite association is regulated by defense mechanism of the host. A vigorous host response to a "new" invader may have selectively been diminished toward the "old" and more familiar parasite to the point where the host has become immunologically tolerant. It is also feasible to suppose that a selective obliteration of some provocative parasite antigen has taken place, to the advantage of parasite, through the failure of the host's recognition processes to awaken. The intracellular position of *Leishmania* parasites, while ensuring them of ready access to their metabolic needs, may have two immunological significances. First, the parasite is protected from deleterious effects of antibodies and complement components. Second, the parasite antigens are masked inside the host cell, where they are unable to provoke the immune responses of the host.

It should be evident from this rather cursory review that the immunology of leishmanial infections has arrived to a rather inconclusive point. It was seen that lymphocytic responses are vigorous but in vain, macrophages seem incapacitated, and serum antibodies appear to play no role. Part of this situation seems to stem from the fact that we often forget to appreciate the ingenuity of the parasites' survival mechanisms. The exclusive existence of the parasite in macrophages— the cells of prime importance in specific and nonspecific defense mechanism of the host—is one of the most remarkable examples of successful parasitism. The immune machinery of the host seems to be outwitted by the parasite's strategy of hiding inside the macrophages. Conditions such as DCL or PKDL, despite their ugly appearance, are the best examples of a mutual host–parasite adaptation. The host often becomes a source for dissemination of the parasite, and the parasite-laden lesions do not even ulcerate. Necrotic processes reveal parasite antigens and trigger the host's immune responses; that is why Ridley viewed necrosis as more important than delayed-type hypersensitivity in the healing process and considered the granulomatous reactions a postnecrotic phenomenon. Elucidation of the mechanisms responsible for the necrotic processes would bring more useful information to this aspect of leishmanial diseases.

ACKNOWLEDGEMENTS. We gratefully acknowledge support from the UNDP/World Bank/WHO Special Programme for Research and Training in Tropical Diseases and from the Swiss National Foundation. We would also like to thank Robert Etges for his editorial comments.

REFERENCES

Abdalla, R. E., 1977, Immunodiffusion, counterimmunoelectrophoresis and immunofluorescence in diagnosis of Sudan mucosal leishmaniasis, *Am. J. Trop. Med. Hyg.* 26:1135–1138.

Abdalla, R. E., El Hadi, A., Ahmed, M. A. and El Hassan, A. M. 1975, Sudan mucosal leishmaniasis, *Trans. Roy. Soc. Trop. Med. Hyg.* 69:443–449.

Adler, S., 1940, Attempts to transmit visceral leishmaniasis to man, *Trans. Roy. Soc. Trop. Med. Hyg.* 33:419–437.

Adler, S., 1964, Leishmania, in: *Advances in Parasitology*, Volume 2 (B. Dawes, ed.), Academic Press, New York.

Adler, S., and Nelken, D., 1965, Attempts to transfer delayed hypersensitivity to *Leishmania tropica* by leucocytes and whole blood, *Trans. Roy. Soc. Trop. Med.* 59:59.

Aikat, B. K., Pathania, A. G. S., Sehgal, S., Bhattacharya, P. K., Dutta, U., Pasricha, N., Singh, S., Singh Parmar, R., Sahaya, S., and Prasad, L. S. N., 1979a, Immunological responses in Indian kala-azar, *Indian J. Med. Res.* 70:583–591.

Aikat, B. K., Sehgal, S., Mahajan, R. C., Pathania, A. G. S., Bhattacharya, P. K., Sahaya, S., Choudhury A. B., Pasricha, N., and Prasad, L. S. N., 1979b, The role of counter immunoelectrophoresis as a diagnostic tool in kala-azar, *Indian J. Med. Res.* 70:592–597.

Alencar, J. E., Ilardi, A., and Pampiglione, S., 1966, La reazione di fissazione del complemento nella diagnosi della leishmaniosi viscerale: Antigeni da batteri acido alcool resistenti, *Parassitologia* 8:147–181.

Alencar, J. E., Ilardi, A., and Pampiglione, S., 1968, La reazione di fissazione del complemento con antigen da BCG nella leishmaniosi viscerale, *Parassitologia* 10:33–35.

Alexander, J., and Phillips, R. S. 1978, *Leishmania tropica* and *L. mexicana:* Cross-immunity in mice, *Exp. Parasitol.* 45:93–100.

Allain, D. S., and Kagan, I. G., 1975, A direct agglutination test for leishmaniasis, *Am. J. Trop. Med. Hyg.* 24:232–236.

Anthony, R. L., Christensen, H. A., and Johnson, C. M., 1980, Microenzyme-linked immunosorbent assay (ELISA) for the seradiagnosis of New World leishmaniasis, *Am. J. Trop. Med. Hyg.* 29:190–194.

Araujo, F. G., and Mayrink, W., 1968, Fluorescent antibody test in visceral leishmaniasis: II. Studies on the specificity of the test, *Rev. Inst. Med. Trop. S. Paulo* 10:41–45.

Ardehali, S., Sodeiphy, M., Haghighi, P., Rezai, H., and Vollum, D., 1980, Studies on chronic (lupoid) leishmaniasis, *Ann. Trop. Med. Parasitol.* 74:339–445.

Ashford, R. W., 1970, A possible reservoir for Leishmania tropica in Ethiopia, Correspondence, *Trans. Roy. Soc. Trop. Med. Hyg.* 64:930–937.

Behforouz, N., Rezai, H. R., and Gettner, S., 1976, Application of immunofluorescence to detection of antibody in leishmaniasis infection, *Ann. Trop Med. Parasitol.* 70:293–301.

Behin, R., Mauel, J., Biroum-Noerjasin, and Rowe, D. S., 1975, Mechanisms of protective immunity in experimental cutaneous leishmaniasis of the guinea-pig: II. Selective destruction of different *Leishmania* species in activated guinea-pig and mouse macrophages, *Clin. Exp. Immunol.* 20:351–358.

Behin, R., Mauel, J., and Rowe, D. S., 1977a, Mechanisms of protective immunity in experimental cutaneous leishmaniasis in the guinea-pig: III. Inhibition of leishmanial lesion in the guinea-pig by delayed hypersensitivity reaction to unrelated antigens, *Clin. Exp. Immunol.* 29:320–325.

Behin, R., Mauel, J., Biroum-Noerjasin, and Rowe, D. S., 1977b, Studies on cell-mediated immunity to cutaneous leishmaniasis of guinea-pigs and mice by *Leishmania enriettii* and *Leishmania tropica*, in: *Ecologie des Leishmaniose,* CNRS ed. INSERM, Paris.

Behin, R., Mauel, J., and Sordat, B., 1979, *Leishmania tropica:* Pathogenicity and *in vitro* macrophage function in strains of inbred mice, *Exp. Parasitol.* 48:81–91.

Belehu, A., and Turk, J. L., 1976, Establishment of cutaneous *Leishmania enriettii* infection in hamsters, *Infect. Immunol.* 13:1235–1241.

Belehu, A., Poulter, L. W., and Turk, J. L., 1976, Modification of cutaneous leishmaniasis in the guinea-pig by cyclophosphamide, *Clin. Exp. Immunol.* 24:125–132.

Ben Rashid, M. S., 1967, Action lytique du sérum humain normal vis-à-vis de *Leishmania infantum*, *Arch. Inst. Pasteur, Tunis,* 44:155–161.

Bianchi, A. T. J., Hooijkaas, H., Benner, R., Nordin, A. A., and Sehreier, M. H., 1981, Clones of helper T cells mediate antigen-specific, H2 restricted DTH, *Nature* 290:62–63.

Bittencourt, A. L., and Guimares, N. A., 1968, Immunopatologie da leishmaniose tegumentar difusa, *Med. Calanea.* 2:395–402.

Blackwell, J. M., 1982, Genetic control of recovery from visceral leishmaniasis, *Trans. Roy. Soc. Trop. Med. Hyg.* 76:147–151.

Blewett, T. M., Kadivar, D. M. H., and Soulsby, E. J. L., 1971, Cutaneous leishmaniasis in the guinea-pig: Delayed-type hypersensitivity, lymphocyte stimulation and inhibition of macrophage migration, *Am. J. Trop. Med. Hyg.* 20:546–551.

Bradley, D. J., 1974, Genetic control of natural resistance to *Leishmania donovani*, *Nature [London]* 250:353–354.

Bradley, D. J., 1977, Regulation of *Leishmania* population within the host: II. Genetic control of acute susceptibility of mice to *Leishmania donovani* infection, *Clin. Exp. Immunol.* 30:130–140.

Bradley, D. J., 1979, Regulation of *Leishmania* population within the host: IV. Parasite and host cell kinetics studied by radioisotope labeling, *Acta Tropica.* 36:171–179.

Bradley, D. J., 1980, Genetic control of resistance to protozoal infections, in: *Genetic Control of Natural Resistance to Infections and Malignancy (Perspectives in Immunology)* (E. Skamene, P. Kongshavn, and M. Landy, eds), Academic Press, New York.

Bradley, D. J., 1982, Introduction and genetic of susceptibility to *Leishmania donovani*. *Trans. Roy. Soc. Trop. Med. Hyg.* 76:143–146.

Bradley, D. J., and Kirkley, J., 1977, Regulation of *Leishmania* population within the host: I. The variable course of *Leishmania donovani* infection in mice, *Clin. Exp. Immunol.* 30:119–129.

Bray, R. S., 1970, Serotypes of *Leishmania* in relation geography and disease states, *Ethiopian Med. J.* 8:207–212.

Bray, R. S., 1974, Epidemiology of leishmaniasis: Some reflections on causation, in: *Trypanosomiasis and Leishmaniasis with Special Reference to Chagas' Disease, Ciba Foundation Symposium 20* (new series).

Bray, R. S., and Lainson, R., 1965, Failure to transfer hypersensitivity to *Leishmania* by injection of leucocytes, *Trans. R. Soc. Trop. Med. Hyg.* 59:221–222.

Bray, R. S., and Lainson, R., 1966, The immunology and serology of Leishmaniasis IV. Results of Ouchterlony double diffusion tests, *Trans. Roy. Soc. Trop. Med. Hyg.* 60:605–609.

Bray, R. S., and Lainson, R., 1967, Studies on the immunology and serology of Leishmaniasis. V. The use of particles as vehicles in passive agglutination tests. *Trans. Roy. Soc. Trop. Med. Hyg.* 61:490–505.

Bryceson, A. D. M., 1970a, Diffuse cutaneous leishmaniasis in Ethiopia: II. Treatment, *Trans. Roy. Soc. Trop. Med. Hyg.* 64:369–379.

Bryceson, A. D. M., 1970b, Diffuse cutaneous leishmaniasis in Ethiopia: III. Immunological studies, *Trans. Roy. Soc. Trop. Med. Hyg.* 64:380–387.

Bryceson, A. D. M., Bray, R. S., Wolstencroft, R. A., and Dumonde, D. C., 1970, Immunity in cutaneous Leishmaniasis of the guinea-pig, *Clin. Exp. Immunol.* 7:301–341.

Bryceson, A. D. M., Preston, P. M., Bray, R. S., and Dumonde, D. C., 1972, Experimental cutaneous leishmaniasis: II. Effects of immuno-suppression and antigenic competition on the course of infection with *Leishmania enriettii* in the guinea-pig, *Clin. Exp. Immunol.* 10:305–335.

Bryceson, A. D. M., Bray, R. S., and Dumonde, D. C., 1974, Experimental cutaneous leishmaniasis: IV. Selective suppression of cell-mediated immunity during the response of guinea-pig to infection with *Leishmania enriettii*, *Clin. Exp. Immunol.* 16:189–202.

Buchmüller, Y., and Mauel, J., 1979, Studies of the mechanisms of macrophage activation: II. Parasite destruction in macrophages activated by supernates from concanavalin A-stimulated lymphocytes, *J. Exp. Med.* 150:359–370.

Buchmüller, Y., and Mauel, J., 1981, Studies on the mechanisms of macrophage activation: Possible involvement of oxygen metabolites in killing of *Leishmania enriettii* by activated mouse macrophages, *J. Reticuloend. Soc.* 29:181–192.

Buss, G., 1929, Untersuchungen mit Leishmania-vakzine, *Arch. f. Schiffs u. Tropenhyg.* 33:65–83.

Camargo, M. E., and Rebonato, C., 1969, Cross reactivity in fluorescence tests for *Trypanosoma* and *Leishmania* antibodies: A single inhibition procedure to ensure specific results, *Am. J. Trop. Med. Hyg.* 18:500–505.

Carvalho, E. M., Teixeira, R. S., and Warren, J. J., Jr., 1981, Cell-mediated immunity in American visceral leishmaniasis: Reversible immunosuppression during acute infection, *Infect. Immun.* 33:498–502.

Casali, P., and Lambert, P. H., 1979, Purification of soluble immune complexes from serum using polymethacrylate beads coated with congentinin or C1q, *Clin. Exp. Immunol.* 37:295–309.

Cascio, G., Purpura, A., and Prioslisi, A., 1963, Test dell' emo-agglutinazione condizionata per la recerca delle agglutinin anti *Leishmania, Pediatra Napoli* 71:251–258.

Christensen, H. A., and de Vasquez, A. M., 1981, Susceptibility of *Aotus trivirgatus* to *Leishmania braziliensis* and *L. mexicana, Am. J. Trop. Med. Hyg.* 30:54–56.

Convit, J., 1958, Leishmaniasis tegamentaria difusa: Nueva entidad clinico patologica y parasitaria, *Rev. Sanid. Asist. Soc. Caracas* 23:1–28.

Convit, J., and Pinardi, M. E., 1969, Applying the indirect immunofluorescency test in the study of American cutaneous leishmaniasis, *Derm. Int.* 8:17–20.

Convit, J., Pinardi, M. E., and Rondon, A. J., 1972, Diffuse cutaneous leishmaniasis: A disease due to an immunological defect of the host, *Trans. Roy. Soc. Trop. Med. Hyg.* 66:603–610.

Corradin, G., Etlinger, H. M., and Chiller, J. M., 1977, Lymphocyte specificity to protein antigens: I. Characterization of the antigen-induced *in vitro* T cell-dependent proliferative response with lymph node cells from mice, *J. Immunol.* 119:1048–1053.

Da Cunha, A. M., and Dias, E., 1938, Sur la préparation d'un antigène stable pour la réaction de fixation du complément dans leishmanioses, *C. R. Séance Soc. Biol.* 129:991–993.

Desjeux, P., Santoro, F., Afchain, D., Loyens, M., and Capron, A., 1980, Circulating immune complexes and anti-IgG antibodies in mucocutaneous leishmaniasis, *Am. J. Trop. Med. Hyg.* 29:195–198.

Destombes, P., 1960, Application du concept de "systémisation polaire" aux leishmanioses cutanées, *Bull. Soc. Path. Exot.* 53:299–300.

Djoko-Tamnou, J., Leclerc, C., Modabber, F., and Chedid, L., 1981, Studies on visceral *Leishmania tropica* infection in Balb/c mice: I. Clinical features and cellular changes, *Clin. Exp. Immunol.* 46:493–498.

Dostrovsky, A., and Sagher, F., 1946, The intracutaneous test in cutaneous leishmaniasis, *Ann. Trop. Med. Parasitol.* 40:265–269.

Dostrovsky, A., Sagher, F., and Zuckerman, A., 1952a, Isophasic reaction following experimental super-infection of *Leishmania tropica, Arch. Derm. Syph.* 66:665.

Dostrovsky, A., Zuckerman, A., and Sagher, F., 1952b, Successful experimental superinfection of *Leishmania tropica* in patients with relapsing cutaneous leishmaniasis, *Harefuah* 43:29–30.

Duxbury, J. M., and Sadun, E. H., 1964, Fluorescent antibody test for the serodiagnostic of visceral leishmaniasis, *Am. J. Trop. Med. Hyg.* 13:525–529.

Edrissian, G. H., and Darabian, P., 1979, A comparison of enzyme-linked immunosorbent assay and indirect fluorescent antibody test in the serodiagnosis of cutaneous and visceral leishmaniasis in Iran, *Trans. Roy. Soc. Trop. Med. Hyg.* 73:289–292.

Gardener, P. J., Schory, L., and Chance, M. L., 1977, Species differentiation in the genus *Leishmania* by morphometric studies with the electron microscope, *Ann. Trop. Med. Parasitol.* 71:147–155.

Garnham, P. C. C., 1971, American leishmaniasis, *Bull WHO* 44:521–527.

Ghose, A. C., Haldar, J. P., Pal, S. C., Mishra, B. P., and Mishra, K. K., 1979, Phytohemaglutinin-induced lymphocyte transformation test in Indian Kala-azar, *Trans. Roy. Soc. Trop. Med. Hyg.* 73:725–726.

Ghose, A. C., Haldar, J. P., Pal, S. C., Mishra, B. P. and Mishra, K. K., 1980, Serological investigations on Indian Kala-azar, *Clin. Exp. Immunol.* 40:318.

Girgla, H. S., Marsden, R. A., Singh, G. M., and Ryan, T. J., 1977, Post-Kala-azar dermal leishmaniasis, *Br. J. Dermatol.* 3:307–311.

Gorczynski, R. M., 1982, Nature of resistance to leishmaniasis in experimental rodents, *Develop. Compar. Immunol.* 6:199–207.

Gorczynski, R. M., and MacRae, S., 1982, Analysis of a subpopulation of glass-adherent mouse skin cells controlling resistance/susceptibility to infection with *Leishmania tropica* and correlation with the development of independant proliferative signals to Lyt-1$^+$/Lyt-2$^+$ T lymphocytes, *Cell. Immunol.* 67:74–89.

Grimaldi, G. F., Moriearty, P. L., and Hoff, R., 1980a, *Leishmania mexicana:* Immunology and histopathology in C3H mice, *Exp. Parasitol.* 50:45–56.

Grimaldi, G. F., Moriearty, P. L., and Hoff, R., 1980b, *Leishmania mexicana* in C3H mice-BCG and levamisole treatment of established infections, *Clin. Exp. Immunol.* 41:237–242.

Guimares, M. C. S., Celesle, B. J., de Castilho, E. A., Mineo, J. R., and Paira Diniz, J. M., 1981, Immunoenzymatic assay (ELISA) in mucocutaneous leishmaniasis, Kala-azar, and Chagas' disease: An epimastigote *Trypanosoma cruzi* antigen able to distinguish between anti-*Trypanosoma* and anti-*Leishmania* antibodies, *Am. J. Trop. Med. Hyg.* 30:942–947.

Guirges, S. Y., 1971, Natural and experimental re-infection of men with oriental sore, *Ann. Trop. Med. Parasitol.* 65:197–205.

Haldar, J. P., Saha, K. C., and Ghose, A. C., 1981, Serological profiles in Indian post Kala-azar dermal leishmaniasis, *Trans. Roy. Soc. Trop. Med. Hyg.* 75:514–517.

Hale, C., and Howard, J. G., 1981, Immunological regulation of experimental cutaneous leishmaniasis: 2. Studies with Biozzi high and low responder mice, *Parasite Immunol.* 3:45–55.

Handman, E., and Spira, D. T., 1977, Growth of *Leishmania* amastigotes in macrophages from normal and immune mice, *Z. Parasitenkd.* 53:75–81.

Handman, E., Ceredig, R., and Mitchell, G. F., 1979, Murine cutaneous leishmaniasis: Disease patterns in intact and nude mice of various genotypes and examination of some differences between normal and infected macrophages, *Aus. J. Exp. Biol. Med.* 57:9–30.

Handman, E., Mitchell, G. F., and Goding, J. W., 1981, Identification and characterization of protein antigens of *Leishmania tropica* isolates, *J. Immunol.* 126:508–512.

Herman, R., and Farrell, J. P., 1977, Effects of cyclophosphamide on visceral leishmaniasis in the mouse, *J. Protozool.* 24:429–436.

Hoare, C. A., 1955, Intraspecific biological groups in pathogenic protozoa, *Refuah Veterinaria* 12:258–263.

Hommel, M., 1976, Enzyme Immunoassay in leishmaniasis, *Trans. Roy. Soc. Trop. Med. Hyg.* 70:15–16.

Hommel, M., Peters, W., Ranque, J., Quilici, M., and Lanotte, G., 1978, The micro-ELISA technique in the serodiagnosis of visceral leishmaniasis, *Ann. Trop. Med. Parasitol.* 72:213–218.

Howard, J. G., Hale, C., and Liew, F. Y., 1980, Immunological regulation of experimental cutaneous leishmaniasis: III. The nature and significance of specific suppression of cell-mediated immunity, *J. Exp. Med.* 152:594–607.

Howard, J. G., Hale, C., and Liew, F. Y., 1981, Immunological regulation of experimental cutaneous leishmaniasis: IV. Prophylatic effect of sublethal irradiation due to abrogation of suppressor T cell generation in mice genetically susceptible to *Leishmania tropica*, *J. Exp. Med.* 153:557–568.

Howard, J. G., Hale, C., and Liew, F. Y., 1982, Genetically determined response mechanism to cutaneous leishmaniasis, *Trans. Roy. Sec. Trop. Med. Hyg.* 76:152–154.

Irunberry, J., Bennalègue, A., Grangaud, J. P., Mazonni, M., Khati, B., and Khedair, M., 1968, Etude des immuglobulines plasmatiques dans le Kala-azar *Arch. Inst. Pasteur Alger.* 46:102–113.

Kadivar, D. M., and Soulsby, E. J., 1975, Model for disseminated cutaneous leishmaniasis, *Science* 190:1198–1200.

Kanan, M. W., 1975, Mucocutaneous leishmaniasis in guinea-pigs inoculated intravenously with *Leishmania enriettii:* Preliminary report, *Br. J. Dermatol.* 92:663–673.

Khan, H. M., 1977, Post Kala-azar dermal leishmaniasis (A review of 10 cases), *Bangladesh Med. Res. Council Bull.* 3:55–56.

Lainson, R., and Shaw, J. J., 1972, Leishmaniasis of the New World: Taxonomic problem, *Br. Med. Bull.* 28:44.

Lainson, R. and Shaw, J. J., 1977, Leishmaniasis in Brazil: XVI. Observation on cross-immunity in monkeys and man infested with *Leishmania mexicana mexicana L. m. amazonensis, L. braziliensis braziliensis, L. b. guyanensis* and *L. b. panamensis, J. Trop. Med. Hyg.* 80:29–35.

Lainson, R., and Shaw, J. J., 1978, Epidemiology and ecology of leishmaniasis in Latin America, *Nature [London]* 273:595–600.

Leclerc, C., Modabber, F., Deriaud, E., and Chedid, L., 1981, Systemic infection of *Leishmania tropica* (major) in various strains of mice, *Trans. Roy. Soc. Trop. Med. Hyg.* 75:851–854.

Leclerc, C., Modabber, F., Deriaud, E., Djoko-Tamnou, J., and Chedid, L., 1982, Studies on visceral *Leishmania tropica* infection of Balb/c mice: II. Cellular analysis of *in vitro* unresponsiveness to sheep erythrocytes (submitted).

Lemma, A., and Yau, P., 1973, Course of development of *Leishmania enriettii* infection in immunosuppressed guinea-pigs, *Amer. J. Trop. Med. Hyg.* 22:477–481.

Liew, F. Y., Hale, C., and Howard, J. G., 1982, Immunologic regulation of experimental cutaneous leishmaniasis: V. Characterization of effector and specific suppressor T cells, *J. Immunol.* 128:1917–1922.

Lin, Y. L., and Askona, B. A., 1981, Biological properties of an influenza A virus-specific killer T clone: Inhibition *in vivo* and induction of delayed hypersensitivity reactions, *J. Exp. Med.* 154:225–234.

Louis J. A., Moedder, E., Behin, R., and Engers, H., 1979, Recognition of protozoan parasite antigens by murine T lymphocytes: I. Induction of specific T lymphocyte dependent proliferative responses to *Leishmania tropica. Eur. J. Immunol.* 9:841–847.

Louis, J. A., Moedder, E., MacDonald, H. R., and Engers, H. D., 1981, Recognition of protozoan parasites by murine T. lymphocytes. II: Role of the H-2 gene complex in interactions between antigen-presenting macrophages and *Leishmania*-immune T lymphocytes, *J. Immunol.* 126:1661–1666.

Louis, J. A., Lima, G. M., and Engers, H. D., 1982a, Murine T lymphocytes responses specific for the protozoan parasite *Leishmania tropica* and *Trypanosoma brucei, Clin. Immunol. Allerg.* 2:597–612.

Louis, J. A., Zubler, R. H., Coutinho, S. G., Lima, G., Behin, R., Mauel, J., and Engers, H. D., 1982b, The *in vitro* generation and functional analysis of murine T cell populations and clones specific for a protozoan parasite, *Leishmania tropica, Immunol. Rev.* 61:215–243.

Lumsden, W. H. R., 1974, Leishmaniasis and trypanosomiasis: The canative organisms compared and contrasted, in: *Trypanosomiasis and Leishmaniasis with Special Reference to Chagas' Disease,* Ciba Foundation Symposium 20 (new series).

Lysenko, A. J., 1971, Distribution of leishmaniasis in the world, *Bull. WHO* 44:515–520.

Mannweiler, E., Lederer, I., and Zum Felde, I., 1978, Das Antikörperbild bei Patienten mit Leishmaniasen, *Zentralbl. Bakteriol. Parasitendk. Infectionskr. Hyg. Abt. 1 Reihe A.* 240:397–402.

Manson-Bahr, P. E. C., 1961, Immunity in Kala-azar. *Trans. Roy. Soc. Trop. Med. Hyg.* 5:550–555.

Manson-Bahr, P. E. C., 1963, Active immunization in leishmaniasis, in: *Immunity to Protozoa* (P. C. C. Granham, A. E. Pierce, and I. Roitt, eds.), Blackwell, Oxford, England.

Mauel, J., Behin, R., Biroum-Noerjasin, and Rowe, D. S., 1975, Mechanisms of protective immunity in the guinea-pig: I. Lack of effects of immune lymphocytes and of activated macrophages, *Clin. Exp. Immunol.* 20:339–350.

Mayrink, W., Melo, M. N., Da Costa, C. A., Magalhaes, P. A., Dias, M., Coelho, M. V., Araujo, F. G., Williams, P., Figueiredo, Y. P., and Batista, S. M., 1976, Intradermo reaçaô de Montenegro na leishmaniose tegumentar americana apos terapeutica antimonial. *Rev. Med. Trop. S. Paulo* 18:182–185.

Mayrink, W., da Costa, C. A., Magalhaes, P. A., Melo, M. N., Dias, M., Oliveira Lima, A., Michalick, M. S., and Williams, P., 1979, A field trial of a vaccine against American dermal leishmaniasis, *Trans. Roy. Soc. Trop. Med. Hyg.* 73:385–388.

Mendes, E., 1979, Transfer of delayed hypersensitivity to leishmanin (Montenegro reaction), *Cell. Immunol.* 42:424–427.

Menzel, S., and Bienzle, U., 1978, Antibody response in patients with cutaneous leishmaniasis of the Old World, *Tropenmed. Parasitol.* 29:194–197.

Miller, H. C., and Twohy, D. W., 1969, Cellular immunity to *Leishmania donovani* in macrophages in culture, *J. Parasitol.* 55:200–207.

Mitchell, G. F., Curtis, J. M., Handman, E., and MacKenzie, I. F. C., 1980, Cutaneous leishmaniasis in mice: Disease pattern in reconstiluted nude mice of several genotypes infected with *Leishmania tropica, Aust. J. Exp. Biol. Med. Sci.* 58:521–532.

Modabber, F. Z., Alimohammadian, M., Khamesipour, A., Pourmand, M. H., Kamali, M., and Nasseri, M., 1980, Studies on the genetic control of visceral leishmaniasis in Balb/c mice by *L. tropica,* in: *Genetic Control of Natural Resistance to Infection and Malignancy* (E. Skamene, P. A. L. Kongshavn, and M. Landy, eds.), Academic Press, New York.

Montenegro, J., 1926, Cutaneous reaction in leishmaniasis, *Arch. Derm. Syph.* 13:187–194.

Moriearty, P. L., Grimaldi, G., Jr., Galvao-Castro, B., Oliveira Neto, M. P., and Marzochi, M. C. A., 1982, Intralesional plasma cells and serologica responses in human cutaneous leishmaniasis, *Clin. Exp. Immunol.* 47:59–64.

Moses, A., 1919, Da fixaçâ do complemento na leishmaniose tegumentar, *Brazil Med.* 33:107–108.

Muniz, J., and Medina, H., 1948, Leishmaniose tegumentar do Cobaio *Leishmania enriettii n.* spp., *Arq. Biol. Tec. Curitiba,* 3:13–30.

Murray, H. W., 1981a, Susceptibility of *Leishmania* to oxygen intermediates and killing by normal macrophages, *J. Exp. Med.* 153:1302–1315.

Murray, H. W., 1981b, Interaction of *Leishmania* with a macrophage cell-line: Correlation between intracellular killing and the generation of oxygen intermediates, *J. Exp. Med.* 153:1690–1695.

Murray, H. W., 1982, Cell-mediated immune response in experimental visceral leishmaniasis: II. Oxygen-dependent killing of intracellular killing of *Leishmania donovani* amastigotes, *J. Immunol.* 129:351–357.

Murray, H. W., Masar, H., and Keithly, J. S., 1982, Cell-mediated immune response in experimental visceral leishmaniasis: I. Correlation between resistance to *Leishmania donovani* and lymphokine-generating capacity, *J. Immunol.* 129:344–350.

Naik, S. R., Vinayak, V. K., Talwar, P., Sehgal, S., Mehra, Y. N., Datta, B. N., and Chhuttani, P. N., 1978, Visceral leishmaniasis masquerading as a nasopharyngeal tumor: Report of a case, *Trans. Roy. Soc. Trop. Med. Hyg.* 72:43–45.

Narayanan, K., Rajagopalan, P., Raina, V., Kumur, R., and Malaviya, A. N., 1979, Immunological studies in Kala-azar: Case report, *J. Comm. Dis.* 11:203–208.

Nasseri, M., and Modabber, F., 1979, Generalized infection and lack of delayed hypersensitivity in Balb/c mice infected with *L. tropica* major, *Infect. Immunol.* 26:611–614.

Neva, F. A., Wyler, D., and Nash, T., 1979, Cutaneous leishmaniasis. A case with persistent organisms after treatment in presence of normal immune response. *Am. J. Trop. Med. Hyg.* 28:467–471.

Packchanian, A., 1979, Experimental cutaneous leishmaniasis with *L. tropica* in albino hairless mice, *Mus musculus, Trans. Roy. Soc. Trop. Med. Hyg.* 73:31–36.

Pampiglione, S., La Placa, M., and Schlick, G., 1974, Studies on Mediterranean leishmaniasis: I. An outbreak of visceral leishmaniasis in Northern Italy, *Trans. Roy. Soc. Trop. Med. Hyg.* 68:349–359.

Pearson, R. D., and Steigbigel, R. T., 1980, Mechanism of lethal effect of human serum upon *Leishmania donovani, J. Immunol.* 125:2195–2201.

Pérez, H., Arredondo, B., and Machado, R., 1979a, *Leishmania mexicana* and *Leishmania tropica:* Cross immunity in C57 BL/6 mice, *Exp. Parasitol.* 48:9–14.

Pérez, H., Labrador, F., and Torrealba, J. W., 1979b, Variations in the response of 5 strains of mice to *Leishmania mexicana, Int. J. Parasitol.* 9:27–32.

Pérez, H., Pocino, M. and Malave, I. 1981, Nonspecific immunodepression and protective immunity in mice infected with *Leishmania mexicana, Infect. Immun.* 32:415–419.

Pessôa, S. B., and Pestana, B. R., 1940, A intradermo reaçâo de Montenegro nas Campanhas sanitarias Centra a Leishmaniose, *Sâo Paulo Med.* 13:133–151.

Petersen, E. A., Neva, F. A., Oster, C. N., and Bogaert Diaz, H., 1982, Specific inhibition of lymphocyte-proliferation responses by adherent suppressor cells in diffuse cutaneous leishmaniasis, *N. Engl. J. Med.* 306:387–392.

Pettit, J. H. S., 1962, Chronic (lupoid) leishmaniasis, *Br. J. Dermatol.* 74:127–131.

Poulter, L. W., 1979, The kinetics and quality of acquired resistance in self-healing and metastatic leishmaniasis, *Clin. Exp. Immunol.* 36:30–37.

Poulter, L. W., 1980a, Mechanisms of immunity to leishmaniasis: I. Evidence for a changing basis of protection in self-limiting disease, *Clin. Exp. Immunol.* 39:14–26.

Poulter, L., 1980b, Mechanisms of immunity to Leishmaniasis. II. Significance of the intramacrophage localization of the parasite, *Clin. Exp. Immunol.* 40:25–35.

Preston, P. M., and Dumonde, D. C., 1976a, Immunology of clinical and experimental leishmaniasis, in: *Immunology of Parasitic Infections* (S. Cohen and E. H. Sadun, eds.), Blackwell Scientific Publications, Oxford, England.

Preston, P. M., and Dumonde, D. C., 1976b, Experimental cutaneous leishmaniasis: V. Protective immunity in subclinical and self-healing infection in the mouse, *Clin. Exp. Immunol.* 23:126–128.

Preston, P. M., Carter, R. L., Leuchars, E., Davies, A. J. and Dumonde, D. C., 1972, Experimental cutaneous leishmaniasis: III. Effects of thymectomy on the course of infection of CBA mice with *Leishmania tropica, Clin. Exp. Immunol.* 10:337–357.

Preston, P. M., Behbehani, K., and Dumonde, D. C., 1978, Experimental cutaneous leishmaniasis: VI. Anergy and allergy in the cellular immune response during non-healing infection in different strains of mice, *J. Clin. Lab. Immunol.* 1:207–220.

Puguin, P., and Miescher, P. A., 1979, Le Kala-azar: Etude clinique et physiopathologique à propos d'un nouveau cas observé en Suisse, *Schweiz. Med. Wochenschr.* 109:265–269.

Quilici, M., Dunan, S., and Ranque, J., 1968, L'immunofluorescence dans les leishmanioses: Comparaison avec la réaction de fixation du complément, *Med. Trop. Marseille* 28:37–43.

Radwansky, Z. K., Bryceson, A. D. M., Preston, P. M., and Dumonde, D. C., 1974, Immunofluorescence studies of *L. enriettii* infection in the guinea-pig, *Trans. Roy. Soc. Trop. Med. Hyg.* 68:124–128.

Ranque, J., and Quilici, M., 1970, Recent advances in immunodiagnosis of leishmaniasis, *J. Parasitol.* 56(Sec. II):277–278.

Ranque, J., Quilici, M., Dunan, S., and Assadurian, Y., 1969, Réactions d'immunoprécipitation en gélose dans les leishmanioses, *Méd. Trop. Marseille* 29:70–75.

Rezai, H. R., Haghighi, P., and Ardehali, S., 1972a, Histological appearance of the site of inoculation and lymph nodes of guinea-pigs at various times after infection with *Leishmania enriettii, Trans. Roy. Soc. Trop. Med. Hyg.* 66:225–234.

Rezai, H., Gettner, S., and Behforouz, N., 1972b, Anti-leishmanial activity of immune guinea-pig serum, *J. Med. Microbiol.* 5:371–375.

Rezai, H. R., Behforouz N., Amirhakimi, G., and Kohanteh, J., 1977, Immunofluorescescence and counter-immunoelectrophoresis in the diagnosis of Kala-azar, *Trans. Roy. Soc. Med. Hyg.* 71:149–151.

Rezai, H. R., Ardehali, S. M., Amirhakimi, G., and Kharazmi A., 1978, Immunological features of Kala-azar, *Amer. J. Trop. Med. Hyg.* 27:1079–1083.

Rezai, H. R., Farrell, J., and Soulsby, E. L., 1980, Immunological responses of *L. donovani* infection in mice and significance of T cell in resistance to experimental leishmaniasis, *Clin. Exp. Immunol.* 40:509–514.

Ridley, D. S., 1979, The pathogenesis of cutaneous leishmaniasis, *Trans. Roy. Soc. Trop. Med. Hyg.* 73:150–180.

Ridley, D. S., 1980, A histological classification of cutaneous leishmaniasis and its geographical expression, *Trans. Roy. Soc. Trop. Med. Hyg.* 74:515–522.

Ridley, D. S., Marsden, P. D., Cuba, C. C., and Barreto, A. C., 1980, A histological classification of mucocutaneous leishmaniasis in Brazil and its clinical evaluation, *Trans. Roy. Soc. Trop. Med. Hyg.* 74:508–515.

Roffi, J., Dedet, J. P., Despend, P., and Garré, M. L., 1980, Detection of circulating antibodies in cutaneous leishmaniasis by enzyme-linked immunosorbent assay (ELISA), *Am. J. Trop. Med. Hyg.* 29:183–189.

Sagher, F., 1947, Leishmania vaccine test in leishmaniasis of the skin (Oriental sore), *Arch. Dermatol. Syph.* 55:658–663.

Sayles, P. C., Hunter, K. W., Stafford, E. E., and Hendricks, L. D., 1981, Antibody response to *Leishmania mexicana* in African white-tailed rat (Mystromys albicandatus) *J. Parasitol.* 67:585–586.

Schmunis, G. A., and Herman, R., 1970, Characteristics of so-called natural antibodies in virious normal sera against culture form of *Leishmania*. *J. Parasitol.* 56:889–896.

Schwartz, R. H., Yano, A., and Paul, W. E., 1978, Interaction between antigen-presenting cells and primed T lymphocytes: An assessment of gene expression in the antigen presenting cells, *Immunol. Rev.* 40:153–180.

Scott, P. A., and Farrell, J. P., 1981, Experimental cutaneous leishmaniasis: Nonspecific immunodepression in Balb/c mice infected with *Leishmania tropica*, *J. Immunol.* 127:2395–2400.

Sen Gupta, P. C., 1943, A complement fixation test for Kala-azar, *Indian Med. Gaz.* 78:336–339.

Sen Gupta, P. C., and Bhattacharjee, B., 1953, Intradermal test with *Leishmania donovani* antigen in post-Kala-azar dermal leishmaniasis, *J. Trop. Med. Hyg.* 56:110–116.

Sen Gupta, P. C., and Mukherjee, A. M., 1962, Intradermal test with *Leishmania donovani* antigen in post kala-azar dermal leishmaniasis, *Ann. Broch. Exp. Med.* 22:63–66.

Simon, H. B., and Sheagran, J. N., 1971, Immunologically mediated enhancement of macrophages bactericidal capacity, *J. Exp. Med.* 133:1377–1389.

Skov, C. B., and Twohy, D. W., 1974a, Cellular immunity to *Leishmania donovani:* I. The effect of T cell depletion on resistance to *L. donovani* in mice, *J. Immunol.* 113:2002–2011.

Skov, C. B., and Twohy, D. W., 1974b, Cellular immunity to *Leishmania donovani:* II. Evidence for synergy between thymocytes and lymph node cells in reconstitution of acquired resistence to *L. donovani* in mice, *J. Immunol.* 113:2012–2019.

Smrkovski, L. L., and Larson, C. L., 1977a, Effect of treatment with BCG on the course of visceral leishmaniasis in Balb/c mice, *Infect. Immun.* 16:249–257.

Smrkovski, L. L., and Larson, C. L., 1977b, Antigenic cross-reactivity between mycobacterium bovis (BCG) and *Leishmania donovani, Infect. Immun.* 18:561–562.

Smrkovski, L. L., Larson, C. L. and Sogandares-Bernal, F., 1974, Fatal visceral leishmaniasis in a strain of Swiss mice, *J. Parasitol.* 60:718–719.

Smrkovski, L. L., Larson, C. L., and Reed, S. G., 1979, Effect of visceral leishmaniasis on congenitally athymic mice, *Infect. Immun.* 25:1078–1080.

Sordat, B., and Behin, R., 1977, Cutaneous leishmaniasis of the guinea-pig: A sequential study by light and electron microscopy, in: *Ecologie des Leishmanioses,* INSERM, Paris.

Southgate, B. A., and Manson-Bahr, P. E. C., 1967, Studies on the epidemiology of East-African Kala-azar: I. The significance of the positive leishmanin test, *J. Trop. Med. Hyg.* 70:29–33.

Sprent, J. F. A., 1963, *Parasitism,* The William and Wilkins Co., Baltimore.

Stauber, L. A., 1955, Leishmaniasis in the hamster, in: *Some Physiological Aspects and Conse-*

quences of Parasitism (W. H. Cole, ed.), Rutgers University Press, New Brunswick, N.J., pp. 76–90.

Stauber, L. A., 1958, Host resistance to the Khartoum strain of Leishmania donovani, Rice Inst. Pamph. 45:20–96.

Stauber, L. A., 1962, Some recent studies in experimental leishmaniasis, Sci. Rep. Inst. Sup. Sanita 2:68–75.

Stauber, L. A., 1963, Immunity to Leishmania, Ann. N.Y. Acad. Sci. 113:409–417.

Stauber, L. A., 1964, Characterization of strains of Leishmania donovani, in: Proceedings of the Seventh International Congress of Tropical Medicine and Malaria, Rio de Janeiro, pp. 324–325.

Stauber, L. A., McConnel, E., and Hoogstraal, H., 1966, Leishmaniasis in the Sudan republic: 25. Experimental visceral leishmaniasis in the Nile grass rat, Arvicanthus niloticus niloticus Dollman, Exp. Parasital. 18:35–40.

Tremonti, L. and Walton, B. C., 1970, Blast transformation and migration-inhibition in Toxoplasmosis and Leishmaniasis, Amer. J. Trop. Med. and Hyg. 19:49–56.

Turk, J. L., and Bryceson, A. D. M., 1971, Immunological phenomena in leprosy and related diseases, Adv. Immunol. 13:209–266.

Ulrich M., Ortiz, D. T., and Convit, J., 1968, The effect of fresh serum on the leptomonads of Leishmania: I. Preliminary report. Trans. Roy. Soc. Trop. Med. Hyg. 62:628–630.

Veress, B., OMer, A., Satir, A. A., and El Hassan, A. M., 1977, Morphology of the spleen and lymph nodes in fatal visceral leishmaniasis, Immunology 33:606–610.

Von Kretschman, W., 1965, Immunität bei der Leishmania enriettii infection des Meerschweinchens, Zeitschr. Tropenmed. Parasitol. 16:277–283.

Wagener, E. M., 1923, A skin reaction to extract of Leishmania tropica and Leishmania infantum, Univ. Calif. Pub. Zool. 20:477–488.

Walton, B. C., 1970, Indirect fluorescent antibody test for evaluation of effectiveness of chemotherapy in American leishmaniasis, J. Parasitol. 56:480–481.

Walton, B. C., Brooks, W. H. and Arjona, I., 1972, Serodiagnosis of American Leishmaniasis by indirect immunofluorescent antibody test, Amer. J. Trop. Med. Hyg. 21:296–299.

Weintraub, J. and Weinbaum, F. I., 1977, The effect of BCG on experimental cutaneous leishmaniasis in mice, J. Immunol. 118:2288–2290.

Wilson, H. R., Diekmann, B. S., and Childs, G. E., 1979, Leishmania braziliensis and Leishmania mexicana: Experimental cutaneous infection in golden hamsters, Exp. Parasitol. 47:270–283.

Witztum, E., Spira, D. T., and Zuckerman, A., 1978, Blast transformation in different stages of cutaneous leishmaniasis, Isr. J. Med. Sci. 14:244–248.

Wolf, R. E., 1976, Immune response to Leishmania tropica in Maccaca mulata, J. Parasitol. 62:209–214.

Wyler, D. J., Weinbaum, F. I., and Herrod, H. R., 1979, Characterization of in vitro proliferative responses of human lymphocytes to leishmanial antigens, J. Infect. Dis. 140:215–221.

Zubler, R. H., and Louis, J. A., 1981, Clonal assay for T-helper cells (TH) and conditions for H-2 restricted linked cooperation between TH and hapten-primed B cells: Application to the quantitation of hemocyanin or Leishmania tropica-specific TH in primed mice, J. Immunol. 127:1924–1930.

Zuckerman, A., 1975, Current status of the immunology of blood and tissue Protozoa: I. Leishmania, Exp. Parasitol. 38:370–400.

Zuckerman, A., and Lainson, R., 1977, Leishmania, in: Parasitic Protozoa: I. Taxonomy, Kinetoplastid, and Flagellates of Fish (J. P. Kreier, ed.), Academic Press, New York.

7

Immunological Alterations in Chagas' Disease

J. A. O'DALY AND J. AZOCAR

1. THE PARASITE AND THE DISEASE

Chagas' disease is caused by infection with *Trypanosoma cruzi,* a flagellate parasite discovered in Brazil by Carlos Chagas (1909), who described (1911) the clinical, pathological and epidemiological features of the disease that was to bear his name. The *T. cruzi* life cycle is a complex one, with several stages of development in vertebrate and invertebrate hosts. In the vertebrates, *T. cruzi* undergoes intracellular multiplication (amastigote). The emerging nonmultiplying trypomastigotes are found in the bloodstream of the infected vertebrates. In the invertebrate (insect) host, the life of *T. cruzi* is characterized by morphological transformations that take place along the digestive tract. Different strains of *T. cruzi* show differences in morphology during their life cycles (Brener, 1971). The most usual mode of transmission is by means of the invertebrate (hematophagus) intermediary host (Hoare, 1972). After feeding on the infected vertebrates, bloodstream trypomastigotes differentiate in the digestive tracts of the *Triatoma* bugs. Metacyclic forms of the parasite, eliminated in the insect feces, are considered responsible for infection in the vertebrate host (Zeledon, 1977).

Chagas' disease is widely prevalent in Central and South America. It is difficult to establish the exact prevalence mainly because the statistics for the rural population in the affected areas are limited. Chagas' disease is often lethal; widely applicable chemotherapy is unavailable so far. It has been estimated that in Brazil alone, more than 10 million people are infected by *T. cruzi* (Barreto,

J. A. O'DALY AND J. AZOCAR • Center for Microbiology and Cellular Biology, Venezuelan Institute for Scientific Research, Caracas 1010A, Venezuela.

1979). Infection can also occur by blood transfusion, and congenital cases of *T. cruzi* infection have been described (Bittencourt, 1976). These two forms of transmission, together with the migration of infected rural populations to urban areas, have changed the epidemiology of Chagas' disease, which is no longer limited to rural areas.

Upon infection by *T. cruzi,* infected humans undergo a period of incubation characterized by proliferation of amastigotes within the infected cells. This period is asymptomatic and lasts for about 1–3 weeks. During the acute phase, clinical manifestations of Chagas' disease include fever, lymphadenopathy, and hepatosplenomegaly. About 50% of the patients develop unilateral painless periorbital swelling (Romaña's sign). Fewer develop a nodular lesion or chagoma in the skin at the portal of entry. These skin lesions, characterized by mononuclear infiltrates, are not seen in patients who acquire Chagas' disease by transfusion. Some patients present with myocarditis, edema, and meningoencephalitis. After 10 years of the acute phase, signs and symptoms of chronic Chagas' disease may appear in 10% of serologically positive patients. These include cardiomyopathy and enlargement of various organs such as the esophagus, colon, bronchi, stomach, duodenum, and ureter as well as destruction of autonomic ganglia or myositis. During the chronic stage, some patients may also present peripheral polyneuropathy due to generalized neuronal destruction (Spina-Franca and Mattosinho-Franca, 1978; Tafuri, 1979). Experimental Chagas' disease can be induced in animals, where some alterations resemble those observed in infected humans.

Although there is much evidence that *T. cruzi* provokes an immune response in the infected host, there is no evidence for sterilizing immunity against the parasite. The mechanisms that allow *T. cruzi* to escape complete destruction by the immune system are unclear. During the acute phase there are humoral and cellular immune responses against the parasite, which may be responsible for the decreased parasitemia observed after the acute phase in both human and experimental animals. Also, the findings that immunosupression is associated with recrudescent parasitemia in chronically infected patients and experimental animals (Brener and Chiari, 1971; Kohl *et al.,* 1982) strongly suggest that an immune-mediated mechanism may be responsible for the low level of parasitemia observed after the acute phase of Chagas' disease.

It has been postulated that an immunosupressive effect is induced by *T. cruzi* antigens during the acute phase of Chagas' disease at the time when parasitemia reaches the maximum (Corsini *et al.,* 1980; Albright and Albright, 1981; Clayton *et al.,* 1979; Ramos *et al.,* 1978). Paradoxically, the main clinical and pathological alterations observed in the chronic phase of Chagas' disease are seen to have an autoimmune background (Santos-Buch and Texeira, 1974; Cossio *et al.,* 1974; Mosca and Plaja, 1981). These contrasting immunological alterations observed after *T. cruzi* infection present Chagas' disease as an attractive and complex model of host–parasite immunorelationship (For review see Brener, 1980).

Antigenic Makeup of *T. cruzi*

Using agglutination and precipitation tests in agar gel, Nussenszweig, Deane, and Loetzel (1963) established the heterogeneity of populations of cultured forms of *T. cruzi*. As opposed to the salivarian trypanosomes, where antigenic variation occurs (Gray and Luckins, 1976; Vickerman, 1978; Cross *et al.*, 1980), in *T. cruzi* infections this has not yet been shown. *T. cruzi* strains have been separated according to antigenic makeup, but no geographical distribution or particular animal species has been associated with a given antigenic group (Nussenzweig and Goble, 1966).

Immunoelectrophoretic analysis of soluble extract from cultured *T. cruzi* detects at least 30 antigenic fractions by rabbit anti-*T. cruzi* immune serum, with some fractions exhibiting greater antigenicity than others (Afchain *et al.*, 1978). However, when human immune serum is used, a significantly lower number of antigenic determinants are specific for *T. cruzi* (Afchain *et al.*, 1979). Antibodies to specific *T. cruzi* fraction have been detected in experimental animals and in chagasic patients (Afchain *et al.*, 1978, 1979). Surface antigenic determinants common to epimastigote and trypomastigote forms of *T. cruzi* have been identified in the carbohydrate-containing fraction of the parasite obtained by different techniques (Gottlieb, 1977, 1978; Repka *et al.*, 1980).

T. cruzi-derived circulating antigen has been detected in the infected hosts (Gottlieb, 1977; Dzbenski, 1974). The origin of this circulating antigen, as well as its significance in the immunological aspects of Chagas' disease, is unclear. Kidneys of rats chronically infected with *T. cruzi* presented alterations suggesting immunocomplex nephropathy. Although C3B, fibrinogen, and immunoglobulin deposits were found in the mesangial areas and basement membrane, specific antigens were not detected in the kidneys (Castro and Ribeiro Dos Santos, 1977).

2. IMMUNITY TO *T. CRUZI*

2.1. Natural Immunity

Over 100 mammalian species have been reported to be susceptible to infection by *T. cruzi* (Brener, 1973). However, amphibians and birds are refractory to *T. cruzi* infection (Dias, 1944). Kierszenbaum *et al.* (1976) have found chickens' resistance to be a complement-dependent phenomenon, unrelated to antibody or cell-mediated immunity.

Different inbred mice strains have shown differences in natural resistance to *T. cruzi* infection. Animals with low antibody-forming capacity have been found to be more susceptible, as compared to high-responder mice, to infection (Kierszenbaum and Howard, 1976). The age (Culberston and Kessler, 1941) and sex

(Hauschka, 1947) of mice have been found to influence their resistance. It is likely that the immunoresponsiveness related to mice strain is the main factor determining natural resistance to *T. cruzi* infection (Kierszenbaum and Howard, 1976; Pécora and Barcinski, 1979; Nogeira *et al.*, 1980).

2.2. Acquired Immunity

2.2.1. Humoral Immunity

Experimental infection of mice by *T. cruzi* is followed by an increase in the size of spleen and lymph nodes. There are controversies about an absolute increase of immunoglobulin levels during the acute or chronic phase of naturally or laboratory-acquired Chagas' disease in humans (Lelchuck *et al.*, 1970; Vattuone *et al.*, 1973; Hanson *et al.*, 1974; Schmunis *et al.*, 1978). Nevertheless, there is agreement that specific immunoglobulin reactive with *T. cruzi* antigens appears after infection by this parasite in humans and experimental animals. Guerreiro and Machado (1913) detected complement-fixing antibodies in humans with Chagas' disease. Further studies demonstrated the presence of specific antibodies (precipitins and agglutinins) during the acute and chronic phases of Chagas' disease (Muniz and Freitas, 1944; Krettli and Brener, 1976). During the last years, several immunological techniques (immunofluorescence, hemagglutination, ELISA) have been adopted as diagnostic tools for Chagas' disease, based on the presence of anti-*T. cruzi* antibodies in the serum of infected humans and animals (Cerisola, 1970; Kagan, 1974; Voller *et al.*, 1975).

Antiserum from infected or immunized animals has been shown to be able to lyse cultured and blood-forms of *T. cruzi* in complement-dependent reactions (Budzko *et al.*, 1975; Kierszenbaum, 1976). Protection against potentially lethal infections can be obtained in passively immunized animals by the transfer of immune plasma from animals that survived the acute phase of *T. cruzi* infection (Kierszenbaum and Howard, 1976; Krettli and Brener, 1976). Correlation between increased total IgG and decreased circulating and intracellular forms of *T. cruzi* in mice adds support to the role of humoral immunity in protection against *T. cruzi* (Hanson, 1977). The specific role that antibodies play in host resistance to *T. cruzi* needs further study. However, some of the observations mentioned already suggest that immunoglobulins may be important in limiting the parasitemia and the pathological and clinical manifestations that occur during the acute phase of Chagas' disease.

2.2.2. Interferon

Rytel and Marsden (1970) and Sonnenfeld and Kierszenbaum (1981) reported an antiviral factor with interferon-like characteristics in mice infected with

T. cruzi, which reached the peak during the first days postinfection. Schmunis *et al.* (1977) suggested that interferon was produced at the time of cell penetration by the parasite. *In vivo* detection of interferon-like activity has been found only during the acute phase of *T. cruzi* infection in mice (Sonnenfeld and Kierszenbaum, 1981). A protective effect by interferon in the infectious process has been described *in vitro* in *Toxoplasma* (Remington and Merigan, 1968), *Eimeria* (Fayer and Baron, 1971), species and *in vivo* during *Plasmodium berghei* infection in mice (Jachiel *et al.*, 1968). Martínez-Silva *et al.* (1970) observed that in mice treated with the interferon-inducer polyinosinic-polycytidylic acid (poly I-C), the parasitemia and mortality were higher after *T. cruzi* infection than in infected mice untreated with poly I-C. Similar findings were reported by Kumar *et al.* (1971). Recently Kierszenbaum and Sonnenfeld (1982) have shown that *in vivo* administration of interferon in mice is associated with enhancement of host resistance to *T. cruzi* infection. The same authors suggested that the effect of interferon was a direct one on the immune system of the host and had no effect itself on the parasite motility, infectivity, or virulence.

2.2.3. Cell-Mediated Immunity

Although cell-mediated immunity develops in both humans and experimental animals with Chagas' disease (González-Cappa *et al.*, 1968; Seah, 1970; Schmunis *et al.*, 1973; Lelchuck *et al.*, 1974; Splitter *et al.*, 1977), it is not yet clear to what extent it may contribute to host defense against the parasite or to the parasite's pathogenicity. Several *in vitro* tests provide evidence for the existence of cell-mediated immunity. Inhibition by *T. cruzi* antigens of cell migration is exhibited by peripheral leukocytes derived from patients with chronic Chagas' disease (Yanofsky and Albado, 1972; Lelchuck *et al.*, 1974). In experimentally infected mice, inhibition of migration of peritoneal mononuclear cells is also induced by *T. cruzi* antigens (Schmunis *et al.*, 1973).

A comprehensive evaluation of cellular immunity in patients with chronic Chagas' disease has been done by Montufar *et al.* (1977). The percentage and absolute number of peripheral T lymphocytes, the lymphocytes' responsiveness to phytohemagglutinin, and rates of sensitization to chlorodinitrobenzene were similar in patients and controls. However, migration of peripheral leukocytes derived from patients was inhibited by *T. cruzi* antigens. Lelchuck *et al.* (1977), found that, in patients with chronic Chagas' disease who had been treated with nitrofuran, the peripheral leukocyte migration index was similar to that of normal controls (as compared with the migration index of untreated patients with Chagas' disease). Tschudi *et al.* (1972) found that peripheral blood lymphocytes from patients with chronic Chagas' disease responded to specific *T. cruzi* antigens with transformation; this was not observed when lymphocytes from healthy controls were used.

Positive delayed skin reactions elicited by *T. cruzi* antigens have been reported in patients with chronic Chagas' disease (Amato-Neto *et al.*, 1964) and in experimental animals (Seah *et al.*, 1974; Teixeira *et al.*, 1975). Earlier reports of negative delayed skin tests in Chagas' disease reviewed by Goble (1970) may have been associated with the diversity of antigens used. Some *T. cruzi* antigens elicit more intense, delayed-type reactions than others (Teixeira *et al.*, 1975; Zeledon and Ponce, 1974).

Antibody-dependent cell-mediated cytotoxicity (ADCC) has been shown against epimastigote forms of cultured *T. cruzi*. Eosinophils or lymphoid mouse cells have been identified as effector cells in ADCC against *T. cruzi* (Abrahamsohn and Diaz Da Silva, 1977; Sanderson *et al.*, 1977). Antibody-coated trypomastigote forms of *T. cruzi* are susceptible to cytotoxic activity by human lymphoid, neutrophil, and eosinophil cells (Kierszenbaum, 1979). Recently, Rimaldi *et al.* (1981) put forward the suggestion, based on *in vitro* studies, that human polymorphonuclear leukocytes may collaborate in the destruction of epimastigote forms of *T. cruzi* in the presence of specific antiparasite antibodies. Evidence that specific antibodies enhance the ability of macrophages to take up both epimastigote and trypomastigote forms of *T. cruzi* had been presented earlier (Hoff, 1975; Alcantara and Brener, 1978; Sanderson and De Souza, 1979). Reed *et al.* (1982) have demonstrated that although extensive destruction of epimastigote is observed by peritoneal macrophages from normal or previously immunized mice, lysing of trypomastigotes was typically seen only in the presence of both immune macrophages and specific antibodies.

2.2.4. Evaluation of Cell-Mediated Immunity in Resistance to *T. cruzi* Infection

Several cell-mediated reactions have been implicated as effector mechanisms in immunity against *T. cruzi* infection. The participation of macrophage in acquired immunity to acute infections of *T. cruzi* was suggested earlier by Taliaferro and Pizzi (1955), who reported that macrophages in immune animals were more efficient in destroying these parasites than were macrophages in nonimmunized animals. The importance of macrophages in *T. cruzi* infection has long been appreciated and is perhaps the best characterized mechanism concerning killing of epimastigotes and trypomastigotes (Goble and Boyd, 1962; Hoff, 1975; Nogeira and Cohn, 1977). Agents known to be specifically toxic to macrophages, such as silica, have been associated with increased parasitemia and mortality in experimentally infected mice (Tanowitz *et al.*, 1980). In contrast, nonspecific stimulation of the reticuloendothelial system enhances resistance to *T. cruzi* in experimental animals (Brener and Cardozo, 1976; Kierszenbaum and Ferraresi, 1979; Abrahamsohn *et al.*, 1981). Adoptive transfer of protection against *T. cruzi* with lymphocytes and macrophages from syngeneic donors that had recovered from the acute infection by *T. cruzi* has been reported (Burgess and Hanson, 1979).

Previous studies in mice and rats suggest that a regulatory role is exerted by the thymus in the development of immunity during primary infection with *T. cruzi*. The thymic dependence of the primary response to *T. cruzi* has been suggested earlier by Schmunis *et al.* (1971), who reported that neonatal thymectomy of Rockland mice resulted in exacerbations of *T. cruzi* infection, thymectomized animals dying earlier than unoperated controls. Adult thymectomy followed by antithymocyte serum treatment also resulted in high mortalities and parasitemias in mice (Behbehani, 1971). Robertson *et al.* (1973) reported that neonatally thymectomized rats and antithymocyte-serum–treated mice had greater parasitemias than sham operated or normal-serum–treated mice respectively. Trischman *et al.* (1978) found that congenitally athymic ("nude") BALB/c mice suffered high parasitemias and died, while normal littermates frequently survived and had much lower parasitemias. Kierszenbaum and Pienkowski (1979) also reported similar findings. In addition, the same authors found that transplantation of neonatal thymus into athymic mice reestablished normal levels of resistance to *T. cruzi*, comparable to those of normal littermates. Kierszenbaum (1980) reported that congenitally athymic nude mice recipients of immune serum from mice that had recovered from *T. cruzi* infection show lower parasitemia after inoculation with *T. cruzi* as compared with littermate recipients of normal mouse serum. Although significantly delayed, mortality of the athymic mice could not be prevented by the administration of specific antibodies. In previous experiments with the Biozzi antibody–low-responder mice, Liacopapalous-Briot *et al.* (1972) and Kierszenbaum and Howard (1976) reported that passive antibody transfer led to prevention of mortality after *T. cruzi* infection. This comparison between low-responder and athymic mice would support the concept that cellular immunity contributes to host defense against *T. cruzi*.

Recently Burgess and Hanson (1980) reported that exacerbation of *T. cruzi* infections were induced in thymectomized, irradiated, bone marrow-reconstituted (TX) mice as compared with sham thymectomized, irradiated, bone marrow-reconstituted (STX) mice. The same authors reported that reconstitution of TX mice with thymocytes restored the resistance to the level of STX mice. The effects of T-cell depletion on immunological memory to the parasite were also studied by Burgess and Hanson (1980), who reported that immunological memory against *T. cruzi* present in spleen cells in mice recovered from *T. cruzi* infections could be ablated by treatment with rabbit anti-brain-associated theta serum but not with rabbit anti-mouse immunoglobulin serum. Trischman and Bloom (1980) reported the protection of *T. cruzi*-infected mice by passive transfer of T cells as well as T-cell-depleted populations of spleen cells from *T. cruzi*-immunized syngeneic mice.

Although effector mechanisms of T-cell-mediated immunity against *T.*

cruzi are still unclear, thymus-derived lymphocytes could play a crucial role in immunity against parasites in several ways. Direct cellular toxicity against *T. cruzi*-infected cells has been reported in an allogeneic (Santos-Buch and Teixeira, 1974) and syngeneic system (Kuhn and Murnane, 1977), although the specific cytotoxic effector cell was not identified in those studies. T-cell-mediated direct cytotoxicity has already been shown to exist against viral infected (Doherty *et al.*, 1974) and tumor cells (Dennert, 1976). Also, through T-helper-cell activity, T lymphocytes may be necessary for a competent humoral immune response (Aune and Pierce, 1981, 1982). The correlation of high levels of antibodies with higher resistance to *T. cruzi* infection has been shown earlier (Kierszenbaum and Hayes, 1976). Another mechanism by which T lymphocytes may influence the immunoresponse to *T. cruzi* or other parasites may be through the production of soluble mediators. Activation of T lymphocytes by the mitogen concanavalin A induces the production of a soluble factor by T-suppressor cells; this has an inhibiting effect on macrophages, acting through these cells, suppressing primary and secondary humoral immunoresponses (Aune and Pierce, 1981).

A recently described subset of lymphocytes with the ability to recognize and lyse tumorigenic and virus-infected cells without prior sensitization have attracted considerable interest because of their possible roles in host resistance to infection and neoplasia (Herberman and Holden, 1978). Effector cells with these characteristics have been called natural killer (NK) cells. Morphological evidence has associated NK cell activity with large granular lymphocytes in humans (Timonen *et al.*, 1979), rats (Herberman *et al.*, 1980) and mice (Luini *et al.*, 1981). Hatcher and Kuhn (1982) reported that mice infected with *T. cruzi* or uninfected mice stimulated with poly I-C showed enhanced *in vitro* NK activity against epimastigote or trypomastigote forms of *T. cruzi*, as opposed to uninfected, unstimulated controls. No direct relation was found between susceptibility to *T. cruzi* infection and NK activity against the parasite. The actual contribution of NK cells to resistance against *T. cruzi* infection needs further evaluation.

3. IMMUNITY TO *T. CRUZI* AND PATHOGENESIS

3.1. Autoimmunity in *T. cruzi* Infections

Common manifestations during the chronic phase of Chagas' disease include cardiomyopathy, megaesophagus, and megacolon. Infiltration of the heart by lymphoid cells is associated with myofibrillar degradation and fibrosis. Direct evidence of heart muscle cell lysis has been obtained by electron microscopic studies (reviewed by Amorin *et al.*, 1979). An additional pathogenic mechanism involving the destruction of neuronal cells in both the heart and digestive system has been proposed by Koberle (1974), who suggested that the major pathological features associated with cardiopathy and megasyndromes are of neurologic origin and may be initiated by the immune response. Although there is much evidence suggesting that chronic-stage alterations have an immunological basis where immune mechanisms might produce both direct myopathic and neuropathic lesions, the mechanisms by which the autoimmunity is generated and operates are unclear.

The role of humoral immunity during the chronic phase of Chagas' disease is unclear. It has been suggested that during this phase humoral immunity could be responsible at least in part for the pathogenicity of manifest late-stage Chagas' disease. By immunofluorescence techniques, Cossio et al. (1974) have demonstrated immunoglobulins reactive with endocardium, vascular structures, and interstitium of striated muscle (EVI antibody) in the serum of chronically infected patients. EVI antibodies have also been demonstrated in acute and congenital cases of Chagas' disease (Szarfman et al., 1975, 1977). The higher incidence of EVI antibodies in patients with Chagas' cardiomiopathy as compared with asymptomatic patients gives further support to the idea that a humoral autoimmune mechanism operates in the pathogenesis of manifest Chagas' disease (Cossio et al., 1974). The antigenic determinants to which EVI antibodies are directed needs further definition. The possibility that cross-reacting antigens are expressed by T. cruzi and some tissues of the vertebrate host seems likely. Recently, a monoclonal antibody generated against mammalian dorsal root ganglia had specificity for subpopulation of central and peripheral neurons and also recognized an antigenic determinant of T. cruzi. An interesting finding was that all classes of neurons known to undergo degeneration in Chagas' disease expressed the antigenic determinant recognized by the antibody. In addition, the monoclonal antibody was able to react with cardiac but not with skeletal muscle, suggesting that common antigenic determinants are shared by the parasite and affected host cells (Wood et al., 1982).

The presence of antibodies that react against determinants expressed by neurons has been detected previously in patients with Chagas' disease and mice experimentally infected by T. cruzi (Koberle, 1961; Khoury et al., 1979; Ribeiro Dos Santos and Hudson, 1981). Alcantara (1961) and Koberle and Alcantara (1960) have suggested that the intense central and peripheral denervation seen during the acute and chronic phases of Chagas' disease, both in humans and animals, may be responsible for the megasyndromes and cardiopathy observed in Chagas' disease. Since neurons are only rarely parasitized in T. cruzi infections (Koberle and Alcantara, 1960), the possibility that their destruction may be mediated by an autoimmune response has been suggested (Texeira et al., 1975). Ribeiro Dos Santos and Hudson (1981) have demonstrated that parasite antigens can be absorbed into mammalian cells and have suggested that in this way mammalian cells may become targets for the immunoresponse to *T. cruzi*. Khoury *et al.* (1979) have suggested that an antibody against neurons from acute and chronic cases of Chagas' disease recognized reactive antigens located on the Schwann cells. The same authors reported that the antinerve antibody could be absorbed by *T. cruzi* culture forms, suggesting the existence of cross-reacting antigens between *T. cruzi* and nerve tissue.

Direct cytotoxic mechanisms may also contribute in the pathogenicity that characterizes the chronic phase of Chagas' disease. Santos-Buch and Teixeira (1974) described the destruction of allogeneic parasitized and nonparasitized rabbit heart cells *in vitro* by lymphocytes derived from rabbits immunized with *T. cruzi* antigens or chronically infected by *T. cruzi*. Lymphocytes from a chagasic individual that presented a positive macrophage migration inhibition test with heart antigens were able to destroy murine heart cells (Cossio *et al.*, 1976). The destruction of *T. cruzi*-parasitized mouse cells by syngenic spleen cells derived from *T. cruzi*-infected mice was reported by Kuhn and Murnane (1977). However, Hanson (1977), using similar methods, failed to show lymphocyte-mediated cytotoxicity against kidney cells or macrophages infected by *T. cruzi*. Lysis of *T. cruzi*-infected and uninfected human fetal heart cells by lymphocytes from patients with acute or chronic Chagas' disease was also described (Teixeira *et al.*, 1978). The same authors suggested that autoimmune T lymphocytes may be stimulated to aberrant effector functions due to common antigens shared by *T. cruzi* and neuron and heart host cells. Ribeiro Dos Santos and Hudson (1981), using mice experimentally infected by *T. cruzi*, observed a decrease in neuron numbers between days 10 and 20 postinfection, at the time when parasitemia was resolving. They also reported that antineuron or antimuscle immunity—measured by the development of cytotoxic T lymphocytes or inhibition of migration of peritoneal cells (Ribeiro Dos Santos and Hudson, 1980a)—did not develop until after the 20th day postinfection and increased between the 20th and 90th days postinfection, when no additional reduction in neuron number was observed. Using indirect immunofluorescence techniques, Ribeiro Dos Santos and Hudson (1980a, 1980b, 1981) reported that parasite antigens attach to both infected and uninfected mammalian muscle and heart cells but not to erythrocytes or lymphocytes of human origin. The same authors reported that the binding of parasite antigens to cell membranes renders those cells susceptible to lysis by the elements of the anti-*T. cruzi* immune response. Recently, Mosca and Plaja (1981) have reported that lymphocytes from patients with chagasic cardiomyopathy—as opposed to lymphocytes derived from normal donors or patients with nonchagasic heart disease—were highly sensitive to stimulation by rat heart antigens, suggesting the existence of *in vivo* sensitization against heart antigens in patients with cardiomyopathy.

Whether different *T. cruzi* tissue tropism exists in humans has not yet been shown. However, the existence of *T. cruzi* strains that show selective parasitism for different tissues or organs of animal origin (Badinez, 1945) has been demonstrated. It is possible that if *T. cruzi*-selective parasitism for a given tissue exists, this may be a factor determining the pathologic manifestations of the disease. In congenital human Chagas' disease—where the main manifestations are prematurity, low birth weight, hepatosplenomegaly, anemia, jaundice, edema, and petechial and meningoencephalitic signs (Bittencourt, 1976; Szarfman *et al.*, 1975)—parasites are found predominantly in muscle and reticuloendothelial cells (Bittencourt, 1976).

3.2. *T. cruzi*-Induced Immunosuppression

In mammalian hosts infected by parasites, immunologic control mechanisms are thought to contribute to the homeostatic features of many host–parasite relationships (Greenwood, 1974). It has usually been found that parasite-infected hosts exhibit a markedly diminished ability to mount immune responses (Ogilve and Wilson, 1976). During active infection of *T. cruzi* in mice, suppression of the humoral (Clinton *et al.*, 1975; Cunningham *et al.*, 1978) and cellular (Reed *et al.*, 1977; Rowland and Kuhn, 1978) immune responses to heterologous antigens has been observed. The significance of the observed immunosuppression for the development of protective immunity against *T. cruzi* is not known.

Experimental infection of mice with *T. cruzi* is followed by parasitemia, enlargement of lymph nodes and spleens, and immunosuppression (Clinton *et al.*, 1975; Rowland and Kuhn, 1978). O'Daly *et al.* (1984) infected C57BL/6 and C3H/He mice with strain Y of *T. cruzi* and found suppression of humoral immunity to sheep erythrocytes, as determined by hemolytic plaque assay to detect antibody-producing cells during the acute phase of infection. In their study, the time of greater humoral suppression coincided with the time of maximum splenomegaly and parasitemia (about 10–17 days postinfection, Figure 1), and was followed by recovery of humoral immunity during the chronic phase of infection. Cunningham and Kuhn (1978) described decreased humoral response during the acute and chronic phase of *T. cruzi* infection; this is probably related to the stronger parasite inoculum used by the last authors.

Cellular immunity in mice determined *in vitro* by lymphocyte responsiveness to T-dependent and -independent mitogens is also decreased during the acute phase of *T. cruzi* infection (Rowland and Kuhn, 1978; Kierszenbaum and Hayes, 1980); controversy exists about the mechanism and identity of the suppressor cell. Ramos *et al.* (1979) reported that spleen cells from late *T. cruzi*-infected mice inhibited the ability of normal spleen cells to respond to mitogens. The cells mediating immunosuppression were susceptible to treatment with antithymus serum plus complement, suggesting a T-cell origin for the suppressor spleen cells. Reed *et al.* (1977) suggested that parasite-harboring macrophages could present changes in their surface receptor sites, which would interfere with

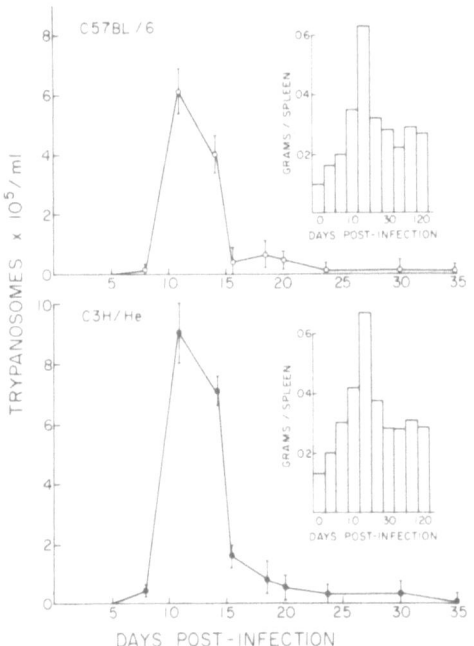

Figure 1. Parasitemia and splenomegaly in *Trypanosoma cruzi* infected mice. C57BL/6 (O——O) and C3H/He (●——●) mice were infected intraperitoneally with 5×10^2 blood-form try-pomastigotes, strain Y of *Trypanosoma cruzi*. Parasitemia and spleen size were determined at different days post-infection. Each value represents the average of three experiments ± S.D.

T-cells and affect their responsiveness. However, macrophages from *T. cruzi*-infected mice show increased phagocytic activity (Clinton *et al.*, 1975). O'Daly *et al.* (1984) found that decreased spleen cell responsiveness to T- and B-cell mitogens was a finding limited to the acute phase of *T. cruzi* infection in mice during the time of maximum parasitemia and splenomegaly. The same authors found that spleen cells with macrophage-like characteristics induced decreased responsiveness to mitogens in spleen cells from normal mice. They reported that while lymphocyte responsiveness was completely recovered by C57BL/6 mice during the chronic infectious phase, the recovery of lymphocyte responsiveness to B-cell mitogens by C3H/He mice, which are more sensitive to *T. cruzi* infection, was only partial (Figure 2).

Humoral immunosuppression during *T. cruzi* infection was described by Cunningham *et al.* (1978). They reported the presence of suppressor substance in the serum of *T. cruzi*-infected mice. The suppressor substance was characterized as having a molecular weight of 196,000–210,000 and sensitivity to trypsin treatment; it was absorbed or inactivated by syngeneic T but not B lymphocytes

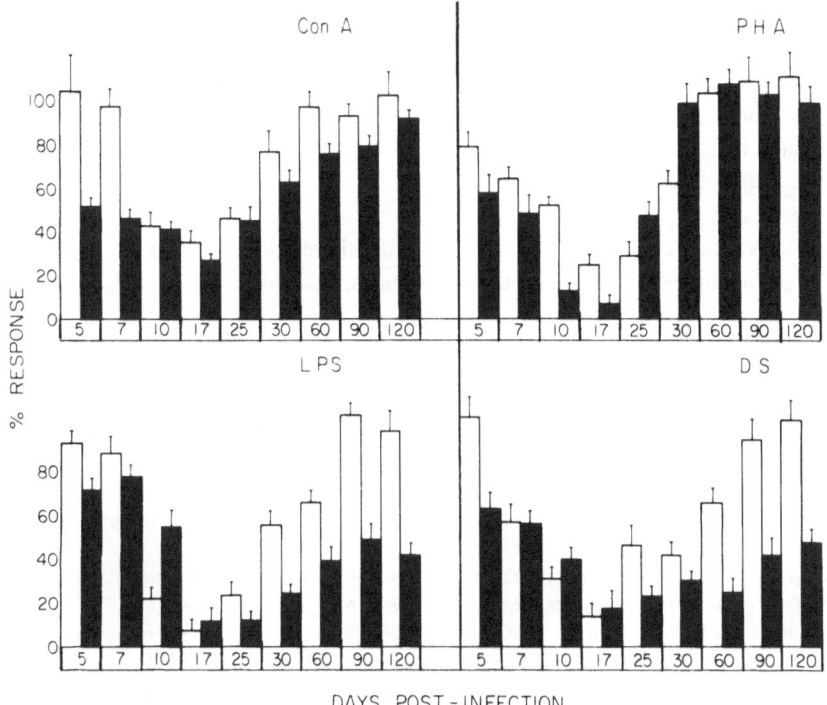

Figure 2. Blastogenic response of splenic cells to Con A, PHA, LPS and DS, determined at different days post-infection in both C57BL/6 (open bars) and C3H/He (filled bars) mice (as indicated in Figure 1). Results are expressed as percent of C.P.M. obtained with uninfected controls. Each value represents the average of three experiments ± S.D.

(Cunningham and Kuhn, 1980a). Further studies by the same authors (1980b) indicated that transfer of decreased responsiveness by the suppressor substance was related to the H-2 haplotype of the recipient mice. Clinton *et al.* (1975) mentioned that interferon, which is produced early during the *T. cruzi* infection, may have an immunosuppressive effect.

In vivo suppression of cell-mediated immunity has also been reported during *T. cruzi* infection. Reed *et al.* (1977) observed decreased skin-test reactivity to BCG protoplasm or oxazolone during the stage of marked parasitemia. Corsini *et al.* (1980), on the other hand, found no impairment of delayed-type hypersensitivity reactions to 2,4-dinitro-1-fluorobenzene. These authors used a smaller parasite inoculum than Reed *et al.* (1977). Allogenic skin-grafting experiments in mice also showed decreased T-cell responsiveness during *T. cruzi* infection; this is consistent with the lack of cytotoxic lymphocytes generated from mixed lymphocyte cultures that contained spleen cells from infected animals (Pearson *et al.*, 1978).

Teixeira *et al.* (1978) studied cell-mediated responsiveness *in vivo* in patients with acute Chagas' disease as determined by delayed-type skin response to *T. cruzi* antigens. Patients with apparent acute Chagas' disease, with symptoms and signals of acute illness, and showed positive responses; patients with asymptomatic acute Chagas' disease were negative for delayed-type skin reactions to the same parasite antigens.

ACKNOWLEDGMENTS. We thank Ms. Miriam Pérez de León and Ms. Amanda Suarez for their excellent secretarial assistance.

REFERENCES

Abrahamsohn, I. A., and Dias Da Silva, W., 1977, Antibody-dependent cell mediated cytotoxicity against *Trypanosoma cruzi*, *J. Parasitol.* 60:1037–1038.

Abrahamsohn, I. A., Blotta, M. H. S. L., and Curotto, M. A., 1981, Enhancement of delayed type hypersensitivity to *Trypanosoma cruzi* in mice treated with mycobacterium bovis B.C.G. and cyclophosphamide, *Infect. Immun.* 31:1145–1151.

Afchain, D., Fruit, J., Yarzabal, L., and Capron, A., 1978, Purification of a specific antigen of *Trypanosoma cruzi* for culture forms, *Am. J. Trop. Med. Hyg.* 27:478–482.

Afchain, D., Le Ray, D., Fruit, J., and Capron, A., 1979, Antigenic make-up of *Trypanosoma cruzi* culture forma: Identification of a specific component, *J. Parasitol.* 65:507–514.

Albright, J. W., and Albright, J. F., 1981, Inhibition of murine humoral immune response by substances derived from trypanosomes. *J. Immunol.* 126:300–303.

Alcantara, F. G., 1961, Sistema neurovegetativo do coracao na molestia de Chagas experimental, *Rev. Goiana Med.* 7:111–115.

Alcantara, H., and Brener, Z., 1978, The *in vitro* interaction of *Trypanosoma cruzi* blood stream forms and mouse peritoneal macrophages, *Acta Trop.* 35:209–219.

Amato-Neto, V., Magaldi, C., and Pessoa, S. B., 1964, Intradermorreacao para o diagnostico da doenca de Chagas' con antigeno de *Trypanosoma cruzi* obtenido de cultura de tecido, *Rev. Gioana Med.* 10:121–126.

Amorin, D. S., Mango, J. C., Gallo, L., and Neto J. A. M., 1979, Forma crónica cardiaca, in: *Trypanosoma cruzi e doenca de Chagas* (Z. Brener and Z. A. Andrade eds.), R. Guana Bara Koogan, Rio de Janeiro.

Aune, T. M., and Pierce, C. W., 1981, Monoclonal soluble immune response suppressor derived from T cell hybridomas, in: *Monoclonal Antibodies and T Cell Hybridomas* (G. J. Nammerling and J. Kearney, eds.), Elsevier, New York, pp. 516–530.

Aune, T. M., and Pierce C. W., 1982, Activation of a suppressor T cell pathway by interferon, *Proc. Nat. Acad. Sci. U.S.A.* 79:3808–3812.

Badinez, O. S., 1945, Contribución a la anatomía patológica de la enfermedad de Chagas, *Biología* 3:3–52.

Barreto, M. P., 1979, *Trypanosoma cruzi* e doenca de Chagas, in: *Epidemiología* (Z. Brener and Z. Andrade, eds.), Editora Guanabara, Rio de Janeiro, Brazil.

Behbehani, M. K., 1971, *Trypanosoma* (Schizotrypanum) *cruzi* infections in x-irradiated and in thymectomized mice, *Trans. Roy. Soc. Trop. Med. Hyg.* 65:265.

Bittencourt, A. L., 1976, Congenital Chagas' disease, *Am. J. Dis. Child.* 130:97–103.

Brener, Z., 1971, Life cycle of *Trypanosoma cruzi, Rev. Inst. Med. Trop. Sao Paulo* 13:171–178.

Brener, Z., 1973, Biology of *Trypanosoma cruzi, Annu. Rev. Microbiol.* 27:347–383.

Brener, Z., 1980, Immunity to *Trypanosoma cruzi*. *Adv. Parasitol.* 18:247–298.

Brener, A., and Cardozo, J. E., 1976, Nonspecific resistance against *Trypanosoma cruzi* enhanced by *Corynebacterium parvum, J. Parasitol.* 62:645–646.

Brener, Z., and Chiari, E., 1971, The effects of some immunosuppressive agents in experimental Chagas' disease, *Trans. Roy. Soc. Trop. Med. Hyg.* 65:629–636.

Budzko, D. B., Pizzimenti, M. C., and Kierszenbaum, F., 1975, Effects of complement depletion in experimental Chagas' disease: Immunoanalysis of virulent blood forms of *Trypanosoma cruzi, Infect. Immun.* 11:86–91.

Burgess, D. E., and Hanson, W., 1979, Adoptive transfer of protection against *Trypanosoma cruzi* with lymphocytes and macrophages, *Infect. Immun.* 25:838–843.

Burgess, D. E., and Hanson, W. L., 1980, *Trypanosoma cruzi:* The T-cell dependence of the primary immune response and the effects of depletion of T cells and Ig-bearing cells on immunological memory, *Cell. Immunol.* 52:176–186.

Castro, A. C. L., and Ribeiro Dos Santos, R., 1977, Immunopatología do rim na forma cronica da molestia de Chagas experimental. *Rev. Goiana Med.* 23:1–13.

Cerisola, J. A., 1970, Immunodiagnosis of Chagas' disease: Hemagglutination and immunofluorescence test, *J. Parasitol.* 56:409–410.

Chagas, C., 1909, Neve Trypanosomen, *Arch. Schiff Tropenhyg.* 13:120–122.

Chagas, C., 1911, Nova entidade morbida do homen resumo feral do Estudos etiológicos e clinicos, *Memórias do Instituto Oswaldo do Cruz* 3:219–275.

Clayton, C. E., Sacks, D. L., Ogilvie, B. M., and Askonas, B. A., 1979, Membrane fractions of trypanosomas mimic the immunosuppressive and mitogenic effects of living parasites on the host, *Parasitol. Immunol.* 1:241–249.

Clinton, B. A., Ortiz-Ortiz, L., García, W., Martínez, T., and Capin, R., 1975, *Trypanosoma cruzi:* Early immune response in infected mice, *Exp. Parasitol.* 37:417–425.

Corsini, A. C., Costa, M. G., Oliveira, O. L. P., Camargo, I. I. B., and Rangel, H. A., 1980, A fraction (F.A.d.) from *Trypanosoma cruzi* epimastigotes depresses the immunoresponse in mice, *Immunology* 4O:505–511.

Cossio, P. M., Diaz, C., Szarfman, A., Krentzen, E., Candiolo, B., and Arana, R. M., 1974, Chagasic cardiopathy, demonstration of a serum gamma globulin factor which reacts with endocardium in vascular structures, *Circulation* 49:13–21.

Cross, G. A. M., Holder, A. A., Gleen, G., and Boothroyd, J. C., 1980, An introduction to antigenic variation in trypanosomes, *Am. J. Trop. Med. Hyg.* 29:1027–1032.

Culbertson, J. T., and Kessler, W. R., 1941, Age resistance of mice to *Trypanosoma cruzi, J. Parasitol.* 28:155–158.

Cunningham, D. S., and Kuhn, R. E., 1980a, *Trypanosoma cruzi* induced suppressor substance: I. Cellular involvement and partial characterization, *J. Immunol.* 124:2122–2129.

Cunningham, D. S., and Kuhn, R. E., 1980b, *Trypanosoma cruzi* induced suppressor substance: II. Regulatory activity, *Immunogenetics* 10:557–571.

Cunningham, D. S., Kuhn, R. E., and Rowland, E. C., 1978, Suppression of humoral response during *Trypanosoma cruzi* infections in mice, *Infect. Immun.* 22:155–160.

Dennert, G., 1976, Thymus derived killer cells: Specificity of function and antigen recognition. *Transplant. Rev.* 29:59–124.

Dias, E., 1944, Nao receptividade do pombo domestico a infeccao por Schiotrypanum, *Memorias do Instituto Oswaldo Cruz* 40:191–193.

Doherty, P. C., Zinkernagel, R. M., and Ramshaw, I. A., 1974, Specificity and development of cytotoxic thymus-derived lymphocytes in lymphocytic choriomeningitis, *J. Immunol.* 112:1548–1552.

Dzbenski, T. H., 1974, Exoantigens of *Trypanosoma cruzi in vivo, Tropenmed. Parasitol.* 25:485–491.

Fayer, R., and Baron, S., 1971, Activity of interferon and inducer against development of *Eimeri tenella*, *J. Protozool.* 18:12–17.

Goble, F. C., 1970, South American trypanosomisis, in: *Immunity to Parasitic Animals* (G. J. Jackson, R. Herman, and I. Singer, eds.), Appleton-Century-Crofts, New York, pp. 597–689.

Goble, F. C., and Boyd, J. L., 1962, Reticuloendothelial blockade in experimental Chagas' disease, *J. Parasitol.* 48:223–228.

González-Cappa, S. M., Schmunis, G. A., Traversa, O. C., Yousky, J. F., and Parodi, A. S., 1968, Complement fixation tests, skin tests and experimental immunization with antigens of *Trypanosoma cruzi* prepared under pressure, *Am. J. Trop. Med. Hyg.* 17:709–715.

Gottlieb, M., 1977, A carbohydrate-containing antigen from *Trypanosoma cruzi* and its detection in the circulation of infected mice, *J. Immunol.* 119:465–470.

Gottlieb, M., 1978, *Trypanosoma cruzi:* Identification of a cell surface polysaccharide, *Exp. Parasitol.* 45:183–189.

Gray, A. R., and Luckins, A. G., 1976, Antigenic variation in salivarian trypanosomes, in: *Biology of the Kinetoplastida* (W. A. R. Lumsden and D. A. Evans, eds.), Academic Press, London, pp. 493–542.

Greenwood, B. M., 1974, Immunosuppression in malaria and trypanosomiasis, in: *Parasites in the Immunized Host: Mechanisms of Survival*, Ciba Foundation Symposium (new series) 25.

Guerreiro, C., and Machado, A., 1913, Da reacao de Bordet e Gengouna molestia de Carlos Chagas como elemento de diagnostico, *Brasil Medico* 27:225–226.

Hanson, W. L., 1977, Immune response and mechanisms of resistance in *Trypanosoma cruzi*, *Pan Am. Health Org. Sci. Pub.* 347:22–34.

Hanson, W. L., Devli, R. F., and Robertson, E. L., 1974, Immunoglobulin levels in a laboratory acquired case of human Chagas' disease, *J. Parasitol.* 60:532–533.

Hatcher, F. M., and Kuhn, R. E., 1982, Destruction of *Trypanosoma cruzi* by natural killer cells, *Science* 218:295–296.

Hauschka, T. S., 1947, Sex of host as a factor in Chagas' disease, *J. Parasitol.* 33:339–404.

Herberman, R. B., and Holden, T. H., 1978, Natural cell-mediated immunity, in: *Advances in Cancer Research, Vol. 27* (G. Klein and S. Weinhouse, eds.), Academic Press, New York, pp. 305–377.

Herberman, R. B., Timonen, T., Reynolds, C., and Ortaldo, J. R., 1980, in: *Natural Cell-Mediated Immunity against Tumors* (R. B. Herberman, ed.), Academic Press, New York.

Hoare, G. A., 1972, *The Trypanosomes of Mammals: A Zoological Monograph*, Blackwell Scientific Publications, Oxford, England.

Hoff, B., 1975, Killing *in vitro* of *Trypanosoma cruzi* by macrophages from mice immunized with *T. cruzi* or BCG and absence of cross-immunity on challenge *in vivo*, *J. Exp. Med.* 142:299–311.

Jachiel, R. I., Nussenzweigh, R., Vilcek, J., and Vanderberg, J., 1968, Protective effect of interferon inducers on *Plasmodium berghei* malaria, *Am. J. Trop. Med. Hyg.* 18:823–835.

Kagan, I. G., 1974, Advances in the immunodiagnosis of parasitic infections, *Z. Parasitenkd.* 45:163–195.

Khoury, E. L., Ritacco, V., Cossio, P. M., Laguens, R. P., Szarfman, A., Dez, C., and Arana, R. M., 1979, Circulating antibodies to peripheral nerve in American trypanosomiasis (Chagas' disease), *Clin. Exp. Immunol.* 36:8–15.

Kierszenbaum, F., 1976, Cross-reactivity of lytic antibodies against blood forms of *Trypanosoma cruzi*, *J. Parasitol.* 62:134–135.

Kierszenbaum, F., 1979, Antibody-dependent killing of blood stream forms of *Trypanosoma cruzi* by human blood leukocytes, *Am. J. Trop. Med. Hyg.* 28:968–973.

Kierszenbaum, F., 1980, Protection of congenitally athymic mice against *Trypanosoma cruzi* infection by passive antibody transfer, *J. Parasitol.* 66:673–675.

Kierszenbaum, F., and Ferraresi, R. W., 1979, Enhancement of host resistance against *Trypanosoma cruzi* infection by the immunoregulatory agent muramyl dipeptide. *Infect. Immun.* 25:273–278.

Kierszenbaum, F., and Hayes, M. M., 1980, Evaluation of lymphocyte responsiveness to polyclonal activators during acute and chronic experimental *Trypanosoma cruzi* infection, *Am. J. Trop. Med. Hyg.* 29:708–710.

Kierszenbaum, F., and Howard, J. G., 1976, Mechanisms of resistance against experimental *Trypanosoma cruzi* infection: The importance of antibodies and antibody forming capacity in the Biozzi high and low response mice, *J. Immunol.* 116:1208–1211.

Kierszenbaum, F., and Pienkowski, M. M. 1979, Thymus-dependent control to the host defense mechanism against *Trypanosoma cruzi* infection, *Infect. Immun.* 24:117–120.

Kierszenbaum, F., and Sonnenfeld, G., 1982, Characterization of the antiviral activity produced during *Trypanosoma cruzi* infection and protective effects of exogenous interferon against experimental Chagas' disease, *J. Parasitol.* 68:194–198.

Kierszenbaum, F., Ivann, J., and Budzco, D. B., 1976, Mechanisms of natural resistance to trypanosomal infection: Role of complement in avian resistance to *Trypanosoma cruzi* infection, *Immunology* 30:1–6.

Kumar, R., Worthington, M., Tilles, J. G., and Abelmann, W. A., 1971, Effect of the interferon inducer polynosinic-polycytidylic acid on experimental *Trypanosoma cruzi* infection, *Proc. Soc. Exp. Biol. Med.* 137:884–888.

Koberle, F., 1961, Patología y anatomía patológica de la enfermedad de Chagas, *Boletin de la Oficina Sanitaria Panamericana* 51:404–428.

Koberle, F., 1974, Pathogenesis of Chagas' disease, in: *Trypanosomiasis and Leishmaniasis with Special Reference to Chagas' Disease*, Ciba Foundation Symposium (new series) 20.

Koberle, F., and Alcantara, F. G., 1960, Mecanismo da destruiao neuronal do sistema nervoso periferico na moslestia de Chagas, *Hospital (Rio de Janeiro)* 57:1057–1062.

Kohl, S., Pickering, L. K., Frankel, L. S., and Yagar, R. G., 1982, Reactivation of Chagas' disease during therapy of acute lymphocytic leukemia, *Cancer* 50:827–828.

Krettli, A. U., and Brener, Z., 1976, Protective effects of specific antibodies in *Trypanosoma cruzi* infections, *J. Immunol.* 116:755–760.

Kuhn, R. E., and Murnane, J. E., 1977, Trypanosoma cruzi: Immune destruction of parasited mouse fibroblasts in vivo, *Exp. Parasitol.* 41:66–73.

Lelchuck, R., Dalmasso, A. P., Inglesini, C. L., Alvarez, M., and Cerisola, J. A., 1970, Immunoglobulin studies of patients with American trypanosomiasis (Chagas' disease), *Clin. Exp. Immunol.* 6:547–555.

Lelchuck, R., Patrucco, A., and Manni, J. A., 1974, Studies of cellular immunity in Chagas' disease: Effect of glutaraldehyde-treated specific antigen on inhibition of leukocyte migration, *J. Immunol.* 112:1578–1581.

Lelchuck, R., Cardoni, R. L., and Fuks, A. S., 1977, Cell-mediated immunity in Chagas' disease: Alterations induced by treatment with a trypanocidal drug (nifurtimox), *Clin. Exp. Immunol.* 110:959–967.

Liacopapoulos-Briot, M., Biouthillier, Y., Mouton, D., Decreuscfond, C., Lambert, F., Stiffel, C., and Biozzi, G., 1972, Comparison of skin allograft rejection and cytotoxic antibody production in two lines of mice genetically selected for high and low humoral antibody synthesis, *Transplantation* 14:590–596.

Luini, W., Boraschi, D., Alberti, S., Aleotti, A., and Tagliaboe, A., 1981, Morphological characterization of a cell population responsible for natural killer activity, *Immunology* 43:663–668.

Martínez-Silva, R., López, V. A., and Chiriboga, J., 1970, Effect of poly I-C on the course of infection with *Trypanosoma cruzi*, *Proc. Soc. Exp. Biol. Med.* 134:885–888.

Montufar, O. M. B., Musatti, C. C., Mendes, E., and Mendes, N. F., 1977, Cellular immunity in chronic Chagas' disease, *J. Clin. Microbiol.* 5:401–404.

Mosca, W., and Plaja, J., 1981, Delayed hypersensitivity to heart antigens in Chagas' disease as measured by *in vitro* lymphocyte stimulation, *J. Clin. Microbiol.* 14:1–5.

Muniz, J., and Freitas, G., 1944, Contribucao para o diagnostico da doenca de Chagas pelas reacoes de imunidade: I. Estudio comparativo entre as recoes de aglutinacao e de fixacao de complemento, *Memorias do Instituto Oswaldo Cruz* 41:303-333.

Nogeira, N., and Cohn, Z., 1977, *Trypanosoma cruzi:* Modification of macrophage functions during infection, *J. Exp. Med.* 146:157-170.

Nogeira, N., Ellis, J., Chaplan, S., and Cohn, Z., 1980, *Trypanosoma cruzi: In vivo* and *in vitro* correlation between T-cell activation and susceptibility in inbred strains of mice. *Exp. Parasitol.* 51:325-334.

Nussenzweig, V., Deane, L. M., and Loetzel, J., 1963, Differences in antigenic constitution of strains of *Trypanosoma cruzi, Exp. Parasitol.* 14:221-232.

Nussenzweig, V., and Goble, F. C., 1966, Further studies on the antigenic constitution of strains of *Trypanosoma* (Schizotrypanum) *cruzi, Exp. Parasitol.* 18:224-230.

O'Daly, J. A., Simonis, S., De Rolo, N., and Caballero, H., 1984, Suppression of humoral immunity and lymphocyte responsiveness during experimental *Trypanosoma cruzi* infections, *Rev. Inst. Med. Trop. Sao Paulo* (in press).

Ogilve, B. M., and Wilson, R. J. M., 1976, Evasion of the immune response by parasites, *Br. Med. Bull.* 32:177-184.

Pearson, T. W., Roelands, G. E., Lundin, L. B., and Mayor-Withey, K. S., 1978, Immune depression in Trypanosome-infected mice: I. Depressed T. lymphocyte responses, *Eur. J. Immunol.* 8:723-727.

Pécora, I. L., and Barcinski, M. A., 1979, Genetic control of the mechanisms of resistance against experimental *Trypanosoma cruzi* Infection: I. role of the macrophages in resistance and susceptible strains of mice, *Rev. Brasil Biol.* 39:445-450.

Ramos, C., Lomoyi, E., Feoli, M., Rodríguez, M., Pérez, M., and Ortiz-Ortiz, L., 1978, *Trypanosoma cruzi:* Immunosuppressed response to different antigens in the infected mouse, *Exp. Parasitol.* 45:190-199.

Ramos, C. I., Schadtler-Siwon, I., and Ortiz-Ortiz, L., 1979, Suppressor cells present in the spleens of *Trypanosoma cruzi* infected mice, *J. Immunol.* 122:1243-1247.

Reed, S. G., Larson, C. L., and Speer, C. A., 1977, Suppression of cell mediated immunity in experimental Chagas' disease, *Z. Parasitend.* 52:11-17.

Reed, S. G., Douglas, T. G., and Speer, C. A., 1982, Surface interactions between macrophages and *Trypanosoma cruzi, Am. J. Trop. Med. Hyg.* 31:723-729.

Remington, J. S., and Meringan, T. C., 1968, Interferon: Protection of cells infected with an intracellular protozoan (*Toxoplasma gondi*). *Science* 161:804-806.

Repka, D., Camargo, I. J. B., Santana, E. M., Cunha, W. M., De Souza, O. C., Sakurada, J. K., and Rangel, H. A., 1980, Surface antigenic determinant of epimastigote forms common to trypomastigote and amastigote forms of different strains of *Trypanosoma cruzi. Tropenmed. Parasitol.* 31:239-246.

Ribeiro Dos Santos, R., and Hudson, L., 1980a, *Trypanosoma cruzi:* Immunological consequences of parasite modification of host cells, *Clin. Exp. Immunol.* 40:36-42.

Ribeiro Dos Santos, R., and Hudson, L., 1980b, *Trypanosoma cruzi:* Binding of parasite antigen to mammalian cells in culture. *Parasit. Immunol.* 2:1-7.

Ribeiro Dos Santos, R., and Hudson, L., 1981, Denervation and the immune response in mice infected with *Trypanosoma cruzi. Clin. Exp. Immunol.* 44:349-354.

Rimaldi, M. T., Olabuenga, S. E., and Bracco, M. M. De E., 1981, Phagocytosis of *Trypanosoma cruzi* by human polymorphonuclear leukocytes. *J. Protozool.* 28:351-354.

Robertson, E. L., Hanson, W. L., and Chapman, W. L., 1973, *Trypanosoma cruzi:* Effects of antithymocyte serum in mice and neonatal thymectomy in rats, *Exp. Parasitol.* 34:168-180.

Rowland, E. C., and Kunn, R. E., 1978, Suppression of anamnestic cellular response during experimental American trypanosomiasis, *J. Parasitol.* 64:741-742.

Rytel, M. W., and Marsden, P. D., 1970, Induction of an interferon-like inhibitor by *Trypanosoma cruzi* infection in mice, *Am. J. Trop. Med. Hyg.* 19:929–931.

Sanderson, C. J., and De Souza, W., 1979, A morphological study of the interaction between *Trypanosoma cruzi* and rat eosinophils, neutrophils and macrophages in vitro, *J. Cell. Sci.* 37:275–286.

Sanderson, C. J., Lopez, A. F., and Moreno, M. M. B., 1977, Eosinophils and not lymphoid K cells kill *Trypanosoma cruzi* epimastigote, *Nature* 268:340–341.

Santos-Buch, C. A., and Texeira, A. R. L., 1974, The immunology of experimental Chagas' disease: III. Rejection of allogeneic heart cells in vitro, *J. Exp. Med.* 140:38–53.

Schmunis, G. A., González-Cappra, S. M., Traversa, O. C., and Janousky, J. F., 1971, The effect of immuno-depression due to neonatal thymectomy on infections. *Trans. Roy. Soc. Trop. Med. Hyg.* 68:338–342.

Schmunis, G. A., Vattuone, H., Szarfman, A., and Pesce, U. J., 1973, Cell mediated immunity in mice inoculated with epimastigote or trypomastigote of *Trypanosoma cruzi, Tropenmed. Parasitol.* 24:81–85.

Schmunis, G. A., Baron, S., Gonzalez-Cappa, S., and Weissenbacher, M. C., 1977, El *trypanosoma cruzi* como inductor de interferon, *Medicina* 37:429–430.

Schmunis, G. A., Szarfman, A., Coanasa, L., and Vainstok, C., 1978, Immunoglobulin concentration in treated human acute Chagas' disease, *Ann. J. Trop. Med. Hyg.* 27:473–477.

Seah, S., 1970, Delayed hypersensitivity in *Trypanosoma cruzi* infection, *Nature* 225:1256–1257.

Seah, S., Marsden, P. V., Voller, A., and Pettit, L. E., 1974, Experimental *Trypanosoma cruzi* infection in rhesus monkeys—the acute phase, *Trans. Roy. Soc. Trop. Med. Hyg.* 27:473–477.

Sonnenfeld, G., and Kierszenbaum, F., 1981, Increased serum levels of an interferon-like activity during the acute period of experimental infection with different strains of *Trypanosoma cruzi, Am. J. Trop. Med. Hyg.* 30:1189–1191.

Spina-Franca, A., and Mattosinho-Franca, L. C., 1978, American trypanosomiasis (Chagas' disease), in: *Handbook of Clinical Neurology* (P. Virken and J. Bruyn eds.), Elsevier North Holland, Amsterdam.

Splitter, G. A., McGuire, T. C., and Davis, W. C., 1977, The differentiation of bone marrow cells to functional T-lymphocytes following implantation of thymus graft and thymic stroma in nude and ATxBM mice, *Cell. Immunol.* 34:93–103.

Szarfman, A., Cossio, P. M., Arana, R. M., Urman, J., Kreutzer, E., Laguens, R. P., Segal, A., and Coarasa, L., 1975, Immunologic and immunopathological studies in congenital Chagas' disease, *Clin. Immunol. Immunopathol.* 4:489–499.

Szarfman, A., Cossio, P. M., Schmunis, G. A., and Arana, R. M., 1977, The EVI antibody in acute Chagas' disease, *J. Parasitol.* 63:149–151.

Tafuri, W. L., 1979, Pathogenesis of *Trypanosoma cruzi* infections, in: *Biology of the Kinetoplastida* (W. H. R. Lumsden and D. A. Evans, eds.), Academic Press, London.

Taliaferro, W. H., and Pizzi, T., 1955, Connective tissue reactions in normal and immunized mice to a reticulotropic strain of *Trypanosoma cruzi, J. Infect. Dis.* 96:199–226.

Tanowitz, H. B., Rager-Zisman, B., and Wittner, M., 1980, The effect of silica on resistance to the "Brazil" strain of *Trypanosoma cruzi* in C57BL/6 (B10) mice, *Trans. Roy. Soc. Trop. Med. Hyg.* 74:820–822.

Teixeira, A. R. L., Teixeira, M. L., and Santos-Buch, C. A., 1975, The immunology of experimental Chagas' disease: IV. Production of lesions in rabbits similar to those of chronic Chagas' disease in man, *Am. J. Pathol.* 80:163–168.

Teixeira, A. R. L., Teixeira, G., Macedo, V., and Prata, A., 1978, *Trypanosoma cruzi*-sensitized T-lymphocyte mediated ^{51}Cr release from human heart cells in Chagas' disease, *Am. J. Trop. Med. Hyg.* 27:1097–1108.

Timonen, T., Saksela, E., Ranki, A., and Hayri, P., 1979, Fractionation morphological and functional characterization of effector cells responsible for human natural killer activity against cell-line targets, *Cell. Immunol.* 48:133–148.

Trischman, T. M., and Bloom, B. R., 1980, *Trypanosoma cruzi:* Ability of T-cell-enriched and -depleted lymphocyte populations to passively protect mice, *Exp. Parasitol.* 49:225–232.

Trischmann, T., Tanowitz, H., Wittner, M., and Bloom, B., 1978, *Trypanosoma cruzi:* Role of the immune response in the natural resistance of inbred strains of mice, *Exp. Parasitol.* 45:160–168.

Tschudi, E. I., Anziano, D. F., and Dalmasso, A. P., 1972, Lymphocyte transformation in Chagas' disease, *Infect. Immun.* 6:905–908.

Vattuone, N. H., Szarfman, A., and González-Cappa, S. M., 1973, Antibody response and immunoglobulin levels in humans with acute or chronic *Trypanosoma cruzi* infections (Chagas' disease), *Am. J. Trop. Med. Hyg.* 76:45–47.

Vickerman, K., 1978, Antigenic variation in trypanosomes, *Nature* 273:613–617.

Voller, A., Draper, C. C., Bidwell, D. E., and Bartlett, A., 1975, Microplate enzyme-linked immunoabsorbent assay for Chagas' disease, *Lancet* 1:426–428.

Wood, J. N., Hudson, L., Jessell, T. M., and Yamamoto, M., 1982, A monoclonal antibody defining antigenic determinants on subpopulations of mammalian neurones and *Trypanosoma cruzi* parasites, *Nature* 296:34–37.

Yanofsky, J. F., and Albado, E., 1972, Humoral and cellular responses to *Trypanosoma cruzi,* *Infect. Immunol.* 109:1159–1161.

Zeledon, R., 1977, Epidemiology, modes of transmission and reservoir host of Chagas' disease, in: *Trypanosomiasis and Leishmaniasis with Special Reference to Chagas' Disease,* Vol. 20, Ciba Foundation Associated Scientific Publishers, Basel, pp. 51–62.

Zeledon, N., and Ponce, C., 1974, A skin test for diagnosis of Chagas' disease, *Trans. Roy. Soc. Trop. Med. Hyg.* 68:414–415.

8

Immunity to Helminths and Prospects for Control

Derek Wakelin

1. INTRODUCTION

The helminths—that is, the parasitic worms belonging to the Platyhelminthes and Nematoda—collectively constitute one of the major causes of morbidity and mortality in man and his domestic animals. The prevalence of infection is, to a great extent, determined by climatic conditions and by standards of hygiene and sanitation; together, these influence the availability of vectors (where required), the survival of infective stages, and the ease of transmission. The impact of infections upon the health of the population is, in turn, determined by nutritional levels and by the presence of intercurrent infections. For all these reasons helminth infections are commonest and most serious in tropical and subtropical regions of the world, although some are widespread also in temperate regions and may be a source of major economic loss in domestic stock.

Three major groups of helminth parasites affecting man can be identified: the schistosomes, the filarial nematodes (both designated as target diseases in the UNDP/World Bank/WHO Special Programme), and the gastrointestinal nematodes. Other helminths, though they may cause serious local problems (e.g., lung and liver flukes, larval tapeworms, *Trichinella,* Guinea worm, and visceral larval migrans), are of lesser global significance and space does not permit any detailed treatment here. Accurate figures for the prevalence of the major infections are, of course, impossible to obtain, but the estimates quoted below (taken from Peters and Gilles, 1977) give some idea of the scale of the problem.

Derek Wakelin • Department of Zoology, University of Nottingham, Nottingham NG7 2RD, England.

Schistosomes, the blood flukes, are estimated to infect some 300 million people. The adult parasites live within veins around the intestine or bladder and may survive for several years. The females release eggs into the small capillaries; thus transmission depends upon passage of the eggs through the walls of the organ concerned and their release from the body in feces or urine (Figure 1a). Eggs hatch rapidly once in contact with fresh water and the released miracidium has a short period in which to contact and penetrate a suitable snail intermediate host. Once this is achieved the larval parasite undergoes prolonged asexual reproduction and development so that infected snails may release large numbers of the infective cercarial stages over prolonged periods. Infection occurs when the cercaria, which remain viable in water for only 24 hr or so, come into contact with the skin of a suitable host, penetrate into the dermis and commence the migration that ultimately takes them as adult worms into veins around the intestine and bladder. Three species of the genus *Schistosoma* are responsible for the major foci of infection in man, namely *Schistosoma mansoni* and *Schistosoma haematobium* in Africa, South and Central America, and *Schistosoma japonicum* in Asia. In all, the major causes of disease are the pathophysiological effects arising from tissue hypersensitivity reactions to the eggs.

Filarial nematodes, all of which are transmitted to man by arthropod vectors, are estimated to infect some 300 million people. A number of species, notably *Wuchereria bancrofti* and *Brugia malayi,* invade the lymphatic system; *Onchocerca volvulus* lives within dermal tissues. The adults of all filariids are long, slender worms capable of surviving for many years; the females liberate vast numbers of live microfilaria larvae (Figure 1b). In the lymphatic species, the microfilaria circulate around the body in the blood, from which they are taken up by blood-feeding mosquitoes. In *Onchocerca,* the microfilaria migrate away from the subcutaneous nodules, in which the adults live, and move in the dermal tissues. For this species the vectors are the blood pool feeding *Simulium* flies. In both cases the larval nematodes undergo developmental stages in the vector, the infective stages being once more introduced into the mammalian host when infected vectors feed. Lymphatic filariasis is characterized by inflammatory reactions and by pathological changes in the parasitized tissues, sometimes extending to involve extremities of the body, as in elephantiasis. Onchocerciasis causes severe dermal pathology, probably as a result of chronic hypersensitivity responses to the microfilaria, but may also involved the eye and lead to blindness.

Despite the very large numbers of people infected with schistosomes or with filariids, it is probable that, because of the widespread occurrence of multiple infections, there is a considerably greater total number of infections with gastrointestinal nematodes, perhaps in excess of 1000 million. There are several species that parasitize the intestine, but four in particular are responsible for the majority of recorded infections: *Ascaris lumbricoides, Trichuris trichiura,* and the hookworms *Ancylostoma duodenale* and *Necator americanus.* To these may be added *Strongyloides stercoralis* and the pinworm *Enterobius vermicularis,* although the latter is reputedly commoner in temperate than in tropical regions.

Unlike the filariids, these nematodes do not require vectors and their transmission is effected either by direct larval penetration of skin or mucous membranes (hookworms, *Strongyloides*) or by accidental ingestion of infective eggs (Figures 1c and 1d). The group as a whole is designated the "soil-transmitted helminths," and their high prevalence reflects the ease with which transmission occurs when the climate favors survival of the infective stages and socioeconomic conditions discourage adequate standards of hygiene and sanitation.

The gastrointestinal worms are associated with chronic and insidious disease rather than with acute symptoms. They may cause a variety of nutritional and intestinal disturbances; hookworms may, in addition, through their blood-feeding activities, be associated with blood loss and anemia. *Ascaris*, hookworms and *Strongyloides* undertake extensive parenteral migrations before maturing in the small intestine, and infections are commonly associated with hypersensitivity responses.

Present strategies for controlling helminth infections in man rely on treatment of infected individuals by chemotherapy and on breaking transmission cycles by vector control, improvement of sanitation and hygiene, and health-education programs. Immunoprophylaxis is not yet a practical proposition for man, though it is the goal of much current research and would have many advantages. This chapter will review current knowledge of immunity and immune responses to helminth parasites and consider present and future prospects of immunologically based methods for controlling these widespread and important infectious organisms. In a review of this kind, the choice of topic areas and the depth of treatment is necessarily limited; the reader is therefore referred to the following articles for more extended accounts of both general and specific aspects of immunity to helminths:

1. *General Reviews:* Mitchell (1979a); Mansfield (1981); Cohen and Warren (1982).
2. *Schistosomiasis:* McLaren (1980); Butterworth et al. (1982); Capron et al. (1982).
3. *Filariasis:* Nelson (1970); Denham and McGreevy (1977); Ogilvie and Mackenzie (1982); Mansfield (1982).
4. *Gastrointestinal Helminths:* Marsden (1978); Befus and Bienenstock (1982).
5. *Effector Mechanisms:* Butterworth (1977); Askenase (1979); Mitchell (1979b, 1980); Santoro et al. (1979a).
6. *Antigens:* Pery and Luffau (1979); Maizels et al., (1982); Mitchell and Anders (1982).
7. *Vaccination:* Clegg and Smith (1978); Taylor and Muller (1980); Lloyd (1981).

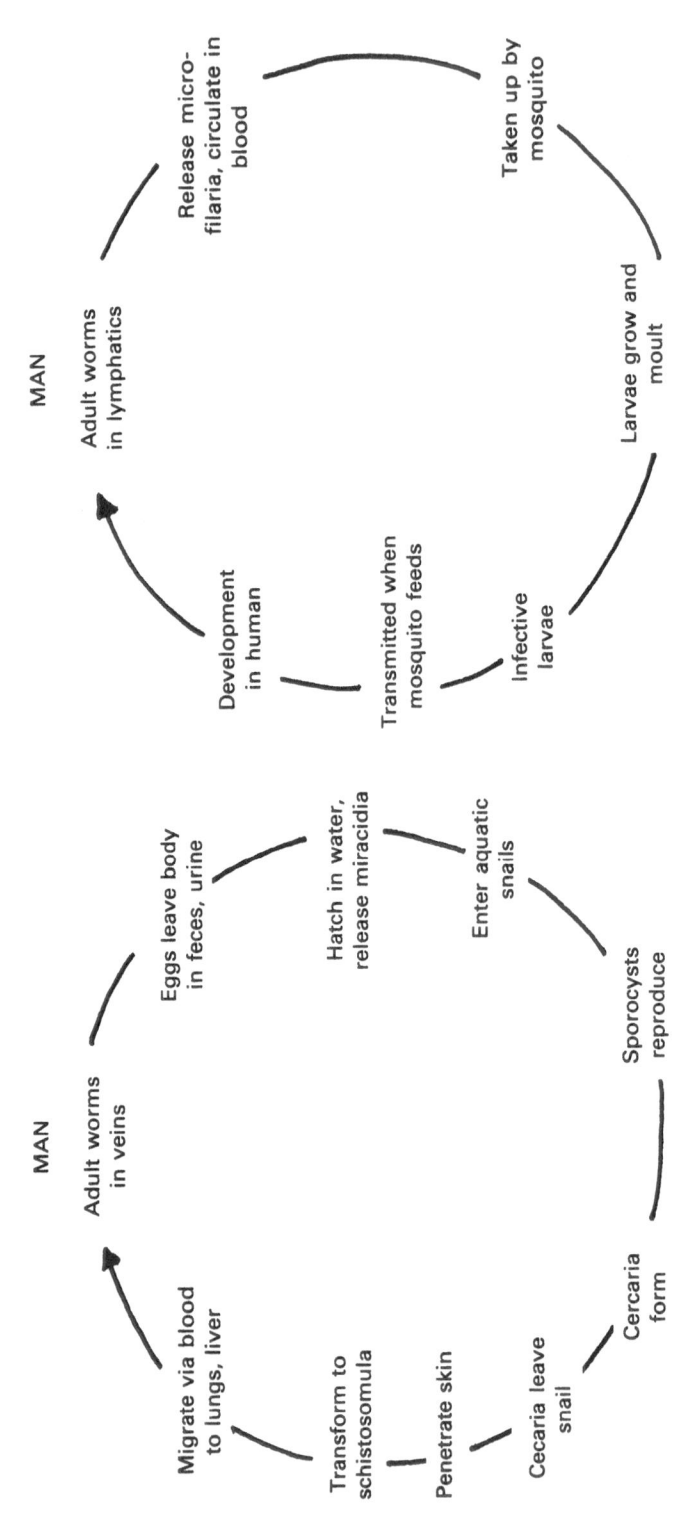

MAN

Release micro-
filaria, circulate in
blood

Taken up by
mosquito

Adult worms
in lymphatics

Larvae grow and
moult

Development
in human

Transmitted when
mosquito feeds

Infective
larvae

b. *Wuchereria*. Cycle takes ≃ 6–12 months.

MAN

Eggs leave body
in feces, urine

Hatch in water,
release miracidia

Enter aquatic
snails

Adult worms
in veins

Sporocysts
reproduce

Migrate via blood
to lungs, liver

Transform to
schistosomula

Cercaria
form

Penetrate skin

Cecaria leave
snail

a. *Schistosoma*. Cycle takes ≃ 2–3 months.

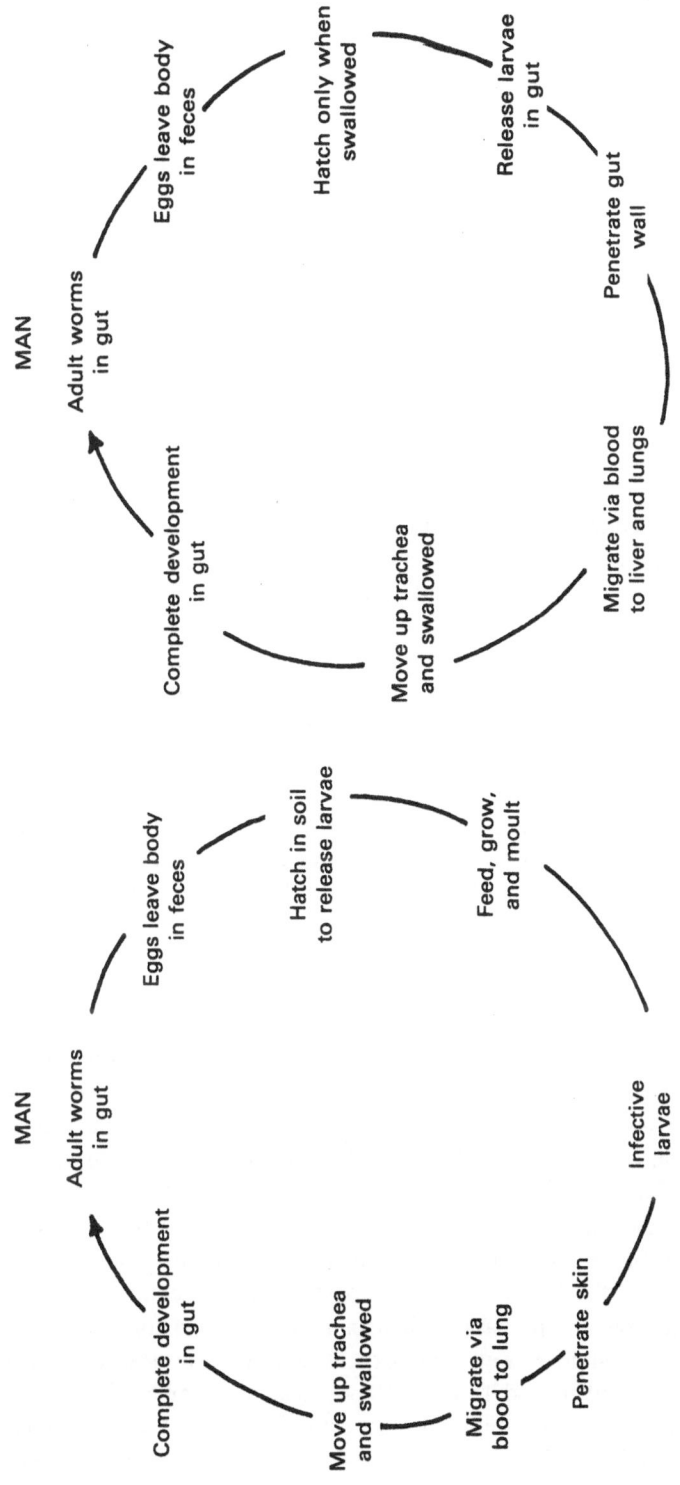

MAN

Adult worms
in gut

Eggs leave body
in feces

Hatch only when
swallowed

Complete development
in gut

Release larvae
in gut

Move up trachea
and swallowed

Penetrate gut
wall

Migrate via blood
to liver and lungs

d. *Ascaris.* Cycle takes ≃ 3 months.

MAN

Adult worms
in gut

Eggs leave body
in feces

Hatch in soil
to release larvae

Complete development
in gut

Feed, grow,
and moult

Move up trachea
and swallowed

Migrate via
blood to lung

Penetrate skin

Infective
larvae

c. Hookworm. Cycle takes ≃ 2 months.

Figure 1. Life cycles of representatives of the major helminth parasites of man: (a) *Schistosoma;* (b) *Wuchereria;* (c) Hookworm; (d) *Ascaris, Trichuris.*

2. IMMUNITY TO HELMINTHS

Man, like other animals, appears to show a certain degree of natural resistance to helminth infections, and this may be more pronounced in some races than in others. Age-related resistance also appears to exist, although, without experimental data, it is not easy to divorce this phenomenon from age-related changes in exposure to infection. There is abundant evidence of immunological responsiveness to infection, much of it reflected in pathological manifestations (reviewed in Cohen and Warren, 1982), but there is only circumstantial evidence for the operation of effective immunologically based mechanisms of resistance to infection—that is, for immunity in a narrow sense (protective immunity). Indeed, the chronic nature of many helminth diseases implies that such mechanisms, if they exist, must operate inefficiently. Experimental studies in man are necessarily limited to *in vitro* work, thus approaches to the question of immunity draw heavily on the extensive data describing immunity to helminths in experimental animals. In the latter, immunity can be identified and quantified by many parameters but most precisely by direct measurement of the *in vivo* development and survival of the worm itself. In man such direct measurements are restricted to those stages that can be assessed in readily accessible specimens such as blood, skin snips, urine, or feces and thus relate only to parasite reproduction; parasite survival cannot be measured directly. Indirect approaches, such as the use of immunological tests designed to assess antibody or cellular responses to worm antigens, show notoriously poor correlation with the presence or absence of viable organisms, although measurement of free antigen or of circulating complexes may be more useful in this respect (Deelder *et al.*, 1980).

2.1. Immunity *in Vivo*

In a number of experimental systems, immunity is apparent during the course of initial (primary) infections and is reflected in a drop in reproductive output and loss of the adult worm population—self- or spontaneous cure. Such immunity is seen in schistosome infections in certain hosts (e.g., the rat) but is less evident in other species. Clearly in this situation immunity is expressed against the adult stages, and there is good evidence that it is the adults that provide the major antigenic stimulus. In other hosts (e.g., rhesus monkey and mouse), immunity is stimulated by the adults from a primary infection but is expressed against the larval stages developing from a second or subsequent challenge infection, the primary adult population surviving for a considerable time after this immunity is well developed. This form of resistance—concomitant immunity (Smithers and Terry, 1969)—probably resembles that which occurs in man and refects the ability of older schistosomes to evade the protective responses that kill larval stages at an early stage of development. In immune mice, for example, 30% of the schistosomula that survive penetration through the skin are killed before leaving the dermis and 43% of those that reach the lungs die before maturation (Smithers and Gammage, 1980).

The course of schistosomiasis in man offers no evidence for the operation of a strong or absolute resistance to reinfection of the kind demonstrable in experimental hosts. Curves of the prevalence and intensity of infection in endemic areas (Figure 2) can be interpreted as showing (1) the slow development of a concomitant immunity that limits superinfection and (2) a slow decline in egg production that follows spontaneous death of the original adult population. There is evidence to suggest that these may well be the correct interpretations; certainly sera taken from patients infected with *S. mansoni* or *S. haematobium* contains antibody that, *in vitro*, can facilitate leukocyte-mediated killing of schistosomula (Butterworth, 1977).

Several studies have demonstrated protective immunity to filarial nematodes in experimental hosts (Ogilvie and Mackenzie, 1982). There is a wide spectrum of responsiveness in terms of the duration and frequency of infections necessary to evoke immunity and in the stage-specificity of the effects of immunity, but comparison between systems is complicated by the fact that in many cases the host–parasite relationship is not one that occurs naturally. Thus physiological incompatibilities may also be involved.

Infections with *Brugia pahangi* in cats are used to model Brugian filariasis in man. In this system immunity develops only slowly and many infections are required before there is immunity to reinfection (Denham *et al.*, 1972). Resistance to challenge is preceded by disappearance of microfilaria from the blood, and amicrofilaremia is associated with the appearance of antimicrofilarial antibodies (Ponnudurai *et al.*, 1974). Antibodies that react with infective larvae or with adults can be detected in both susceptible and resistant cats, but antibodies that kill microfilaria appear only when the host is amicrofilaremic. In the less natural model, *Dipetalonema viteae* in hamsters, microfilaria disappear from the blood even though potentially fecund adults persist for some considerable time afterward. Some workers have demonstrated serum factors that can suppress microfilarial release *in vitro* and *in vivo* in this system (Haque *et al.*, 1978) and others have shown antimicrofilarial antibodies that can cooperate with cells in destroying larvae (Weiss and Tanner, 1979). In mice—which are, overall poorer hosts for *D. viteae*—the survival pattern is reversed, with adults dying long before microfilaria are cleared from the circulation (Haque *et al.*, 1980b).

If the disappearance of microfilaria from the blood and appearance of antimicrofilarial antibodies can be taken as indicators of immunity, it is likely that, in endemic areas, at least a proportion of the population develops immunity to the lymphatic filarias (Piessens *et al.*, 1980). Immunity to *Onchocerca* is suggested by the intensity curve of skin microfilarial burden recorded in endemic areas (Figure 3), but—as with schistosomiasis (see above)—many factors deter-

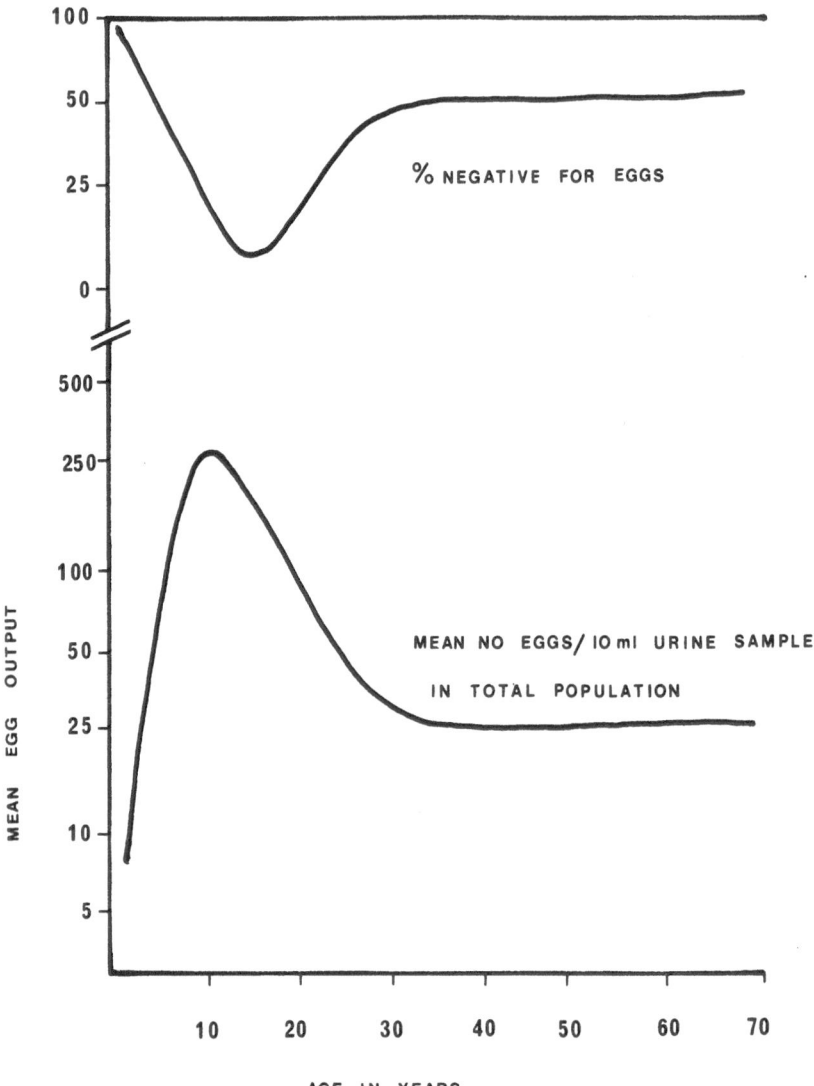

Figure 2.   Prevalence and intensity of infection with a schistosome (*S. haematobium*) in a population living in an endemic area. (Data from Bradley and McCullough, 1973.)

mine such curves and, indeed, some studies have shown apparently unimpeded
reinfection after removal of adult worms by chemotherapy (Duke, 1968).

    Although some parallels do exist between man and experimental hosts when
schistosomes and filariids are considered, there appear to be major differences as
far as the intestinal nematodes are concerned. *Ascaris, Trichuris,* hookworms,

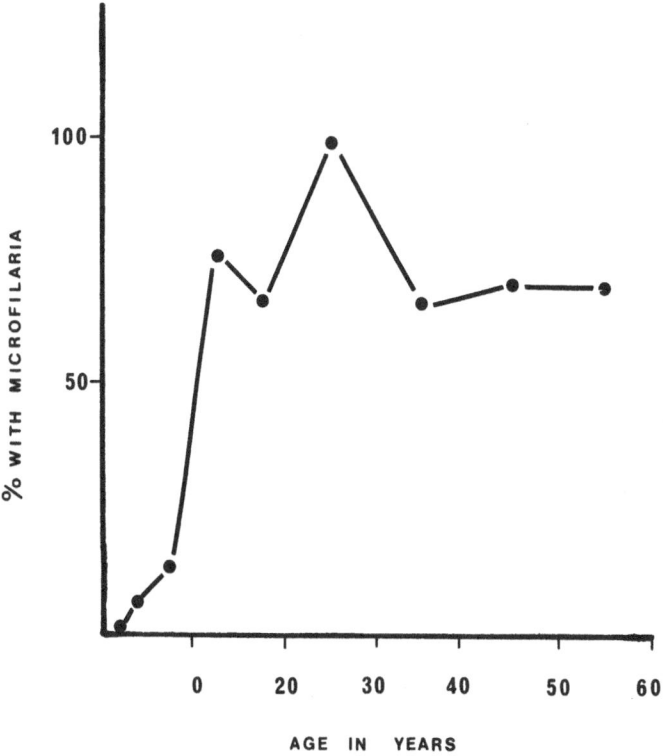

Figure 3.   Prevalence of infection with *Onchocerca* in a population living in an endemic area. (Data from Duke and Moore, 1968.)

and *Strongyloides* are all characterized by their chronicity in man, whereas in the comparable infections in laboratory hosts (e.g., *Trichuris muris* in mice, *Ancylostoma caninum* in dogs, *Strongyloides ratti* in rats) and in other rodent model systems (*Nippostrongylus brasiliensis*, *Trichinella spiralis*, and *Trichostrongylus colubriformis*), strong spontaneous cure responses are stimulated during initial infection and there is a high level of resistance to reinfection (Wakelin, 1978a). Perhaps a closer analogy with the human situation is provided by infections with *Nematospiroides dubius* in mice, in which primary infections are chronic, surviving for many months, and resistance to reinfection develops slowly despite abundant evidence of the capacity of the host to develop and express protective responses under appropriate conditions (Bartlett and Ball, 1972; Behnke and Wakelin, 1977). That there may be some immunity to hookworm is suggested by the fact that levels of infection have been found to plateau in the second to fifth decade of life (Banwell and Schad, 1978), but no evidence for immunity was obtained in experimental human infections (Ball and Bartlett, 1969). Despite the clear-cut immunopathology associated with *Ascaris* infections in man, evidence for protective immunity is equally tenuous. Nothing is known of immunity to *Trichuris* in man, although, as with many parasites, there is greater prevalence and intensity in children than in adults. This may simply reflect greater environmental exposure to infection in the younger age group; indeed, there is good evidence for substantial reinfection after chemotherapy. Immunity to *Strongyloides* is again suggested by the patterns of infections in populations and this interpretation is supported by the dramatic hyperinfections that can follow immunosuppressive treatments (Purtilo *et al.*, 1974).

2.2. Helminths as Antigens

Helminths are complex metazoan organisms and confront their hosts with a wide spectrum of antigenic materials present in structural components or released through metabolic processes (Pery and Luffau, 1979; Mitchell and Anders, 1982). This inherent complexity is compounded by the fact that there may be sequential expression of distinct antigenic specificities as parasitic worms pass through developmental stages. Clearly it would be an enormous task to approach the identification of antigens concerned with immunity through a complete antigenic analysis, but in practice this task is simplified by the fact that comparatively few antigens seem to play a major role in evoking responses that lead to protective immunity. This conclusion originates in the many observations that, although infected or immunized hosts produce marked cellular and serological responses to a variety of parasite antigens, there is little if any correlation with immune status. In addition, experimental evidence from model systems such as *Ascaris, Trichinella,* and *Trichuris* in rodents has shown that the capacity of complex antigen preparations (such as whole-worm homogenates) to stimulate immunity can be associated almost entirely with specific, defined fractions. Thus many immunological responses to parasite antigens are quite irrelevant to the continued survival and well-being of the parasite concerned. Indeed, although sometimes useful in diagnosis, such responses may be harmful to the host through their immunopathological potential. Reactivity to helminth antigens in man can be measured *in vitro* by serological means or by lymphocyte transformation and *in vivo* by intradermal injection to generate hypersensitivity responses, but correlation of particular antigens with protective immunity can only be explored in laboratory systems.

2.2.1. Schistosomes

In schistosome infections, a battery of antigens—protein, glycoprotein, and carbohydrate—is released from the adult worms during their metabolism and feeding. In addition the eggs, with the enclosed miracidia, constantly release a variety of highly immunogenic materials. However, there seems little doubt that the antigens of prime importance for immunity are located at the body surface of the worm. Many *in vitro* studies using schistosomula stages have shown specific antibody binding to the outer membranes of the tegument, and such antibodies can mediate attachment of potentially destructive leukocytes. More direct demonstration of these antigens has come from radiolabeling and polyacrylamide gel electrophoresis studies (Snary *et al.*, 1980; Taylor and Butterworth, 1982), which have identified a number of proteins of molecular weights 14,000 to 185,000 in the tegument of *S. mansoni* schistosomula. Four of these proteins were precipitated by sera from immune mice and from infected patients. Monoclonal antibodies directed against surface antigens present on schistosomula and adult worms have been shown to mediate cytotoxicity *in vitro* and to transfer immunity *in vivo* (Capron *et al.*, 1980; Smith *et al.*, 1982). In addition to its antigenic properties, the schistosome surface has other properties relevant to the operation of protective mechanisms. Receptors for the Fc portion of IgG have been identified (Torpier *et al.*, 1979a), and it is well known that there is surface activation of complement via the alternative pathway (Ramalho-Pinto *et al.*, 1978; Santoro *et al.*, 1979b). The tegument of the parasite is therefore a particularly vulnerable site and strong selective pressures exist for the worms to render themselves less open to immunologically mediated attack. This is achieved in two ways: by acquisition of host molecules (host antigens), which render the surface less foreign, and by intrinsic changes in tegumental organization, which reduce the accessibility of antigenic determinants (McLaren and Terry, 1982). Some of the consequences of the molecular changes involved in these protective strategies have been revealed in elegant freeze-fracture studies of schistosomes taken at intervals throughout their development (McLaren *et al.*, 1978; Torpier *et al.*, 1979b).

2.2.2. Nematodes

In contrast to the schistosomes—which as Platyhelminthes are characterized by the possession of a plasma-membrane-bounded cytoplasmic outer surface—nematodes possess a complex, tough, collagenous external cuticle. For many years it was considered that this surface was relatively inert and played no important part in stimulating immune responses, despite some evidence for antibody binding and antibody-mediated cellular attachment. Recent studies, however, have shown in several species, including filariids, that distinct antigens are expressed on the cuticular surface and that these antigens elicit antibodies capable of combining with the antigens and of mediating attachment of leukocytes (Maizels *et al.*, 1982). Additional evidence suggests that there may be constant turnover of such antigens with release into the surrounding environment (Philipp *et al.*, 1980; Smith *et al.*, 1981). The composition and structure of surface antigens is under active investigation; in one of the best-studied model nematodes, *T. spiralis,* it is known that the antigenic moieties are proteins and glycoproteins (Parkhouse *et al.,* 1981).

A variety of immunization procedures have failed to show any protection with antigens derived from internal structures in filariids, and it is considered that in these species surface antigens play the major role (Ogilvie and MacKenzie, 1982). Their importance in initiating focusing protective responses is reflected in the ready adherence of leukocytes to antibody-coated stages, in the *in vitro* demonstrations that parasites can be killed under such circumstances, and in the appearance of antibodies with surface specificity in infected hosts, human as well as experimental. It is particularly striking that amicrofilaremia in the host is associated with the appearance of antibodies directed against microfilarial antigens (e.g., Piessens *et al.,* 1980). There is accumulating evidence that, in certain filariids, the cuticle plays an important role in nutrient uptake (Howells and Chen, 1981) and is therefore a vulnerable target. In this context it is interesting that whereas microfilaria taken directly from the uteri of female *Litomosoides carinii* can be shown to have a number of protein components on their cuticle, these are not detectable in microfilariae from the blood. The major protein present on the latter appears to be host serum albumin, which may therefore have some parasite-protective role (Philipp *et al.,* 1982). Recent studies suggest that a similar phenomenon occurs in *Wuchereria.*

The relevance of surface antigens to protective responses against gastrointestinal species other than those with parenteral stages is less apparent. Indeed, in those systems in which antigens capable of stimulating immunity have been identified, their origin is from intestinal structures, such as the stichocytes of *Trichinella* and *Trichuris* (Jenkins and Wakelin, 1977; Despommier and Lacetti, 1981); the gland cells concerned with production of factors necessary for moulting (e.g., in *Ascaris;* Stromberg, 1979); or enzymes with a putative role in feeding (Thorson, 1963). Such antigens may well evoke antibody responses that directly interfere with the feeding, growth, and reproduction of the worm, but it is likely that an equally significant role lies in generating inflammatory changes that alter the worm's immediate environment.

2.3. Immune Responses

Immunity to helminths in experimental animals is without exception associated with the development and expression of T-cell-dependent responses (Mitchell, 1980). The most fruitful analyses of the relationship of particular responses to this immunity have involved transfer of serum or cells *in vivo* or the testing of antibody and cellular components *in vitro* for their capacity to recognize and destroy parasitic stages. With some important exceptions there is remarkably little evidence that antibodies acting alone or with complement components alone can directly mediate immunity. Equally there is little evidence for any direct interaction with worms of cytotoxic T lymphocytes. Effective immunity almost always involves the cooperation of antibodies with effector leukocytes or the generation of antibody- and T-cell-mediated inflammatory responses.

2.3.1. Antibodies

Helminth infections elicit pronounced antibody responses in all major immunoglobulin classes and characteristically result in elevated levels of IgE. In certain cases infection potentiates levels of both specific and nonspecific reaginic antibody and stimulates marked hypergammaglobulinemia (see section 2.5). Successful passive transfer of immunity with serum from immune animals has been recorded in experimental systems related to each of the major groups of helminths considered here,—for example, *S. mansoni* in mice and rats (Phillips *et al.*, 1975; Sher *et al.*, 1977a; Mangold and Knopf, 1981), filarial infections in rodents (Wong, 1964; Haque *et al.*, 1978), hookworm in dogs (Miller, 1967), *Ascaris* and *Trichuris* in rodents (Selby and Wakelin, 1973; Khoury and Soulsby, 1977)—as well as in the extensively used model systems of *N. brasiliensis*, *T. spiralis*, and *T. colubriformis* (Wakelin, 1978a).

Interpretation of such transfers in terms of antibody function is difficult because the contribution of the recipient to the observed response is unknown. In none of the above is there any clear evidence for a direct role of antibody; indeed, there is evidence against such a role in that, where it has been examined, passive transfer is relatively ineffective when the recipient has been irradiated. Only in isolated experimental systems, such as infections with the larvae of the cestode *Taenia taeniaformis* in rodents, has a direct role been proposed, with IgA preventing mucosal invasion by oncospheres and complement-fixing IgG isotypes participating in the destruction of early cystic stages in the liver (Mitchell *et al.*, 1977; Lloyd and Soulsby, 1978).

Because of the difficulty of interpreting the results of *in vivo* transfer, many workers have used *in vitro* systems to analyze the role of antibodies in immunity. Here again there are few cases where antibody alone or antibodies with complement brings about parasite destruction. Such lethal antibody is, however, present in sera from humans, monkeys, and rodents infected with or immunized against schistosomes. This antibody (known to be IgG) will kill schistosomule stages in the presence of complement but has no effect when passively transferred *in vivo* (Clegg and Smithers, 1972; Sher *et al.*, 1974).

An old concept of direct antibody-mediated effects upon nematodes was the inactivation of enzymes used in metabolic antivities. Antibodies with such specificities have been identified (e.g., against malate dehydrogenase in *Ascaris;* Rhodes *et al.*, 1965), and there is evidence that antibodies raised against enzymes released by adult hookworms have antienzyme activity (Thorson, 1956).

Equal effects might be expected against the enzymes used by skin-penetrating larvae of both nematodes and schistosomes. Circumstantial evidence for direct antiworm activities of antibodies comes from those experiments where antisera have been passively transferred into recipients that have been irradiated to prevent cellular cooperation with the antibody concerned. Under these conditions worms may show cytopathological damage, stunting of growth, and impaired fecundity (Jones and Ogilvie, 1971; Wakelin, 1975). Reduced fecundity in the *Trichinella* model system has been achieved by *in vitro* incubation of adult females in serum and intestinal antibody fractions (Jacqueline *et al.*, 1978).

Despite these examples of direct antiworm activity, there is overwhelming evidence, from both *in vitro* and *in vivo* studies, that antibody-dependent protective activity requires the cooperation of cellular elements.

2.3.2. T Lymphocytes

The central role of T cells in antihelminth immunity appears to be expressed through helper function, both in antibody production and in the generation of hypersensitivity and inflammatory reactions. Direct, cytolytic interactions with helminths, of the kind that effect immunity against viruses, do not occur even when, as in the case of schistosome larvae, the parasite surface presents both parasite antigen and host MHC determinants (Sher *et al.*, 1978; Butterworth *et al.*, 1979).

2.3.3. Cooperative Responses between Antibody and Cells

In vitro evidence for cooperative interactions between antibodies and leukocytes that lead to killing of parasites has been obtained with schistosomes, filariids, the parenteral stages of gastrointestinal nematodes, and several other species.

Damage and destruction of the schistosomulum stage of schistosomes can be brought about by cooperation between a variety of immunoglobulins and a variety of leukocytes (see Table 1). A great deal of research has been carried out on this aspect of immunity (much of it in the rat—*S. mansoni* model) and only an outline can be given here. Fuller accounts are given in McLaren (1980) and Capron *et al.* (1982).

In those interactions involving IgG antibody, there is specific recognition of tegumentally expressed antigens followed by adherence of effector cells through their Fc and C3b receptors. Since the tegument can itself activate complement, adherence through C3b receptors can occur in the absence of antibody, but under these circumstances killing is less efficient (Figure 4). Eosinophils are particularly efficient at *in vitro* killing, adhering closely to the tegument and releasing a variety of factors, including lysosomal peroxidase enzymes and cationic pro-

Table I

Antibody–Cell Effector Mechanisms Capable
of Killing Schistosomula *in Vitro*

Cell	Antibody	Species
Neutrophil	IgG	Rat, guinea pig, man
Eosinophil	IgG	Rat, mouse, baboon, man
Macrophage	IgG	Rat
Macrophage	IgE	Rat, baboon, man
Eosinophil	IgE	Rat, ?man

teins, that cause local destruction of the worm's surface. There are complex interactions between the worm, the effectors, and other cells. For example, killing efficiency of eosinophils can be increased by the presence of mast cells, possibly through the enhancement of receptors on the eosinophil surface brought about by soluble mediators (Anwar and Kay, 1978). Susceptibility to *in vitro*

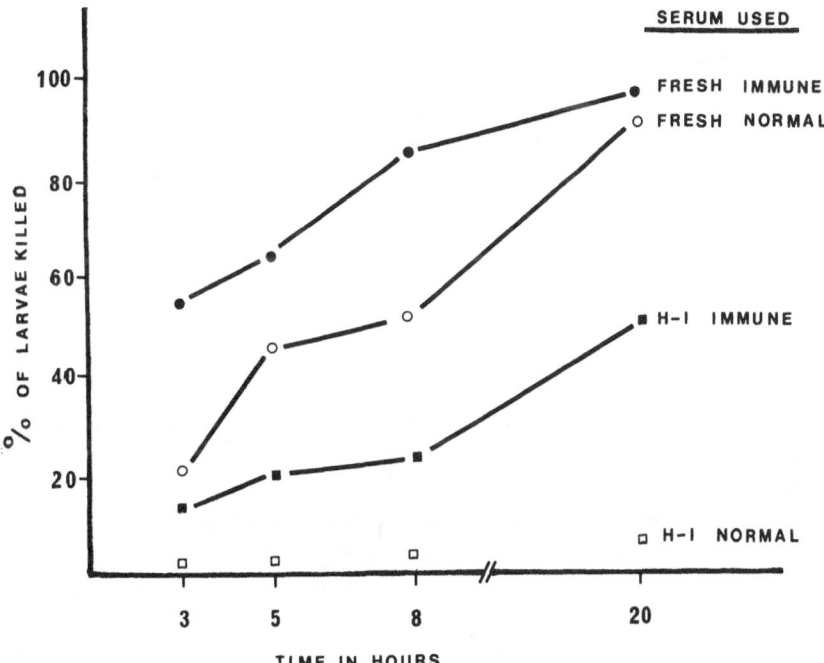

Figure 4.   Survival *in vitro* of *Schistosoma mansoni* schistosomula when incubated with eosinophils and fresh or heat-inactivated (H-I), immune or normal rat serum. (Data from McLaren, 1980.)

killing is restricted to early schistosomules; later stages, recovered after migration *in vivo* or maintained *in vitro,* are much more resistant. The precise reasons for this change in susceptibility are not understood, but there is growing evidence that biochemical and structural alterations in the tegument itself lead to reduced accessibility of antigenic determinants and greater resistance to the action of lytic complement and leukocyte factors. These changes can occur independently of the acquisition of host antigens, although *in vivo* the two events may occur concurrently. Thus, when 3-hr and 5-day schistosomula are labeled with a hapten, only the former are killed by antihapten antibody in combination with complement or eosinophils (Moser *et al.,* 1980). Similarly, when lung-stage and adult *S. mansoni* recovered from mice are reacted with rat anti-mouse antibody, both bind the antibody strongly, but only the latter are killed in the presence of eosinophils (McLaren and Terry, 1982).

An important observation has been that schistosomule killing can be facilitated by reaginic (IgE) and IgG anaphylactic antibodies, both of which show marked increases in schistosome infections (Capron *et al.,* 1982). IgE acts as an opsonizing antibody, allowing adherence of eosinophils, and, in the form of complexes, also activates macrophages, greatly enhancing their killing activity. IgG isotypes act primarily by allowing eosinophil adherence.

A major question regarding *in vitro* studies on schistosomule killing has been their relevance to immunity *in vivo* and particularly to immunity in man. Schistosomule susceptibility to immune effectors forms the basis of concomitant immunity and destruction of larvae *in vivo* and is strongly associated with the activity of eosinophils and other leukocytes (Lichtenberg *et al.,* 1976). Passively transferred antisera can transfer immunity if the host can mount myeloid responses, but they are ineffective if the host cannot (Sher, 1977a). Absorption of sera to reduce levels of IgE and IgG decreases the level of immunity transferred (Capron *et al.,* 1980). Treatment of animals to prevent normal antibody production (Bazin *et al.,* 1980) or to reduce eosinophil levels (Mahmoud *et al.,* 1975) is associated with reduced immunity on infection. The antibody–leukocyte systems that bring about killing *in vitro* have been largely studied in the rat but do operate with components taken from infected humans (Butterworth *et al.,* 1982). Despite this strong circumstantial evidence, there are still difficulties in unrestricted extrapolation from these experimental *in vitro* observations into the normal human situation.

In vitro killing of helminths has been investigated most intensively with schistosomes, but similar interactions involving antibody and leukocytes have been demonstrated with a variety of nematode parasites, primarily using larval stages as targets. Much of this work has been concerned with model systems, particularly *Trichinella* (Mackenzie *et al.,* 1980); but there is good evidence for the operation of identical mechanisms against parasites of clinical significance, such as filariids and hookworms (Higashi and Chowdhury, 1970; Rudin *et al.,*

1980; Mackenzie, 1980; Klaver-Wesseling et al., 1982). As with schistosomes, cell adherence may result from direct activation of complement or from the recognition of antigenic determinants present on the cuticle by specific antibody, being mediated through C3b and Fc receptors. Little if any killing occurs in the absence of specific antibody, however. In the case of filariids, it has been demonstrated that both IgM (Weiss and Tanner, 1979) and IgG (Subrahmanyam et al. 1978) can participate in destructive in vitro interactions with microfilarial stages; Haque et al. (1981a) have shown that IgE and IgE complexes can enable eosinophils and macrophages to kill microfilaria of D. viteae. Formal demonstration of a direct recognition role for IgE in in vivo antinematode responses has not so far been made, but it is significant that rats rendered incapable of mounting IgE responses develop much greater muscle larval burdens of Trichinella (Dessein et al., 1981). Together with the data gained from the use of antieosinophil serum by Grove et al. (1977) in this system, this implies that an IgE–eosinophil interaction is important in controlling the number of parenteral larvae that successfully encyst in the muscles.

Although eosinophils can function as effective killer cells against nematodes, it is clear that, unlike schistosomes, a variety of other cells can act equally effectively in this role. Neutrophils (Rudin et al., 1980), macrophages (Haque, et al., 1980a) and even lymphocytes (Chaicumpa et al., 1977) have all been shown to damage larval stages.

The in vivo relevance of data gained from in vitro studies with nematodes rests largely on evidence that antibodies capable of mediating cell adherence appear in the sera of hosts, including man, infected with a variety of filariid parasites. Antibodies with specificity for infective larvae and adult worms appear before those reacting with microfilaria, and antimicrofilarial antibodies only appear when the host becomes amicrofilaremic (e.g., Subrahmanyam et al., 1978; Piessens et al., 1980). In hosts unable to make adequate antibody, microfilaremia is prolonged (Thompson et al., 1979). Direct evidence for an in vivo effector role of leukocytes in combination with antibody has come from Weiss and Tanner (1979), who have shown that larval D. viteae implanted into immune hosts survive well if contained within micropore chambers that do not allow entry of cells but are killed rapidly if cells have access.

Eosinophilia is a common phenomenon in human filariasis, and the syndrome of tropical pulmonary eosinophilia has been associated with the immune destruction of microfilaria larvae (Mackenzie, 1980). Eosinophils also appear prominently in tissue reactions against filariids and the skin-penetrating or tissue-migrating larvae of gastrointestinal nematodes such as Strongyloides (Moqbel, 1980) and Ascaris (Pawlowski, 1978). Although static studies of histopathological responses cannot confirm an effector role for these cells, the evidence from many studies strongly suggests that such a role is of considerable importance in protective immunity.

2.3.4. T-Cell–Myeloid Interactions

T cells regulate the production of eosinophils and influence the behavior and kinetics of mast cells and macrophages. The *in vivo* correlates of the *in vitro* killing of helminths, discussed above, therefore represent one example of T-cell–myeloid interactions involved in protective immunity, but the full extent of such interactions is much more comprehensive. Askenase (1977, 1979) has suggested a pivotal role for T cells and amine-containing cells in the initiation and development of delayed hypersensitivity and other inflammatory responses relevant to helminth immunity. The ability of T cells to promote the production of amine-containing cells, and to attract them to sites of antigenic stimulus, is seen as an important step in allowing the accumulation of potential effector cells such as eosinophils, neutrophils, and macrophages. The interaction of antigen-bearing mast cells or basophils with specific IgE or IgG isotypes results in amine release, thus facilitating extravasation of effector cells at areas of lowered vascular permeability.

There is some evidence to support the operation of such mechanisms in *in vivo* immunity to schistosomes (Dean *et al.*, 1976; Askenase, 1977), and it is likely that they will be found to operate against other helminths with tissue-migratory stages.

Interaction of T lymphocytes with myeloid cells is also thought to underlie protective immunity against nematodes living in the intestine (Wakelin, 1978a). While there is almost no evidence to suggest that such worms are susceptible to the direct activity of effector leukocytes, a great deal of circumstantial evidence suggests that expulsion of worms from the gut is induced by the pathophysiological consequences of T-cell-mediated inflammatory events. In its simplest form, worm expulsion may occur as a result of exposure to factors released from degranulating amine-containing cells, as is the case with *T. colubriformis* in guinea pigs (Rothwell *et al.*, 1974). However, no immunologically mediated inflammatory event in the intestine can be described in simple terms; amine release will affect a variety of physiological parameters (e.g., permeability, peristalsis, mucus release), each of which may also have deleterious effects on the helminths present. It is probable that, in the majority of cases, worm loss represents the consequence of a complex interaction of T cells, myeloid cells, and antibody that leads to substantial environmental fluctuations within the intestine.

2.4. Restrictions on Immunity

Under optimum conditions the responses described in section 2.3 can operate to provide a highly effective immunity. It is clear, however, that in many situations immunity is only partially effective or may not exist at all. A variety of factors arising from both host and parasite can restrict the effective operation of immune responses, and these must be taken into account in considering strategies for immunological control of helminth infections.

A major factor influencing the level of immunity expressed is the host's genetically determined capacity to respond. There is a great deal of circumstantial evidence in man—and direct evidence in domestic stock and experimental animals—for individual, race, and strain variation in susceptibility and resistance to helminth infection. This has been extensively reviewed (Wakelin, 1978b; Dargie, 1982). Variation can be detected at almost every phase of the host–parasite relationship and may involve mechanisms of natural as well as acquired resistance. Only the latter is considered here.

Genetic variation in protective immunity can arise in all of the components of the response described in section 2.3, as has been demonstrated in several experimental systems. For example, variation in antibody production determines the ability of mouse strains to express immunity during primary infections with the larval stages of the cestode *T. taeniaeformis* (Mitchell *et al.*, 1980). Mice are known also to vary in their capacity to recognize and make antibodies against the surface antigens of the nematode *T. spiralis* (Jungery and Ogilvie, 1982). Since these antibodies can mediate adherence of eosinophils, there may well be variations in control of the parenteral stages of infection. Recent evidence has shown the existence of genetically determined variation in capacity to mount both mast cell and eosinophil responses after infection (Alizadeh and Wakelin, 1982; Vadas, 1982; Wakelin and Donachie, 1983). Variation in the myeloid component of protective immunity is thought to underlie the clearly marked strain variation in immunity to the intestinal stages of *Trichinella* (Wakelin, 1980) and will obviously be of significance in immunity against larval helminths mediated by interactions between antibodies and leukocytes. Indeed, Claas and Deelder (1979) have shown that there is genetic variation in eosinophil responses in mice infected with *S. mansoni,* and Bickle *et al.* (1980) as well as Dean *et al.* (1981) have shown strain-dependent difference in immunity to reinfection in this system. Genetic factors also influence the course of filarial infections, as demonstrated with *D. viteae* in both mice and hamsters (Neilson, 1978; Haque *et al.* 1980b).

Extrapolation of these experimental observations to infections in man is very difficult. It is significant, however, that in endemic areas, where approximately uniform levels of exposure to infection might be predicted, there are marked differences within populations in the levels of infection observed and in the pathological consequences of infection (e.g., see Mahmoud, 1981; Ogilvie and Mackenzie, 1982). Some association between HLA type and the occurrence of hepatosplenomegaly caused by schistosomiasis has been reported (Salam *et al.,* 1979), but the basis of this correlation is unknown.

Although it is axiomatic that genetically determined differences in susceptibility and resistance must occur in genetically heterogeneous populations, their detection is made more difficult by the fact that, in endemic areas, it is likely that intercurrent infections will be common and nutritional standards inadequate; both of these factors can also exert depressive influences on the initiation and expression of protective immunity.

Even if attention is confined only to intercurrent parasitic infections, it is well documented that common protozoal infections, such as malaria and trypanosomiasis, can exert profound immunodepressive effects (Greenwood, 1974). It has been shown in several experimental models that there can be marked interference with protective responses against helminth infections (e.g., Phillips *et al.*, 1974). Similar interactions have also been described for concurrent infections between different species of helminth, a most significant observation being the depression of natural resistance to the establishment of *D. viteae* in rats when the host is also infected with *S. mansoni* (Haque *et al.*, 1981b). However, concurrent infections with gastrointestinal nematodes may also induce, not immunodepression, but enhanced resistance through the nonspecific effects of intestinal inflammatory responses (see Wakelin, 1978a).

Immunodepression induced by inadequate nutrition, both protein calorie malnutrition and trace-element deficiency, is also a well defined phenomenon, and there is good experimental evidence for decreased resistance to helminths in malnourished animals (Bolin *et al.*, 1977). Strong circumstantial evidence suggests that this may also be true in man.

The mechanisms of resistance to helminths appear to be particularly susceptible to the physiological changes associated with reproduction in the female. Several workers have shown in rodents that lactating animals develop less immunity during primary infections and express less immunity during challenge (e.g., Selby and Wakelin, 1975). This effect is also well described in sheep and other domestic stock, particularly in the context of gastrointestinal nematode infections. A further hazard associated with reproduction is the possibility of transplacental transmission of parasite antigens or parasite stages, with associated depression of responsiveness (tolerization) in the offspring. That this can occur has been most strikingly demonstrated by Haque and Capron (1982), who have shown transplacental transfer of microfilaria larvae of *D. viteae* in rats and subsequent unresponsiveness to *D. viteae* antigens in litters born to infected mothers.

All the major helminthiases can be associated with marked depression of immune responsiveness to both parasite-specific and unrelated antigens. The mechanisms underlying this depression are many and various and have been extensively investigated, particularly in schistosomiasis and filariasis (see section 2.5). In both patients and experimental systems, there is strong evidence in these infections that depression can be related to the presence of suppressor cell subsets, to circulating immune complexes, and to disruption of lymphoid organization.

The hyporesponsiveness associated with chronic infections, which is mediated through the host's responses to the long-term presentation of antigens by the parasite, may play an important role in assisting the evasion of immune recognition, but there are many other ways by which this can be achieved. The classical example of helminth evasion must be the acquisition by schistosomes of host material (glycolipid, glycoprotein, blood group antigen, MHC molecules, immunoglobulin) which effectively disguises the tegumental antigens from the immune effectors of the host (Smithers *et al.,* 1969). As has already been discussed, this disguise is, *in vivo,* acquired concurrently with tegumental changes that quite independently reduce antigenicity, but the most recent evidence still suggests that host antigens remain a major protective device for the adult worms (McLaren and Terry, 1982). In addition to these tegumental alterations, schistosomes reduce the impact of immune effectors in a variety of ways, including the release of enzymes capable of cleaving immunoglobulin after attachment to the tegument (Auriault *et al.,* 1981) and release of a variety of other factors that interfere with the induction or suppression of the immune response.

Comparable devices in other helminths are less well known, although the chronicity of tissue-dwelling filariids and cestodes implies the existence of similar strategies. Certainly larval cestodes are known to produce anticomplementary factors that help to prevent damage by complement-fixing antibodies (Hammerberg and Williams, 1978), and filarial worms can acquire host serum albumin, possibly as a disguise for cuticular antigens (see section 2.2). It is interesting, in the light of this latter observation, that one of the effects attributed to the microfilarial drug diethylcarbamazine is the exposure, on the microfilarial cuticle, of previously hidden antigenic sites (Mackenzie, 1980) and consequent interaction with the host's immune system.

2.5. Immunopathology

Although parasites are, by popular definition, animals that are harmful to the host, it is only in a few cases that the pathological effects associated with helminths arise as a direct consequence of their activity. Thus hookworms contribute to anemia by their blood-feeding in the intestine, and *Ascaris* may cause nutritional disturbances by physical obstruction of the gut lumen. In the majority of cases, the pathological effects of parasitism result from the host's immune responses. Many infections are associated with immediate hypersensitivity reactions, reflected in skin rashes, pruritus, fevers, respiratory symptoms, and elevated levels of IgE. With species that undergo parenteral migrations before maturing in the intestine (gastrointestinal nematodes) or blood (schistosomes), these immediate reactions are essentially short-term, but they are prolonged in the filariases and may be causally related to some of the long-term pathology seen in patients with lymphatic filariasis and onchocerciasis. [It is interesting in this context that Ottesen *et al.* (1981) have suggested that the production of blocking antibodies in filariasis may be a device for limiting the pathologic potential of such hypersensitivity reactions.]

Pathological conditions arising from delayed hypersensitivity reactions are best known in schistosomiasis, particularly *S. mansoni,* and detailed experimental analysis has conclusively demonstrated the central role of antigens derived from the egg in these responses (Boros and Warren, 1970). The cellular reaction to the antigens is T-cell-mediated and results in formation of a granuloma around each egg trapped in the tissues. In the liver the granulomata may reach a considerable size (up to 100 times the diameter of the egg; Warren, 1973) and contribute directly to blockage of sinusoids, with consequential portal hypertension, hepato- and splenomegaly, and other secondary symptoms (Warren, 1973). Delayed hypersensitivity undoubtedly also plays a major role in the pathogenesis of lymphatic filariasis and onchocerciasis.

In several experimental models it has been shown that helminth infections can lead to hypergammaglobulinemia and to potentiation of IgE antibodies with undetermined specificity (Jarrett and Bazin, 1974; Sher *et al.,* 1977b; Chapman *et al.,* 1979). The first phenomenon may contribute to the raised immunoglobulin levels characteristic of helminth infections. It is possible that high levels of IgE may be associated with some of the hypersensitivity phenomena mentioned above, but there is some evidence against this (Jarrett *et al.,* 1980); indeed, it has been proposed that the converse may be true—that is, that helminth infections are correlated with reduced atopy (see Turner *et al.,* 1978). Circulating antigen–antibody complexes have been demonstrated in both schistosomiasis and filariasis (Phillips and Draper, 1975; Ogilvie and Mackenzie, 1982) and although well-defined immune complex pathology is not normally symptomatic of these infections, it may contribute to glomerulonephritis in the former and to the lesions associated with onchocerciasis. Circulating complexes may also be deleterious to the host in other ways. In experimental schistosomiasis, for example, immune complexes are known to reduce the *in vitro* killing efficiency of effector cells (Capron and Capron, 1980), and this is likely to occur also in filariasis.

The multiple interactive responses elicited by helminth infections involve a complex series of regulatory mechanisms, and immunopathological consequences may arise from the breakdown of normal regulation. One example that can be cited here is the phenomenon of hypereosinophilia, which occurs in tropical regions and may be causally related to helminth infection (Spry *et al.,* 1980). Hypereosinophilia appears to be an abnormal (i.e., malregulated) consequence of the normal eosinophilic responses to infection and can lead to extensive damage to the tissues of the body, in particular to those of the heart.

By comparison with protozoan infections, those due to helminths do not cause major immunodepression, however, there is substantial evidence that infections can lead to reduced responsiveness to both parasite-specific and unrelated antigens (Terry, 1978). In filarial infections, depression of antibody and delayed hypersensitivity to parasite antigens has been described on several occasions, but there is conflicting evidence as to whether this depression can extend to heterologous antigens in man (see Ottesen *et al.*, 1977; Grove and Forbes, 1979). In schistosomiasis, the existence of suppressor cells is well documented; these may depress responses to lymphocyte mitogens as well as to antigens originating from the worm and the eggs (Ottesen, 1979; Ellner *et al.*, 1980; Rocklin *et al.*, 1981). Whether the degree of depression associated with these infections is of clinical significance with respect to unrelated pathogens is debatable, although it clearly contributes to the chronicity and pathogenicity of the infection concerned (see section 2.4). It is significant, however, that the heterologous antigens used by Grove and Forbes (1979) to demonstrate immunodepression in Bancroft's filariasis included tetanus toxoid, typhoid vaccine, and *E. coli* antigens. Some depression of responsiveness to prophylactic vaccinations might therefore be expected to accompany severe helminthiasis.

Immunodepression is known to accompany infection with gastrointestinal helminths in experimental systems, and responses to unrelated antigens may be markedly decreased (Ljungstrom and Huldt, 1977). A potentially significant aspect of such depression, which has been demonstrated in mice infected with *N. dubius*, is its effect upon homologous immunity, that is, existing worms can depress host responsiveness and prevent the operation of protective resistance (Behnke *et al.*, 1983). It is not yet known whether this phenomenon is mediated by antigen overload, blocking antibodies, production of immunomodulatory factors, or antiinflammatory factors, but it is known that the effect is not parasite-specific. Thus, mice infected with this parasite show decreased responsiveness to other gastrointestinal helminths given concurrently (Behnke *et al.*, 1978). A similar phenomenon, with more severe implications in tropical medicine, has been described in mice infected with the adult stages of *T. spiralis* and exposed to cholera toxin. The presence of the helminth not only depressed antitoxin responses strongly but also affected the intestinal response to the toxin and stimulated a much greater secretion of fluid (Ljungstrom, 1979).

3. IMMUNOLOGICALLY BASED CONTROL

3.1. Vaccination against Infection

Whereas it is possible to write at length about experimental investigations of immunity to helminths and our present knowledge of the mechanisms involved, it is difficult to give more than a brief account of vaccination as a practical means of control. Under ideal conditions, vaccination would be the long-term strategy of choice for controlling the major helminth infections of man. If potent, safe vaccines were available, populations could be immunized when most susceptible (i.e., in childhood) and at infrequent intervals thereafter. The stimulation of resistance in this way would reduce the necessity for preventing reinfection from the immediate environment, and the development of "herd immunity" would make transmission less effective and thus help to break the parasites' life cycles.

These theoretical advantages of vaccination can be compared with the social and financial difficulties inherent in improving standards of hygiene and sanitation or of controlling vectors, the logistic and clinical problems sometimes encountered in chemotherapy, and the inadequacy of chemotherapeutic agents for certain infections (notably filariasis). That these advantages can be realized is shown by the success of the vaccine developed for controlling lungworm infection in bovines; the fact that this remains the only commercially available vaccine highlights the difficulties encountered in translating theory into practice (Urquhart, 1980).

A great deal of experimental work has been carried out to develop means of immunizing animals against helminths, and this has been extensively reviewed (Clegg and Smith, 1978; Lloyd, 1981). In certain model systems relevant to man (e.g., *Ascaris* and *Trichuris*), it is possible to raise high levels of immunity against infection by the use of nonviable material prepared from parasite stages (see section 2.2); but such an approach has been largely unsuccessful with helminths such as schistosomes, hookworms, and filariids. With these parasites greater success has been achieved using radiation-attenuated larval stages, which develop sufficiently in the host to generate protective responses but die before maturation, thus avoiding the pathological consequences of infection. In the case of hookworms, a live vaccine using irradiated larvae was developed commercially for use against infections in dogs (Miller, 1971). However, although it gave a very high level of protection against hookworm disease, it did not, in all circumstances, prevent the development of patent infections. For this and other reasons, the vaccine has now been withdrawn (Miller, 1978). In the case of schistosomes, live vaccines based upon the use of irradiated larvae have been used against bovine species in field trials in the Sudan (Bushara *et al.*, 1978; Majid *et al.*, 1980). Again, the vaccine has been successful in terms of preventing disease, but it has not given absolute immunity against infection.

In both instances, development of the vaccines involved the solution of formidable technical problems. In hookworm, for example, procedures for effective sterilization of the irradiated larvae (which, of course, had to be cultured from stages passed in fecal material) were required, and for schistosomes procedures for cryopreserving larvae after irradiation. The fact that these problems were successfully overcome gave some encouragement for the development of equivalent vaccines against the human infections, but the failure to generate complete immunity, coupled with the logistic problems involved in producing irradiated larvae in sufficient quantity and in implementing vaccination programs in the field, render it unlikely that vaccines of this kind will ever be used, although considerable research effort is still directed toward this end (Smithers, 1980).

Filarial infections have presented particular problems for experimentalists concerned with the development of immunization protocols. Not only has it proved difficult to stimulate immunity with antigens prepared from nonviable worm material but there has been little success with attenuated larval vaccines (Ogilvie and Mackenzie, 1982). Even were such approaches successful in the laboratory, the inability to maintain species of human clinical importance in laboratory hosts would provide an insuperable obstacle to the provision of large quantities of parasite stages.

So far, discussion of the difficulties encountered in devising vaccines has centered on the parasitological problems, but there are many immunological problems of equal importance. The infections for which vaccines are required are precisely those where man appears incapable of developing an adequate protective immunity. Some of the factors that might contribute to this lack of immunity have already been considered (section 2.4); those arising from inadequate nutrition, intercurrent infection, and physiological stress would presumably also operate against the effectiveness of immunization procedures. The possibility that man, as a species, is inherently incapable of generating effective immunity against helminths can be dismissed, but there may be major difficulties in realizing the potential for immunity under the conditions existing in areas where helminth diseases are endemic or as observed in animal experience (Urquhart, 1980), in eliciting effective responsiveness in very young individuals. It may be possible to overcome some of these difficulties by using adjuvant material in vaccination, but there are particular problems with the choice of adjuvant in view of the pathological properties that some possess (Chedid, 1978). Related to this problem is the danger of stimulating responses with immunopathological potential when live vaccines or unpurified parasite material is employed. A more optimistic approach may be the identification of protective antigens and the use of modern biological technologies to isolate and synthesize such antigens. The development of the hybridoma technique to produce large quantities of monoclonal antibodies with exquisite specificity makes it possible to identify and purify particular antigens from parasite preparations (Cross, 1982) and to purify them using antibody affinity chromatography. Both the antigen and the antibody can then be assayed for their ability to elicit or to transfer protective immunity against infection. Some progress along these lines has already been made in schistosomiasis (see sections 2.2.1), and it is likely that development in this field will accelerate.

The ability to isolate specific protein antigens with potent immunogenicity makes it possible to consider using DNA recombinant technology to produce large amounts of material that could be incorporated into vaccine preparations. Experiments have already shown that it is feasible *in vitro* to translate messenger RNA from *S. mansoni* (Cordingley *et al.*, 1982), and there are real hopes that such approaches will yield usable quantities of the antigens known to exist on the surface of schistosomula and known to be targets for immune responses. Extrapolation to other helminths would seem reasonable, particularly to those species (e.g., the filariids) where surface antigens are again likely to play a major role in protective immunity. Recent studies using radiolabeling and electrophoretic analysis have demonstrated not only that important antigenic determinants exist on the cuticle of nematodes but that, in general, their number and diversity are comparatively restricted (Maizels *et al.*, 1982). In consequence, isolation and purification is simplified.

If vaccines based upon the techniques of modern molecular biology become readily available, they will, of course, merely provide the prospect of control. The reality will still depend upon many largely imponderable factors in the financing, administration, and execution of vaccination programs and on the behavior and effectiveness of vaccines when used on a large scale in heterogeneous populations. Almost certainly such vaccines would need to be used with adjuvants, and the development of safe, defined, and selective adjuvants would be an essential requirement.

The preparation of defined antigens and a more detailed knowledge of the mechanisms promoting and restricting protective immunity should make it possible not only to consider straightforward vaccination but also to look for more subtle ways of manipulating the immune response in order to increase the effectiveness of particular components (Mitchell and Anders, 1982). For example, if deficient immunity results from defective T-cell recognition of antigen or from defective T-cell help for other components of the response, it may be possible to present antigens in a modified form so that adequate T-cell responsiveness is ensured (Mitchell's "antigen engineering"). In contrast, if the defect is operative in efferent pathways or specific effector functions other than antibody (as hypothesized for the slow response of certain mice to *Trichinella;* Wakelin and Donachie, 1981) remedy of the defect is unlikely to be achieved solely by more effective antigen presentation. One exception to this may be those situations in which effector mechanism deficiencies reflect the activity of parasite-derived factors. Here vaccination against these factors might be used to block their activity and thus potentiate resistance.

3.2. Vaccination against Transmission

Many of the helminthiases discussed in this review show relative or absolute host specificity for man. They may be acquired directly, through ingestion or penetration of infective stages, or indirectly, through invertebrate vectors, but the ultimate source of infection is always another human host. Vaccination as a means of controlling such infections must therefore be aimed at preventing the establishment of infections in man. This is not necessarily the case, however, for those helminthiases which can be transmitted through domestic animals or for which domestic animals are essential intermediate hosts. Here vaccination could be used to limit infections in the animal host and thus reduce the intensity of transmission. Since the requirements (quality control and efficiency) for animal vaccines are less stringent than for those intended for use in man, control using existing approaches might well prove adequate if sufficiently immunogenic vaccines were available. (It is ironic that the one human helminthiasis for which a practical animal vaccine could easily be made available, namely trichinosis, has largely been brought under control by improved husbandry.) Animal vaccination could well play an important role in reducing environmental contamination with *S. japonicum* in Asia, where animal hosts, particularly bovines, play a significant role in the epidemiology of the disease (Pesigan *et al.*, 1958). An irradiated larval vaccine, of the type used in field trials against *Schistosoma bovis* in the Sudan, would help to reduce egg output from these hosts and thus reduce, to some extent, the degree of transmission to man. The control of several other helminthiases would be greatly facilitated by vaccines effective against sources of infection in animal hosts. One specific example is hydatid disease, acquired by man after ingestion of eggs of the tapeworm *E. granulosus,* for which dogs are the final host. This disease is of focal rather than global significance, its distribution being restricted by the epidemiological requirements of close associations between man, dogs, and sheep. This restriction, however, is a potential advantage for control programs and a potent vaccine against adult worms would be a major weapon. Unfortunately, despite some claims of effective immunization in this system (Gemmell, 1962; Herd *et al.*, 1975), stimulation of immunity against intestinal tapeworms is a difficult proposition, and there are many problems in devising vaccination protocols for large-scale programs.

3.3. Vaccination against Pathology

As discussed in section 2.5, immunopathological responses form a major component of the debilitating effects of helminth infection. In schistosomiasis, the major aspect of immunopathology is the delayed-type response to antigens originating from the egg. It is, however, well documented both in mice and men, that the severity of the response is modulated as the infection progresses (Boros *et al.*, 1975). A variety of factors are relevant to this modulation, including serum factors, circulating complexes and suppressor cells (Rocklin *et al.*, 1980). The antigens responsible for the granulomatous response are now well characterized (Pelley *et al.*, 1976; Harrison *et al.*, 1979), and it may well be possible to manipulate immune responsiveness to these antigens so that the pathology resulting from infection is ameliorated (Warren, 1977). Such ''antipathology'' vaccines could, of course, have wider relevance, for example, in preventing the long-term tissue changes associated with filariases. In *Onchocerca* infections, it is possible to envisage an antipathology vaccine that would act through the suppression of microfilaremia without necessarily preventing infection with adult stages. However, there are important ethical considerations in strategies that do not attempt to induce a complete, sterilizing immunity, and these may prevent the employment of such vaccines.

4. SUMMARY AND CONCLUSIONS

A great deal is now known of the ways in which animal hosts mount protective responses against helminth parasites, and the roles of immune and inflammatory components in such responses are increasingly well defined. Progress has been made in identifying those antigens that contribute most to the stimulation of immunity and in analyzing the ways in which parasites can be damaged or killed by immune-mediated responses. Application of the techniques of modern molecular biology will accelerate progress in these fields and, it is hoped, make available defined immunogens that can be considered for use in immunoprophylaxis.

Evidence for strong protective immunity in man remains poor, and the chronicity of the major helminth infections implies inadequate stimulation or expression of the responses known to operate so effectively in experimental model systems. Host genetic, nutritional, physiological, and immunological factors may contribute to this chronicity, as may factors originating directly from the parasites concerned. Understanding of the restrictions operating against protective immune responses is essential if effective countermeasures are to be devised. An important area is clarification of the role of immunological responses to parasite antigens in the generation of pathological changes. Here again, greater understanding of the induction, regulation, and expression of responses with immunopathologic potential is a prerequisite for improved management of helminth disease.

Vaccination would offer many advantages in the control of human helminthiases, not least in short-circuiting the requirements for the social and environmental changes necessary to reduce transmission of infection. However, there are formidable problems in the design and implementation of vaccination programs. As other human vaccines have shown, the availability of defined immunogens and an understanding of their role in stimulating immunity does not guarantee complete protection when used on a large scale in heterogeneous populations. Nevertheless, the limited effectiveness of existing control measures continues to place a high priority on the development of alternative, immunologically based strategies.

REFERENCES

Alizadeh, H., and Wakelin, D., 1982, Genetic factors controlling the intestinal mast cell response in mice infected with *Trichinella spiralis, Clin Exp. Immunol.* 49:331–337.

Anwar, A. R. E., and Kay, A. B., 1978, Enhancement of human eosinophil complement receptors by pharmacologic mediators, *J. Immunol.* 121:1245–1250.

Askenase, P. W., 1977, Immune inflammatory responses to parasites: The role of basophils, mast cells and vasoactive amines, *Am. J. Trop. Med. Hyg.* 26:96–103.

Askenase, P. W., 1979, Immunopathology of parasitic diseases: Involvement of basophils and mast cells, *Springer Sem. Immunopathol.* 4:1–59.

Auriault, C., Ouaissi, M. A., Torpier, G., Eisen, H., and Capron, A., 1981, Proteolytic cleavage of IgG bound to the Fc receptor of *Schistosoma mansoni* schistosomula, *Parasite Immunol.* 3:33–44.

Ball, P. A. J., and Bartlett, A., 1969, Serological reactions to infection with *Necator americanus, Trans. Roy. Soc. Trop. Med. Hyg.* 63:363–369.

Banwell, J. G., and Schad, G. A., 1978, Hookworm, *Clin. Gastroenterol.* 7:129–156.

Bartlett, A., and Ball, P. A. J., 1972, *Nematospiroides dubius* in the mouse as a possible model of endemic hookworm infection, *Ann. Trop. Med. Parasitol.* 66:129–134.

Bazin, H., Capron, A., Capron, M., Joseph, M., Dessaint, J.-P., and Pauwels, R., 1980, Effect of neonatal injection of anti-μ antibodies on immunity to schistosomes (*S. mansoni*) in the rat, *J. Immunol.* 129:2373–2377.

Befus, A. D., and Bienenstock, J., 1982, Factors involved in symbiosis and host resistance at the mucosa-parasite interface, *Progr. Allergy* 31:76–177.

Behnke, J. M., and Wakelin, D., 1977, *Nematospiroides dubius:* Stimulation of acquired immunity in inbred strains of mice, *J. Helminthol.* 57:167–176.

Behnke, J. M., Wakelin, D., and Wilson, M. M., 1978, *Trichinella spiralis:* Delayed rejection in mice concurrently infected with *Nematospiroides dubius, Exp. Parasitol.* 46:121–128.

Behnke, J. M., Hannah, J., and Pritchard, D. I., 1983, *Nematospiroides dubius* in the mouse: Evidence that adult worms depress the expression of homologous immunity, *Parasite Immunol.* 5:397–408.

Bickle, Q., Long, E., James, E., Doenhoff, M., and Festing, M., 1980, *Schistosoma mansoni:* Influence of the mouse host's sex, age and strain on resistance to reinfection, *Exp. Parasitol.* 50:222–232.

Bolin, T. D., Davis, A. E., Cummins, A. G., Duncombe, V. M., and Kelly, J. D., 1977, Effect of iron and protein deficiency on the expulsion of *Nippostrongylus brasiliensis* from the small intestine of the rat, *Gut* 18:182–186.

Boros, D. L., and Warren, K. S., 1970, Delayed hypersensitivity-type granuloma formation and dermal reaction induced and elicited by a soluble factor isolated from *Schistosoma mansoni* eggs, *J. Exp. Med.* 132:488–507.

Boros, D. L., Pelley, R. P., and Warren, K. S., 1975, Spontaneous modulation of granulomatous hypersensitivity in *Schistosomiasis mansoni, J. Immunol.* 114:1437–1441.

Bradley, D. J., and McCullough, F. S., 1973, Egg output stability and the epidemiology of *Schistosoma haematobium:* Part II. An analysis of the epidemiology of endemic *S. haematobium, Trans. Roy. Soc. Trop. Med. Hyg.* 67:491–500.

Bushara, H. O., Hussein, M. F., Saad, A. M., Taylor, M. G., Dargie, J. D., Marshall, T. F. de, and Nelson, G. S., 1978, Immunization of calves against *Schistosoma bovis* using irradiated cercariae or schistosomula of *S. bovis, Parasitology* 77:303–311.

Butterworth, A. E., 1977, Effector mechanisms against schistosomes *in vitro, Am. J. Trop. Med. Hyg.* 26(Suppl.):29–38.

Butterworth, A. E., Vadas, M. A., Martz, E., and Sher, A., 1979, Cytolytic T lymphocytes recognize alloantigens on schistosomula of *Schistosoma mansoni*, but fail to induce damage, *J. Immunol.* 122:1314–1321.

Butterworth, A. E., Taylor, D. W., Veith, M. C., Vadas, M. A., Dessein, A., Sturrock, R. F., and Wells, E., 1982, Studies on the mechanisms of immunity in human schistosomiasis, *Immunol. Rev.* 61:5–39.

Capron, M., and Capron, A., 1980, Schistosomes and eosinophils, *Trans. Roy. Soc. Trop. Med. Hyg.* 74(Suppl.):44–50.

Capron, A., Dessaint, J.-P., Capron, M., Joseph, M., and Pestel, J. 1980, Role of anaphylactic antibodies in immunity to schistosomes, *Am. J. Trop. Med. Hyg.* 29:849–857.

Capron, A., Dessaint, J.-P., Capron, M., Joseph, M., and Torpier, G., 1982, Effector mechanisms of immunity to schistosomes and their regulation, *Immunol. Rev.* 61:41–66.

Chaicumpa, V., Jenkin, C. R., and Fischer, H., 1977, The effect *in vivo* of peritoneal exudate of immune and normal mice on the infectivity of the third stage larvae of *Nematospiroides dubius*, *Austr. J. Exp. Biol. Med. Sci.* 55:561–570.

Chapman, C. B., Knopf, P. M., Hicks, J. D., and Mitchell, G. F., 1979, IgG$_1$ hypergammaglobu-linaemia in chronic parasitic infections in mice: Magnitude of the response in mice infected with various parasites, *Austr. J. Exp. Biol. Med. Sci.* 57:369–387.

Chedid, L., 1978, Therapeutic potential of immunoregulating synthetic compounds, in: *Immunity in Parasitic Diseases*, I.N.S.E.R.M., Paris.

Claas, F. H. J., and Deelder, A. M., 1979, H-2 linked immune response to murine experimental *Schistosoma mansoni* infections, *J. Immunogenet.* 6:167–175.

Clegg, J. A., and Smith, M. A., 1978, Prospects for the development of dead vaccines against helminths, *Adv. Parasitol.* 16:165–218.

Clegg, J. A., and Smithers, S. R., 1972, The effects of immune rhesus monkey serum on schistosomula of *Schistosoma mansoni* during cultivation *in vitro*, *Int. J. Parasitol.* 2:79–98.

Cohen, S., and Warren, K. S. (eds.), 1982, *Immunology of Parasitic Infections*, Blackwell Scientific Publications, Oxford, England.

Cordingley, J. S., McConnell, J., Taylor, D. W., and Butterworth, A. E., 1982, *In vitro* translation of messenger RNA from *Schistosoma mansoni*, *Parasitology* 85(2):xxix.

Cross, G. A. M., 1982, New technologies for parasitology, in: *Parasites—Their World and Ours* (D. F. Mettrick and S. S. Desser, eds.), Elsevier Biomedical Press, Amsterdam, pp. 3–12.

Dargie, J. D., 1982, The influence of genetic factors on the resistance of ruminants to gastrointestinal nematode and trypanosome infections in: *Animal Models in Parasitology* (D. G. Owen, ed.), MacMillan, London, pp. 17–51.

Dean, D. A., Murrell, K. D., Minard, P., and Vannier, W. E., 1976, Evidence for mast cell requirement in immunity of mice to schistosome infection, *Fed. Proc.* 35:228.

Dean, D. A., Bukowski, M. A., and Cheever, A. W., 1981, Relationship between acquired resistance, portal hypertension, and lung granulomas in ten strains of mice infected with *Schistosoma mansoni*, *Am. J. Trop. Med. Hyg.* 30:806–814.

Deelder, A. M., Kornelis, D., Van Marck, E. A. E., Eveleigh, P. C., and Van Egmund, J. G., 1980, *Schistosoma mansoni*: Characterization of two circulating polysaccharide antigens and the immunological response to these antigens in mouse, hamster and human infections, *Exp. Parasitol.* 50:16–32.

Denham, D. A., and McGreevy, P. B., 1977, Brugian filariasis: Epidemiological and experimental studies, *Adv. Parasitol.* 15:243–309.

Denham, D. A., Ponnudurai, T., Nelson, G. S., Rogers, R., and Guy, F., 1972, Studies with *Brugia pahangi*: 2. The effect of repeated infection on parasite levels in cats, *Int. J. Parasitol.* 2:401–407.

Despommier, D. D., and Laccetti, A., 1981, *Trichinella spiralis*: Proteins and antigens isolated from a large-particle fraction derived from the muscle larvae, *Exp. Parasitol.* 51:279–295.

Dessein, A. J., Parker, W. L., James, S. L., and David, J. R., 1981, IgE antibody and resistance to infection: I. Selective suppression of the IgE antibody response in rats diminishes the resistance and the eosinophil response to *Trichinella spiralis* infection, *J. Exp. Med.* 153:423–436.

Duke, B. O. L., 1968, Reinfections with *Onchocerca volvulus* in cured patients exposed to continuing transmission, *Bull. W.H.O.* 39:307–309.

Duke, B. O. L., and Moore, P. J., 1968, The contributions of different age groups to the transmission of onchocerciasis in a Cameroon forest village, *Trans. Roy. Soc. Trop. Med. Hyg.* 62:22–28.

Ellner, J. J., Olds, G. R., Kamel, R., Osman, G. S., Kholy, A. E. and Mahmoud, A. A. F., 1980, Suppressor splenic T lymphocytes in human hepatosplenic *Schistosomiasis mansoni*, *J. Immunol.* 125:308–312.

Gemmell, M. A., 1962, Natural and acquired immunity factors interferring with development during the rapid growth phase of *Echinococcus granulosus* in dogs, *Immunology* 5:496–503.

Greenwood, B. M., 1974, Immunosuppression in malaria and trypanosomiasis, in: *Parasites in the Immunized Host* (R. Porter and J. Knight, eds.), Ciba Foundation Symposium 25, Elsevier, Amsterdam, pp. 137–146.

Grove, D. I., and Forbes, I. J., 1979, Immunodepression in bancroftian filariasis, *Trans. Roy. Soc. Trop. Med. Hyg.* 73:23–26.

Grove, D. I., Mahmoud, A. A. F., and Warren, K. S., 1977, Eosinophils and resistance to *Trichinella spiralis*, *J. Exp. Med.* 145:755–759.

Hammerberg, B., and Williams, J. F., 1978, Interaction between *Taenia taeniaeformis* and the complement system, *J. Immunol.* 120:1033–1038.

Haque, A., and Capron, A., 1982, Transplacental transfer of rodent microfilariae induces antigen specific tolerance in rats, *Nature [London]* 299:361–363.

Haque, A., Lefebvre, M. N., Ogilvie, B. M., and Capron, A., 1978, *Dipetalonema viteae* in hamsters: Effect of antiserum or immunization with parasite extracts on production of microfilariae, *Parasitology* 76:61–75.

Haque, A., Joseph, M., Ouaissi, M. A., Capron, M., and Capron, A., 1980a, IgE antibody-mediated cytotoxicity of rat macrophages against microfilaria of *Dipetalonema viteae in vitro*, *Clin. Exp. Immunol.* 40:487–495.

Haque, A., Worms, M. J., Ogilvie, B. M., and Capron, A., 1980b, *Dipetalonema viteae*: Microfilariae production in various mouse strains and in nude mice, *Exp. Parasitol.* 49:398–401.

Haque, A., Ouaissi, A., Joseph, M., Capron, M., and Capron, A., 1981a, IgE antibody in eosinophil- and macrophage-mediated *in vitro* killing of *Dipetalonema viteae* microfilariae, *J. Immunol.* 127:716–725.

Haque, A., Camus, D., Ogilvie, B. M., Capron, M., Bazin, H., and Capron, A., 1981b, *Dipetalonema viteae* infective larvae reach reproductive maturity in rats immunodepressed by prior exposure to *Schistosoma mansoni* or its products and in congenitally athymic rats, *Clin. Exp. Immunol.* 43:1–9.

Harrison, D. J., Carter, C. E., and Colley, D. G., 1979, Immunoaffinity purification of *Schistosoma mansoni* soluble egg antigens, *J. Immunol.* 122:2210–2217.

Herd, R. P., Chappel, R. J., and Biddel, D., 1975, Immunization of dogs against *Echinococcus granulosus* using worm secretory antigens, *Int. J. Parasitol.* 5:395–399.

Higashi, G. I., and Chowdhury, A. B., 1970, *In vitro* adhesion of eosinophils to infective larvae of *Wuchereria bancrofti*, *Immunology* 19:65–83.

Howells, R. E., and Chen, S. N., 1981, *Brugia pahangi*: Feeding and nutrient uptake *in vitro* and *in vivo*, *Exp. Parasitol.* 51:42–58.

Jacqueline, E., Vernes, A., Bout, D., and Biguet, J., 1978, *Trichinella spiralis*: Facteurs immuntaires inhibiteurs de la production de larves: II. Premier analyse *in vitro* des facteurs humeraux et sécrétoires actifs chez les souris, le rat, et la miniporc infestés ou immunizés, *Exp. Parasitol.* 45:42–54.

Jarrett, E. E., and Bazin, H., 1974, Elevation of total serum IgE in rats following helminth parasite infection, *Nature [London]* 251:613–614.

Jarrett, E. E., McKenzie, S., and Bennich, H., 1980, Parasite-induced "non-specific" IgE does not protect against allergic reactions, *Nature* 283:302–304.

Jenkins, S. N., and Wakelin, D., 1977, The source and nature of some functional antigens of *Trichuris muris, Parasitology* 74:153–161.

Jones, V. E., and Ogilvie, B. M., 1971, Protective immunity to *Nippostrongylus brasiliensis:* The sequence of events which expels worms from the rat intestine, *Immunology* 20:549–561.

Jungery, M., and Ogilvie, B. M., 1982, Antibody response to stage-specific *Trichinella spiralis* surface antigens in strong and weak responder mouse strains, *J. Immunol.* 129:839–843.

Khoury, P. B., and Soulsby, E. J. L., 1977, Immune mechanisms to *Ascaris suum* in inbred guinea pigs: I. Passive transfer of immunity by cells or sera, *Immunology* 32:405–411.

Klaver-Wesseling, J. C. M., Vetter, J. C. M., and Schoeman, E. N., 1982, The *in vitro* interaction between several components of the canine immune system and infective larvae of *Ancylostoma caninum, Parasite Immunol.* 4:227–232.

Lichtenberg, F. von, Sher, A., Gibbons, N., and Doughty, B. L., 1976, Eosinophil-enriched inflammatory response to schistosomula in the skin of mice immune to *Schistosoma mansoni, Am. J. Pathol.* 84:479–500.

Ljungstrom, I., 1979, *Trichinella spiralis:* Formation of specific antibodies and modulation of the immune response, Ph.D. thesis, University of Stockholm, Stockholm.

Ljungstrom, I., and Huldt, G., 1977, Effect of experimental trichinosis on unrelated humoral and cell mediated immunity, *Acta Path. Microbiol. Scand. Sect. C* 85:131–141.

Lloyd, S., 1981, Progress in immunization against parasitic helminths, *Parasitology* 83:225–242.

Lloyd, S., and Soulsby, E. J. L., 1978, The role of IgA immunoglobulins in the passive transfer of protection to *Taenia taeniaeformis* in the mouse, *Immunology* 34:939–945.

Mackenzie, C. D., 1980, Eosinophil leucocytes in filarial infections, *Trans. Roy. Soc. Trop. Med. Hyg.* 74(Suppl.):51–58.

Mackenzie, C. D., Jungery, M., Taylor, P. M., and Ogilvie, B. M., 1980, Activation of complement, the induction of antibodies to the surface of nematodes and the effect of these factors and cells on worm survival *in vitro, Eur. J. Immunol.* 10:594–601.

Mahmoud, A. A. F., 1981, Genetics of schistosomiasis, in: *Modern Genetic Concepts and Techniques in the Study of Parasites,* Volume 4 (F. Michal, ed.), Tropical Diseases Research Series. pp. 303–322, Schwabe and Company, Basel, AG.

Mahmoud, A. A. F., Warren, K. S., and Peters, P. A., 1975, A role for the eosinophil in acquired resistance to *Schistosoma mansoni* infection as determined by antieosinophil serum, *J. Exp. Med.* 142:805–813.

Maizels, R. M., Philipp, M., and Ogilvie, B. M., 1982, Molecules on the surface of parasitic nematodes as probes of the immune response in infection, *Immunol. Rev.* 61:109–136.

Majid, A. A., Bushara, H. O., Saad, A. M., Hussein, M. F., Taylor, M. G., Dargie, J. D., Marshall, T. F. de, and Nelson, G. S., 1980, Observations on cattle schistosomiasis in the Sudan, a study in comparative medicine: Part 3: Field testing of an irradiated *S. bovis* vaccine, *Am. J. Trop. Med. Hyg.* 29:452–455.

Mangold, B. L., and Knopf, P. M., 1981, Host protective humoral immune responses to *Schistosoma mansoni* infections in the rat: Kinetics of hyperimmune serum-dependent sensitivity and elimination of schistosomes in a passive transfer system, *Parasitology* 83:559–574.

Mansfield, J. M. (ed.), 1982, *Parasitic Diseases,* Volume 1, *The Immunology,* Marcell Dekker AG, Basel, Switzerland.

Marsden, P. D. (ed.), 1978, Intestinal parasites, *Clin. Gastroenterol.* 7(1).

McLaren, D. J., 1980, *Schistosoma Mansoni: The Host Surface in Relation to Host Immunity,* Tropical Medicine Research Studies Series, Research Studies Press, Chichester.

McLaren, D. J., and Terry, R. J., 1982, The protective role of acquired host antigens during schistosome migration, *Parasite Immunol.* 4:129–148.

McLaren, D. J., Hockley, D. J., Goldring, O. L., and Hammond, B. J., 1978, A freeze fracture study of the developing tegumental outer membrane of *Schistosoma mansoni, Parasitology* 76:327–348.

Miller, T. A., 1967, Transfer of immunity to *Ancylostoma caninum* infection in pups by serum and lymphoid cells, *Immunology* 12:231–241.

Miller, T. A., 1971, Vaccination against the canine hookworm diseases, *Adv. Parasitol.* 9:153–183.

Miller, T. A., 1978, Industrial development and field use of the canine hookworm vaccine, *Adv. Parasitol.* 16:333–342.

Mitchell, G. F., 1979a, Responses to infection with metazoan and protozoan parasites in mice, *Adv. Immunol.* 28:451–511.

Mitchell, G. F., 1979b, Effector cells, molecules and mechanisms in host-protective immunity to parasites, *Immunology* 38:209–223.

Mitchell, G. F., 1980, T cell dependent effects in parasitic infection and disease, in: *Progress in Immunology,* Volume 4 (M. Fougereau and J. Dausset, eds.), Academic Press, New York.

Mitchell, G. F., and Anders, R. F., 1982, Parasite antigens and their immunogenicity in infected hosts, in: *The Antigens,* Volume 6 (M. Sela, ed.), Academic Press, New York.

Mitchell, G. F., Goding, J. W., and Rickard, M. D., 1977, Studies on immune responses to larval cestodes in mice: Increased susceptibility of certain mouse strains and hypothymic mice to *Taenia taeniaeformis* and analysis of passive transfer with serum, *Austr. J. Exp. Biol. Med. Sci.* 55:165–186.

Mitchell, G. F., Rajasekariah, G. R., and Rickard, M. D., 1980, A mechanism to account for mouse strain variation in resistance to the larval cestode, *Taenia taeniaeformis, Immunology* 39: 481–489.

Moqbel, R., 1980, Histopathological changes following primary, secondary and repeated infections of rats with *Strongyloides ratti,* with special reference to tissue eosinophils, *Parasite Immunol.* 2:11–27.

Moser, G., Wassom, D. L., and Sher, A., 1980, Studies of the antibody-dependent killing of schistosomula of *Schistosoma mansoni* employing haptenic target antigens: I. Evidence that the loss in susceptibility to immune damage undergone by developing schistosomula involves a change unrelated to the masking of parasite antigens by host molecules, *J. Exp. Med.* 152: 41–53.

Neilson, J. T. M., 1978, Primary infections of *Dipetalonema viteae* in an outbred and five inbred strains of golden hamsters, *J. Parasitol.* 64:378–380.

Nelson, G. S., 1970, Onchocerciasis, *Adv. Parasitol.* 8:173–224.

Ogilvie, B. M., and Mackenzie, C. D., 1982, Immunology and immunopathology of infections caused by filarial nematodes, in: *Parasitic Diseases,* Volume 1 (J. M. Mansfield, ed.), Marcel Dekker, Basel, pp. 227–290.

Ottesen, E. A., 1979, Modulation of the host response in human schistosomiasis, *J. Immunol.* 123:1639–1644.

Ottesen, E. A., Weller, P. F., and Heck, L., 1977, Specific cellular immune unresponsiveness in human filariasis, *Immunology* 33:413–421.

Ottesen, E. A., Kumaraswami, V., Paranjape, R., Poindexter, R. W., and Tripathy, S. P., 1981, Naturally occurring blocking antibodies modulate immediate hypersensitivity responses in human filariasis, *J. Immunol.* 127:2014–2020.

Parkhouse, R. M. E., Philipp, M., and Ogilvie, B. M., 1981, Characterization of surface antigens of *Trichinella spiralis* infective larvae, *Parasite Immunol.* 3:339–352.

Pawlowski, Z. S., 1978, Ascariasis, *Clin. Gastroenterol.* 7:157–178.

Pelley, R. P., Pelley, J. R., Hamburger, J., Peters, P. A., and Warren, K. S., 1976, *Schistosoma mansoni* soluble egg antigens: I. Identification and purification of three major antigens, and the employment of radioimmunoassay for their further characterization, *J. Immunol.* 117: 1553–1560.

Pery, P., and Luffau, G., 1979, Antigens of helminths, in: *The Antigens,* Volume 5 (M. Sela, ed.), Academic Press, New York.

Pesigan, T. P., Farooq, M., Hairston, H. G., Jauregui, J. J., Garcia, E. G., Santos, A. T., Santos, B. L., and Besa, A. A., 1958, Studies on *Schistosoma japonicum* infection in the Philippines: I. General considerations and epidemiology, *Bull. W.H.O.* 18:345–455.

Peters, W., and Gilles, H. M., 1977, *A Colour Atlas of Tropical Medicine and Parasitology,* Wolfe Medical Publications Ltd., London.

Philipp, M., Parkhouse, R. M. E., and Ogilvie, B. M., 1980, Changing proteins on the surface of a parasitic nematode, *Nature [London]* 237:538–540.

Philipp, M., Worms, M. J., Maizels, R. M., McLaren, D. J., Parkhouse, R. M. E., Taylor, P. M., and Ogilvie, B. M., 1982, A nematode antigen and a host component on the surface of *Litomosoides carinii, Parasitology* 84:xxx–xxxi.

Phillips, R. S., Selby, G. R., and Wakelin, D., 1974, The effect of *Plasmodium berghei* and *Trypanosoma brucei* infections on the immune expulsion of the nematode *Trichuris muris* from mice, *Int. J. Parasitol.* 4:409–415.

Phillips, S. M., Reid, W. A., Bruce, J. I., Hedlund, K., Colvin, R. D., Campbell, R., Diggs, C. L., and Sadun, E. H., 1975, The cellular and humoral immune response to *Schistosoma mansoni* infections in inbred rats: I. Mechanisms during initial exposure, *Cell. Immunol.* 19:99–116.

Phillips, T. M., and Draper, C. C., 1975, Circulating immune complexes in schistosomiasis due to *Schistosoma mansoni, Br. Med. J.* 2:476–477.

Piessens, W. F., McGreevy, P. B., Ratiwayanto, S., McGreevy, M., Piessens, P. W., Koiman, I., Saroso, J. S., and Dennis, D. T., 1980, Immune responses in human infections with *Brugia malayi:* Correlation of cellular and humoral reactions to microfilarial antigens with clinical status, *Am. J. Trop. Med. Hyg.* 29:563–570.

Ponnudurai, T., Denham, D. A., Nelson, G. S., and Rogers, R., 1974, *Brugia pahangi:* Antibodies against adult and microfilarial stages, *J. Helminthol.* 48:107–111.

Purtilo, D. T., Meyers, W. M., and Connor, D. H., 1974, Fatal strongyloidiasis in immunosuppressed patients, *Am. J. Med.* 56:488–493.

Ramalho-Pinto, F. J., McLaren, D. J., and Smithers, S. R., 1978, Complement-mediated killing of schistosomula of *Schistosoma mansoni* by rat eosinophils *in vitro, J. Exp. Med.* 147:147–156.

Rhodes, M. B., Nayak, D. P., Kelley, G. W., and Marsh, C. L., 1965, Studies in helminth enzymology: IV. Immune responses to malic dehydrogenase from *Ascaris suum, Exp. Parasitol.* 16:373–381.

Rocklin, R. E., Brown, A. P., Warren, K. S., Pelley, R. P., Houba, V., Siongok, T. R. A., Ouma, J., Sturrock, R. F., and Butterworth, A. E., 1980, Factors that modify the cellular-immune response in patients infected by *Schistosoma mansoni, J. Immunol.* 125:1916–1923.

Rocklin, R. E., Tracy, J. W., and Kholy, A. E., 1981, Activation of antigen specific suppressor cells in human *Schistosomiasis mansoni* by fractions of soluble egg antigens nonadherent to con A sepharose, *J. Immunol.* 127:2314–2318.

Rothwell, T. L. W., Prichard, R. K., and Love, R. J., 1974, Studies on the role of histamine and 5-hydroxytryptamine on immunity against the nematode *Trichostrongylus colubriformis:* I. *In vivo* and *in vitro* effects of the amines, *Int. Arch. Allergy* 46:1–13.

Rudin, W., Tanner, M., Bauer, P., and Weiss, N., 1980, Studies on *Dipetalonema viteae* (Filarioidea): 5. Ultrastructural aspects of the antibody-dependent cell-mediated destruction of microfilariae, *Tropenmed. Parasitol.* 31:194–200.

Salam, E. A., Ishaac, S., and Mahmoud, A. A. F., 1979, Histocompatibility-linked susceptibility for hepatosplenomegaly in human *Schistosomiasis mansoni, J. Immunol.* 123:1829–1831.

Santoro, F., Bernal, J., and Capron, A., 1979a, Complement activation by parasites: A review, *Acta Tropica* 36:5–14.

Santoro, F., Lachman, P. J., Capron, A., and Capron, M., 1979b, Activation of complement by *Schistosoma mansoni* schistosomula: Killing of parasites by the alternative pathway and requirement of IgG for classical pathway activation, *J. Immunol.* 123:1551–1557.

Selby, G. R., and Wakelin, D., 1973, Transfer of immunity against *Trichuris muris* in the mouse by serum and cells, *Int. J. Parasitol.* 3:717–722.

Selby, G. R., and Wakelin, D., 1975, Suppression of the immune response to *Trichuris muris* in lactating mice, *Parasitology* 71:77–85.

Sher, A., 1977, Immunity against *Schistosoma mansoni* in the mouse, *Am. J. Trop. Med. Hyg.* 26(Suppl.):20–28.

Sher, A., Kusel, J. R., Perez, H., and Clegg, J. A., 1974, Partial isolation of a membrane antigen which induces the formation of antibodies lethal to schistosomes cultured *in vitro*, *Clin. Exp. Immunol.* 18:357–369.

Sher, A., Smithers, S. R., MacKenzie, P., and Broomfield, K., 1977a, *Schistosoma mansoni:* Immunoglobulins involved in passive immunization of laboratory mice, *Exp. Parasitol.* 41:160–166.

Sher, A., McIntyre, S., and von Lichtenberg, F., 1977b, *Schistosoma mansoni:* Kinetics and class specificity of hypergammaglobulinaemia induced during murine infection, *Exp. Parasitol.* 41:415–422.

Sher, A., Hall, B. F., and Vadas, M. A., 1978, Acquisition of murine major histocompatibility complex gene products by schistosomula of *Schistosoma mansoni, J. Exp. Med.* 148:46–50.

Smith, H. V., Quinn, R., Kusel, J. R., and Girdwood, R. W. A., 1981, The effect of temperature and anti-metabolites on antibody binding to the outer surface of second stage *Toxocara canis* larvae, *Mol. Biochem. Parasitol.* 4:183–194.

Smith, M. A., Clegg, J. A., Snary, D., and Trejdosiewicz, A. J., 1982, Passive immunization of mice against *Schistosoma mansoni* with an IgM monoclonal antibody, *Parasitology* 84:83–91.

Smithers, S. R., 1980, Vaccination against schistosomiasis, in: *New Developments with Human and Veterinary Vaccines,* Liss, New York.

Smithers, S. R., and Gammage, K., 1980, Recovery of *Schistosoma mansoni* from the skin, lungs and hepatic portal system of naive mice and mice previously exposed to *S. mansoni:* Evidence for two phases of parasite attrition in immune mice, *Parasitology* 80:289–300.

Smithers, S. R., and Terry, R. J., 1969, Immunity in schistosomiasis, *Ann. N.Y. Acad. Sci.* 160:826–840.

Smithers, S. R., Terry, R. J., and Hockley, D. J., 1969, Host antigens in schistosomiasis, *Proc. Roy. Soc. Biol.* 171:483–494.

Snary, D., Smith, M. A., and Clegg, J. A., 1980, Surface proteins of *Schistosoma mansoni* and their expression during morphogenesis, *Eur. J. Immunol.* 10:573–575.

Spry, C. J. F., Tai, P.-C., and Ogilvie, B. M., 1980, Hypereosinophilia in rats infected with *Trichinella spiralis* infections, *Br. J. Exp. Pathol.* 61:1–7.

Stromberg, B. E., 1979, The isolation and partial characterization of a protective antigen from developing larvae of *Ascaris suum, Int. J. Parasitol.* 9:307–311.

Subrahmanyam, D., Mehta, K., Nelson, D. S., Rao, Y. U. B. G., and Rao, C. U., 1978, Immune reactions in human filariasis, *J. Clin. Microbiol.* 8:228–232.

Taylor, A. E. R., and Muller, R. (eds.), 1980, *Vaccination Against Parasites,* British Society for Parasitology, Symposium 18, Blackwells, Oxford.

Taylor, D. W., and Butterworth, A. E., 1982, Monoclonal antibodies against surface antigens of schistosomula of *Schistosoma mansoni, Parasitology* 84:65–82.

Terry, R. J., 1978, Immunodepression in parasite infections, *Immun. Parasit. Dis. (INSERM., Paris)* 72:161–178.

Thompson, J. P., Crandall, R. B., Crandall, C. A., and Neilson, J. T., 1979, Clearance of micro-filariae of *Dipetalonema viteae* in CBA/N and CBA/H mice, *J. Parasitol.* 65:966–969.

Thorson, R. E., 1956, Proteolytic activity in extracts of the oesophagus of adults of *Ancylostoma caninum* and the effect of immune serum on this activity, *J. Parasitol.* 42:501–504.

Thorson, R. E., 1963, Physiology of immunity to helminth infections, *Exp. Parasitol.* 13:3–12.

Torpier, G., Capron, A., and Ouaissi, M. A., 1979a, Receptor for IgG (Fc) and human β2 micro-globulin on *S. mansoni* schistosomula, *Nature [London]* 278:447–449.

Torpier, G., Ouaissi, M. A., and Capron, A., 1979b, Freeze-fracture study of immune induced *Schistosoma mansoni* membrane alterations: I. Complement dependent damage in the presence of antisera to host determinants, *J. Ultrastruct. Res.* 67:276–287.

Turner, K. J., Quinn, E. H., and Anderson, H. R., 1978, Regulation of asthma by intestinal parasites: Investigation of possible mechanisms, *Immunology* 35:281–288.

Urquhart, G. M., 1980, Application of immunity in the control of parasitic disease, *Vet. Parasitol.* 6:217–239.

Vadas, M. A., 1982, Genetic control of eosinophilia in mice: Genes expressed in bone marrow-derived cells control high responsiveness, *J. Immunol.* 128:691–695.

Wakelin, D., 1975, Immune expulsion of *Trichuris muris* from mice during a primary infection: Analysis of the components involved, *Parasitology* 70:397–405.

Wakelin, D., 1978a, Immunity to intestinal parasites, *Nature [London]* 273:617–620.

Wakelin, D., 1978b, Genetic control of susceptibility and resistance to parasitic infection, *Adv. Parasitol.* 16:219–308.

Wakelin, D., 1980, Genetic control of immunity to parasites: Infection with *Trichinella spiralis* in inbred and congenic mice showing rapid and slow responses to infection, *Parasite Immunol.* 2:85–98.

Wakelin, D., and Donachie, A. M., 1981, Genetic control of immunity to *Trichinella spiralis:* Donor bone marrow cells determine responses to infection in mouse radiation chimaeras, *Immunology* 43:787–792.

Wakelin, D., and Donachie, A. M., 1983, Genetic control of eosinophilia: Mouse strain variation in response to antigens of parasite origin, *Clin. Exp. Immunol.* 51:239–246.

Warren, K. S., 1973, The pathology of schistosome infections, *Helminth. Abstr.* 42:591–633.

Warren, K. S., 1977, Modulation of immunopathology and disease in schistosomiasis, *Am. J. Trop. Med. Hyg.* 26(Suppl.):113–119.

Weiss, N., and Tanner, M., 1979, Studies on *Dipetalonema viteae* (Filaroidea): 3. Antibody-dependent cell mediated destruction of microfalariae *in vivo. Tropenmed. Parasitol.* 30:73–80.

Wong, M. M., 1964, Studies in microfilaraemia in dogs: II. Levels of microfilaraemia in relation to immunologic responses of the host, *Am. J. Trop. Med. Hyg.* 13:66–77.

9

Structured Vaccines for Control of Fertility and Communicable Diseases

G. P. Talwar

In most tropical countries, a major problem is the alarming rate at which population is growing. It is estimated that the world population will increase from about 4 billion in 1980 to a little above 6 billion at the close of this century (i.e., in 20 years there will be half again as many people on the surface of the earth as had accumulated over the entire previous history of humanity). Of this increase, 90% will occur in the developing countries.

It is interesting to note that with the introduction of immunoprophylaxis and general health services, infant mortality has dropped and life expectancy risen in many countries. Figure 1, an illustrative example of this trend, is from India's census figures. The population growth rate has shown a decline over the years, but the slopes of the two curves are not parallel. The net result is an intensification of the problem. The need for aligning family planning programs with communicable disease control programs is obvious.

Given that population increase has assumed epidemic dimensions, it can be argued that the means employed in the past for combating epidemics of infectious diseases so effectively may also be serviceable for slowing the rate of population growth. Vaccines were the miraculous agents. They are cost-effec-

G. P. Talwar • National Institute of Immunology and Department of Biochemistry, All India Institute of Medical Sciences, New Delhi 110029, India. This article was written during a term as scholar in residence at the John E. Fogarty International Center for Advanced Study in Health Sciences, National Institutes of Health, Bethesda, Maryland 20205.

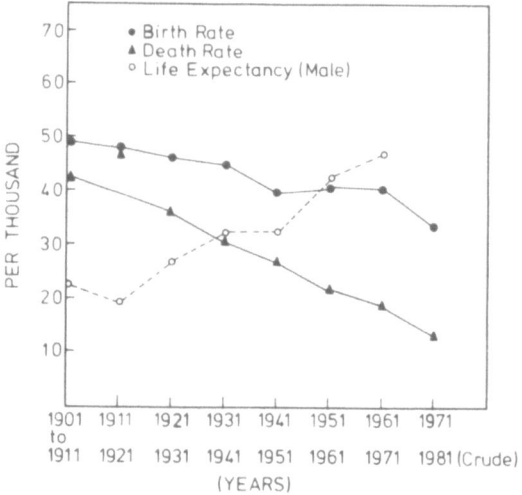

Figure 1.   Census figures on birthrate, death rate, and life expectancy as recorded in India during the past eight decades of the century.

tive. They are amenable to use on a mass scale. They require periodic intake and can be administered by paramedical personnel, obviating the requirement for highly trained personnel. These traits render them particularly suitable to the conditions prevailing in the developing countries. Can vaccines be developed for the control of fertility?

1. FEASIBILITY

Over the past 30 years, a number of clinical cases have been reported in the literature (for review, see Talwar, 1980) in which infertility can be traced to immunological factors. Antibodies that reacted with sperm, egg, or reproductive hormones were observed to be present in these patients in the circulation and or in the genital tract. The manner in which sensitization occurred in these cases is not known. However, these examples of "Nature's experiments" provide concrete examples of the feasibility of immunointerception of fertility.

It is possible to immunize animals experimentally against reproductive tract antigens. The first experiments of this sort were, in fact, carried out independently by two pioneers, Landsteiner and Metchinikoff, and published in 1899. Since then, and more particularly in the last two decades, a number of papers have appeared demonstrating the blocking of fertility in animals, including subhuman primates, after immunization with appropriate reproductive system antigens.

2. ANTIFERTILITY VACCINES

The rationale of these vaccines is to mobilize the body's intrinsic immune system to counteract a hormone or protein critical to the success of reproduction. Mammalian reproduction results from the union of two different gametes, the sperm contributed by the male and the egg by the female of the species. The gametes are produced by the respective gonads under the influence of two gonadotrophic hormones, FSH (follicle-stimulating hormone) and LH (luteinizing hormone). The gonadotropins also stimulate the production of the sex steroid hormones, which play a role in the maturation of the gametes and regulate the metabolic activities of the accessory reproductive organs in a manner essential to reproduction. The gonadotropins are released from the pituitary under the control of another hormone, the gonadotropin-releasing hormone Gn-RH, commonly denoted as LH-RH (luteinizing hormone releasing hormone). Antibodies inactivating the bioactivity of any of these hormones would interfere with fertility. Besides these precursor hormones, vulnerable antigens are also located on gametes. Antibodies against appropriate sperm constituents can agglutinate and immobilize the sperm, resulting in their nonavailability for fertilization. Antibodies against the egg surface antigens, say the zona pellucida glycoproteins, can prevent the binding of the sperm to the egg and thus exercise a prefertilization block. The early embryo carries a number of "stage specific" proteins that disappear with development. Some of these are also present in teratomas and cancers and are referred to as oncofetal antigens. The implanting blastocyst makes and secretes human chorionic gonadotropin (hCG), which has a crucial role in sustaining early pregnancy. It is thus apparent that there are numerous points at which reproduction can be intercepted and that a number of antifertility vaccines are theoretically possible. In this chapter, discussion will be confined to those vaccines that have advanced significantly in the development process.

2.1. The Anti-hCG Vaccine

This is the first and the only vaccine that has reached the stage of early phase I clinical trials so far. The principle of the vaccine is to induce the formation of antibodies reacting with hCG and rendering it biologically inactive. It is believed that hCG is required to sustain the ovarian corpus luteum and maintain the production of progesterone, failing which the uterus will not be receptive to pregnancy and the endometrium will be shed, as in the normal menstrual cycle. Two groups of investigators whose approaches differ in many fundamental respects have been active in developing the anti-hCG vaccines. One group uses the beta subunit of the hormone (Talwar *et al.*, 1976a), and the other a 37 amino acid carboxy-terminal peptide (CTP) of this subunit (Stevens *et al.*,

1981a,b). The modes by which this "self" protein is rendered immunogenic are also different. Our group chose to utilize a carrier, tetanus toxoid, whereas Stevens and co-workers initially advocated haptenic modification of the protein (Stevens, 1976) but have subsequently opted for the carrier approach.

hCG is a glycoproteinic hormone composed of two subunits, alpha and beta. The alpha subunit is common to three other pituitary hormones, the TSH, LH, and FSH. The beta subunit confers in each case the hormonal individuality to these hormones. β-hCG is a glycopeptide of 145 amino acids (Figure 2). It has 12 half cystines but no free SH. The half cystines are thus linked to each other in 6 intrachain S-S bonds. The conformations created by S-S linkages are of paramount importance. When they are opened out, the hormone loses its biological properties and can no longer recognize the receptor on the target organ (Ramak-

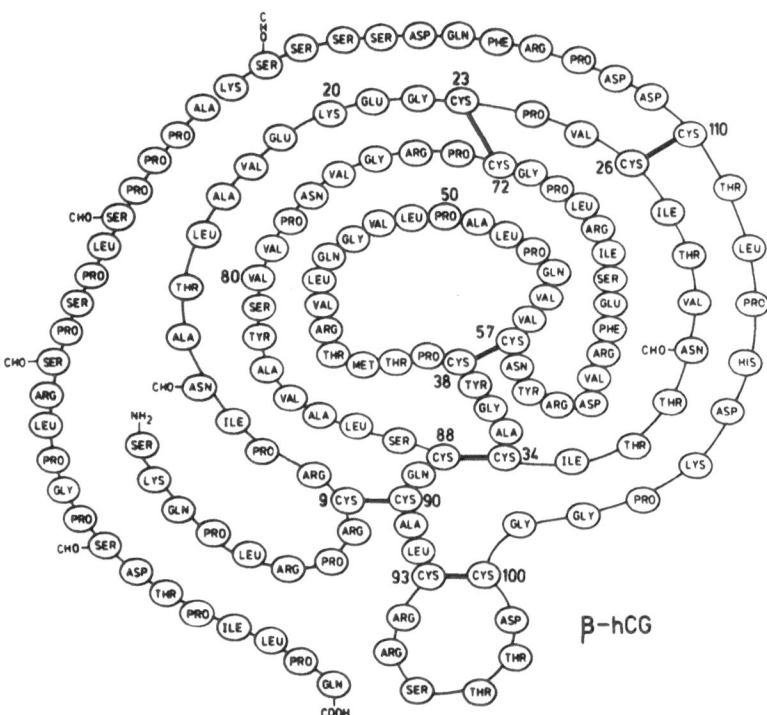

Figure 2. Primary structure of the β-subunit of hCG. It is a glycopeptide of 145 amino acids, in contrast to β-hLH which has 115 amino acids; the carboxy-terminal 30 amino acids constitute the extra piece. This portion is rich in carbohydrates, with four 0-serine residues probably contributing to the longer half-life of hCG in circulation. The 12 half cystines are linked to each other by S-S bonds, the probable position of which are shown in the figure. The carboxy-terminal unique portion has no cystine. The conformations created by S-S linkages are important for biological activity of the native hormone and for the immunodominant epitopes.

rishnan, Das, and Talwar, 1978a). β-hCG and β-hLH have large amino acid homologies, a structural reason why they have very similar biological properties. There are, however, also differences between the beta subunits of the two hormones in 51 amino acid units, 30 of which are located in the CTP portion of the β-hCG molecule. The uniqueness of the 30 amino acid sequence at the CTP end of the molecule makes it an obvious choice as an antigen, since it should not elicit antibodies that cross-react with LH. There are, however, some disadvantages in this choice, as will be evident from the following discussion.

2.1.1. The Immunodominant Epitopes in β-hCG

When an animal is immunized against the native hormone or the non-denatured β-subunit of hCG, the antibodies generated are almost invariably directed against the core part of the molecule and not against the CTP. Of over 500 sera raised in our laboratory, only 2 could be demonstrated to bind with CTP, and that at a low level. The immunodominant epitopes of β-hCG thus reside in the core part of the molecule and not at the CTP end. They are essentially conformational rather than sequential determinants.

The immunogenicity of chemically synthesized CTP and hence its ability to induce anti-hCG antibodies is poor (Ramakrishnan and Talwar, 1980; Chen, Matsuura, and Ohashi, 1980; Birken et al., 1980). Enzymically cleaved peptides with intact carbohydrate residues are better immunogens (Birken et al., 1982). Lengthening of the peptide beyond the 30 amino acid strand unique to β-hCG improves immunogenicity and the neutralization capacity of the antibodies. The 45 amino acid fragment linked to tetanus toxoid as carrier was a better immunogen in rhesus monkeys than the 30 and 35 amino acids peptides (Ramakrishnan, et al., 1979). The antibodies had, however, low affinity when generated against this or other CTP peptides, a finding that others have also observed and reported (Powell et al., 1980; Chen et al., 1980). The association constants Ka of sera raised against the CTPs was of the order of 10^9 M^{-1} in contrast to the values of 10^{10} to 10^{11} M^{-1} usually obtained for sera raised to the beta subunit of hCG (Shastri, et al., 1978). This has an important bearing on the ability of these antibodies to counteract the bioactivity of hCG (Thanavala et al., 1979).

Sera have been raised to the CTPs by (1) linking them with an immunogenic carrier and (2) using a potent adjuvant. Previous studies in rabbits, monkeys, and baboons were carried out by immunization along with Freund's complete adjuvant. All animals immunized did not produce desirable titers of antibodies; for example, Chen et al. (1980) obtained 1 out of 45 rabbits that had a titer of 2 × 10^4. Our own experience in rhesus monkeys is similar (Ramakrishnan et al., 1979). However, Stevens et al. (1981a) have obtained antibodies in mice and rabbits to modified 35 and 37 amino acid peptides coupled to tetanus toxoid and administered with an MDP-derivative in an emulsion containing squalene and water stabilized with Arlacel A. The modification was the introduction of six prolines as a spacer at the N-terminal end of the peptide.

The antigenic sites in the unique carboxy-terminal β-hCG peptide have been mapped to some extent. Two loci, Pro^{144}-Gln^{145}, at the terminus exercise cooperative antigenicity with Arg-Leu-Pro-Gly (residues 133–136) of the β-hCG molecule (Matsuura, Chen, and Hodgen, 1978). This is the main epitope in the CTP portion. Suggestive evidence is also available for an additional antigenic site between 111 and 115. It is, however, not clear whether this site is accessible in the intact hCG. The sedimentation constants of antibody–hCG complexes formed by sera raised against the 45 amino acid CTP indicated at an average of one binding site on the hormone for these antibodies, in contrast to polyvalent attachment of sera raised against the beta subunit of hCG (Ramakrishnan and Talwar, 1980). Lengthening of the CTP by another 8 amino acids opens out perhaps an additional site. Antibodies raised against 53 amino acid CTP have improved bioneutralization capacity (Sahal et al., 1982). The widely utilized NIH serum SB_6 binds only weakly to the 53 CTP, and not at all to the 30 and 35 CTP.

2.1.2. Bioactivity of the Anti-β-hCG and Anti-CTP Antibodies

For fertility regulation, it is imperative that the antibodies produced by the eventual vaccine be competent to neutralize the bioactivity of hCG. The antibodies generated by the vaccine Pr-β-hCG-TT in monkeys and baboons blocked hCG activity in both in vitro and in vivo assays of such factors as uterine weight gain, ventral prostate weight gain, production of testosterone by Leydig cells, and so on (Das et al., 1976). Immunization with β-hCG conferred protection against pregnancy in baboons (Stevens, 1976; Talwar et al., 1980). Marmosets immunized with β-hCG were rendered infertile during the time period when antibody titers were appreciable (Hearn, 1979). A clear demonstration of the ability of the antibodies generated by the vaccine Pr-β-hCG-TT to intercept pregnancy in a subhuman primate species, the baboon, is provided by the experiments of Tandon et al. (1981). Antibodies given to baboons at the time when chorionic gonadotropin (CG) was in circulation reduced both CG activity and progesterone levels, followed by termination of the pregnancy. There is thus evidence from several sources that antibodies against the total β-subunit of hCG are capable of suppressing fertility in more than one species of subhuman primate, as well as in rats (Hulme et al., 1980).

There is less evidence for the effectiveness of the CTPs in controlling fertility. We were unable to obtain protection in baboons after immunization with carboxy-terminal 30, 35, and 45 amino acid peptides conjugated to an otherwise immunogenic carrier, the tetanus toxoid. Louvet et al. (1974) immunized rabbits with a CTP consisting of residues 123 to 145. Although antibodies reacting with

hCG in radioimmunoassays were obtained, these were devoid of hCG neutralization potential. Similar observations were made with the synthetic peptide 116 to
145, the 30 amino acid β-hCG unique peptide. The antibodies had neutralization
potential *in vitro* but not *in vivo* (Ohashi, Matsuura, Chen, and Hodgen, 1980).
This was attributed to the dissociation of the hCG-antibody complexes owing to
the antibody having about 50 times lower affinity for hCG than is the case with
antibodies induced by β-hCG for hCG. According to these investigators, the
association constant of anti-CTP antibodies for hCG was apparently 20 times
lower than that of hCG-gonadal receptor. Our experience is similar. Figure 3
illustrates an experiment in which antibodies from two animals immunized
against the 45 CTP and β-hCG-TT respectively were mixed with ^{125}I-hCG and
the mixture run on a sucrose density gradient. In the case of the β-hCG-TT
antibodies, the entire radioactivity associated with hCG migrated with a sedimentation constant of about 17 S, and hCG was totally scavenged as a firm

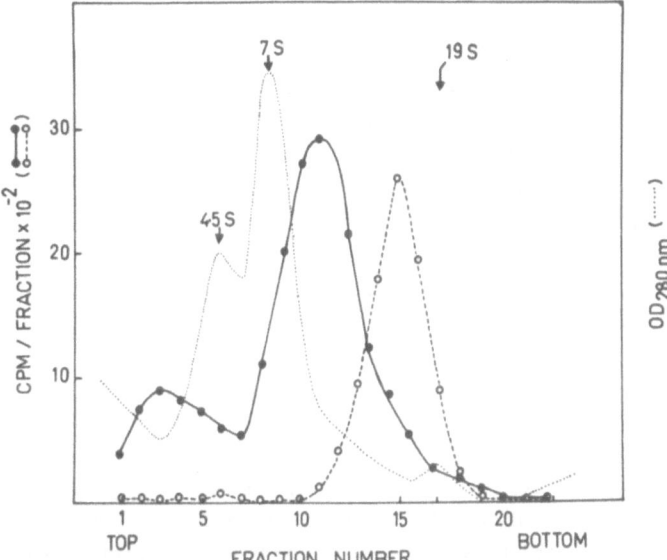

Figure 3. Relative ability of anti-carboxy-terminal peptide and anti β-hCG antibodies to bind
tightly hCG. The two types of antisera were incubated with radioiodinated hCG for 4 hr at room
temperature followed by 17 hr at 4°C. The mixture was then centrifuged on a sucrose density gradient
(5–40%) for 18 hr at 105,000 g. The migration of radioactivity (due to ^{125}I-hCG) is plotted for the
two antibody-hCG mixtures. O----O (anti-Pr-β-hCG-TT + ^{125}I-hCG): note the absence of free ^{125}I-
hCG, the hormone is almost completely bound by antibodies and the complex has a sedimentation
constant of about 17 S; the sedimentation constant of the complex for anti-45 CTP serum and hCG is
about 10 S (●——●); there is, in addition, a peak of radioactivity corresponding to the position of
free dissociated hCG. The continuous dotted line gives the location of marker proteins as determined
by recording of absorbance at 280 nm. (Data from Ramakrishnan *et al.*, 1979.)

complex with the antibodies. With anti-45 CTP sera however, not only was the hCG antibody complex of a lower sedimentation constant but there was also a peak of radioactivity due to free hCG. This had dissociated from the complex owing to largely univalent binding and lower association constants.

The fact that anti-CTP sera have comparatively low association constants for hCG is a common observation of the four laboratories that have worked in this area. The importance of association constants to antifertility effectiveness is illustrated by the findings of Thanavala et al. (1979), who investigated the characteristics of antibodies in β-hCG-immunized marmosets that were either protected or became pregnant. A major difference between the two types of animals was in the association constants of the antibodies. A marmoset having antibodies with Ka of 1.8×10^9 M^{-1} became pregnant, in spite of the fact that it had relatively high antibody titer, whereas marmosets with antibodies having K-a between 9×10^9 and 3.5×10^{10} M^{-1} remained infertile. The same investigators, using essentially the same methodology, have examined sera from rabbits immunized with the terminal 37 amino acid peptide. The affinity constant of antibodies in these animals was between 1 to 4.5×10^9 M (Thanavala, Hay, and Stevens, 1980). This is below the protection limits as judged from observations in marmosets. The fertility was not tested in the animals immunized with the peptide. The investigators, however, reported the ovulation inhibition capability of the sera in rodents. The procedure employed was the prior incubation in vitro of hCG with the sera for an extended period before injection of the complex instead of injecting both the hormone and the antibody in vivo at different sites. It is not clear whether the assay system used would have permitted the titration of a fraction of free hCG had it dissociated from the complex. Usually, CTPs of a greater length can engender bioneutralizing antibodies even though the capacity is low (Ramakrishnan et al., 1979; Chang et al., 1981).

Stevens et al. (1981a) have reported the blocking of fertility in baboons after immunization with the 37 amino acid peptide (109–145) conjugated to a carrier. Out of 42 matings, 4 resulted in pregnancy in the immunized group, whereas 15 became pregnant from 21 matings in the control group. Immunization was carried out with Freund's complete adjuvant. The mean peak titer of antibiodies was 185 moles liter $\times 10^{-10}$ for binding with hCG. The affinity constants of the antibodies are not given. The baboon chorionic gonadotropin has usually 1–10% cross-reaction with anti-hCG antibodies. These findings have yet to be confirmed.

Specificity. The anti-CTP sera are no doubt specific for hCG and devoid of cross-reaction with hLH. They therefore have a special advantage for assays, where a high discrimination is required. Chen, Matsuura, and Ohashi (1980) have discussed the merits and limitations of the hCG-specific antisera generated by the CTP.

Immunization with immunochemically purified β-hCG gives antibodies of high affinity and reactivity with the native hormone hCG. There is cross-reaction with hLH, but it is low and is not material at the tonic and surge levels of hLH encountered in women (Salahuddin *et al.*, 1976). The antibodies had five to tenfold higher affinity for hCG than for hLH (Shastri *et al.*, 1978). The antibodies reacted preferentially with hCG and inhibited hCG-induced ovulation in mice; however, the LH-induced ovulation was not affected (Das *et al.*, 1978). Similar discriminatory action of antibodies was observed on hCG/hLH-induced production of progesterone by the granulosa cells in culture (Mohini *et al.*, 1978). Monkeys immunized with Pr-β-hCG-TT failed to show an increase in progesterone levels on administration of hCG in the late luteal phase of the cycle, whereas hLH action was manifest in such situations (Ramakrishnan *et al.*, 1978a,b). In every laboratory that has worked with β-hCG, the animals immunized (baboons, marmosets, rhesus monkeys, rodents) have continued to ovulate in spite of the anti-hCG antibodies in circulation. It can always be argued that these antibodies may have no cross-reaction with the LH of the species. However, the same observations have been made in women immunized with Pr-β-hCG-TT (Kumar *et al.*, 1976; Hingorani and Kumar, 1979; Shahani *et al.*, 1979; Nash *et al.*, 1980). There was no disturbance in ovulation or menstrual cyclicity. Metabolic and organ functions were not affected.

Fear regarding the effects of immunization with β-hCG on the pituitary pathology has been expressed. This is apparently based on an observed immunofluorescence reaction of baboon serum with pituitary (Thanavala *et al.*, 1978). However, this observation conflicts with considerable other experience. None of the sera raised by us with Pr-β-hCG-TT in rhesus monkeys, baboons, or women reacted with pituitary or other organs (Gupta, Nath, and Talwar, 1978). Several of these sera were examined independently by experts in other well-known centers of immunopathology and a similar conclusion was reached. Autopsy of monkeys hyperimmunized with Pr-β-hCG-TT did not give any evidence of immunopathological lesions (Nath *et al.*, 1976; Gupta *et al.*, 1978). Even when monkeys were immunized with β-ovine LH, which produces frankly cross-reacting antibodies with endogenous LH, no pituitary pathology was observed. These monkeys had received repeated booster shots of β-OLH with Fruend's incomplete adjuvant over several years (Thau *et al.*, unpublished data). Interestingly, Thanavala *et al.* (1979) have subsequently reported the lack of cross-reaction between antisera raised in marmosets against β-hCG and human luteinizing hormone as tested by indirect immunofluorescence on adult human pituitary sections.

2.1.3. Advantages of Cross-Reaction with LH for Control of Fertility

Cross-reaction with hLH and its possible undesirable effects has been a main concern when using β-hCG as an antigen. There have, however, been no concrete data demonstrating the validity of this view. The published data discount any side effects. Every other point is in favor of the total β subunit: it is decidedly more immunogenic than the CTPs; the antibodies generated have high affinity and better reactivity with hCG; the neutralization capacity is distinctly better and demonstrable both *in vivo* and *in vitro;* the antifertility properties have been tested and confirmed by active and or passive approaches in at least three animal species by more than one group of investigators. On the other hand, the CTPs are comparatively poor immunogens, and they generate low-affinity antibodies. Their main advantage is the lack of cross-reactivity with hLH.

An interesting development of recent years is likely to change the entire perception of this issue. A degree of cross-reaction with endogenous LH may, in fact, be beneficial and contributory to the antifertility properties of the antibodies. Eight years back, colleagues at the Population Council immunized rhesus monkeys with beta subunit of ovine LH. The purpose was twofold: (1) to see whether antibodies reactive with the species gonadotropin can indeed prevent fertility and (2) to evaluate the side effects of the antibodies cross-reactive with pituitary LH. β-OLH induced antibodies reactive with rhesus pituitary LH as well as with rhesus chorionic gonadotropin. Infertility was produced in the immunized animals, especially when the antibody titers were >30% (Sundaram *et al.,* 1976; Yamamoto *et al.,* 1982). Effective anti-OLH-β titers did not interfere with ovulation and regular menstrual cycles. The partial cross-reaction of antibodies with the monkey pituitary LH resulted in some shortening of the cycle and in impaired production of progesterone during the luteal phase (Thau *et al.,* 1979; Thau and Sundaram, 1980). This effect, together with the ability of these antibodies to neutralize rhesus chorionic gonadotropin, was apparently responsible for infertility. The shortened luteal phase with high FSH and impaired folliculogenesis may be a dominant factor (Thau *et al.,* 1983). Extensive toxicology studies in these monkeys have not revealed any significant ill effects of heterologous immunization.

3. STRUCTURED VACCINES

3.1. Concept of Linkage with Carriers

hCG, a "self" protein in the female, is produced in large amounts during pregnancy. The female immune system is normally tolerant to it and would not be expected to produce antibodies following injection of the hormone or its subunit. Immunogenicity might be introduced by modifying the molecule either by attaching haptenic groups or by linking it to an immunogenic "carrier" protein. Linkage to tetanus toxoid was proposed for this purpose (Talwar *et al.,* 1976a,b). The choice of this carrier was based on several considerations. Tetanus is still a widespread health hazard in the developing countries, where all births do not take place in hospitals and all children do not receive DPT immunization. Booster immunization is in any case well tolerated and invariably desirable in case of injury. The toxin is among the more purified bacterial proteins in use as a vaccine. It has been administered to millions of humans with advantage and the incidence of hypersensitivity has been low. The protein induces both cell-mediated and humoral immunity. The immune response is of reasonably long duration but reversible.

The vaccine was designed by linking immunochemically purified β-subunit of hCG with tetanus toxoid in discrete molecular proportions (Talwar *et al.* (1976b). This "structured" conjugate was immunogenic in all species of animals tested. It produced antibodies against *both* hCG and tetanus, conferring a double benefit (Talwar *et al.*, 1976a). It overcomes the immunological tolerance in humans, and 61 out of 63 women studied in phase I clinical trials with this vaccine formed anti-hCG and antitetanus antibodies. Figure 4 illustrates the kinetics of the immune response in one of the subjects. The antibodies were of

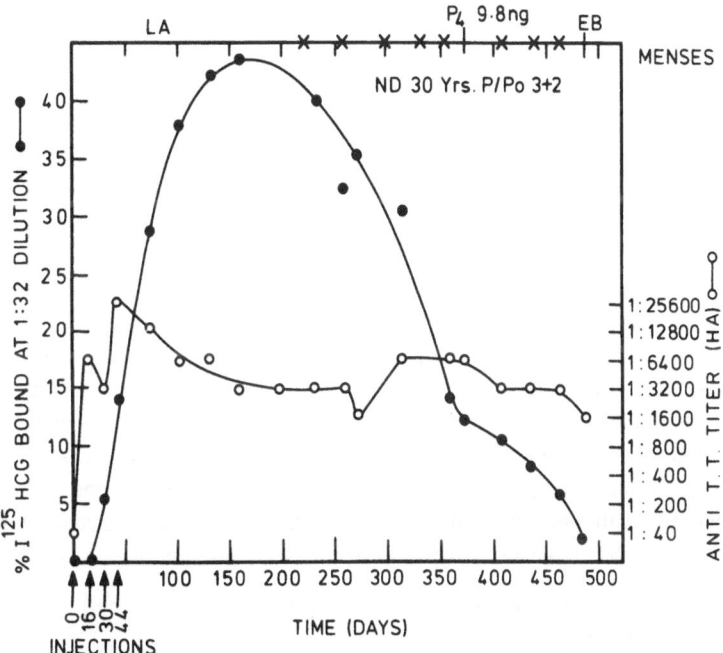

Figure 4. Induction of antibodies to both hCG and tetanus toxoid (TT) following immunization with Pr-β-hCG-TT. The subject was a 30-year-old female, who had five pregnancies. She received four injections I.M. of the vaccine containing 80 μg β-hCG and 10 LF TT at fortnightly intervals. The kinetics of the antibody to hCG and TT are given. Anti-hCG titers declined to near zero levels after 500 days. LA on upper abscissa denotes the period of lactational amenorrhea. X indicates the days of menstruation, P_4 is progesterone in luteal phase.

high affinity and able to neutralize hCG as tested by a variety of *in vitro* and *in vivo* assays. The experience from these trials and the current status of this vaccine is described later in this chapter.

The enhanced immunogenicity conferred by conjugation with tetanus even in animals where β-hCG is antigenic has been confirmed by other investigators. Hulme, Fehilly, and Hearn (1980) immunized female rats with β-hCG-TT to produce, without the use of Freund's complete adjuvant, a high and effective antibody response. Stevens *et al.* (1981a) tested a number of carriers of bacterial origin as well as synthetic polypeptides and confirmed the superiority of tetanus and diptheria toxoids as carriers. β-hCG is a "foreign" protein in rodents; in order to evaluate whether linkage with this carrier as opposed to others indeed gives a better response for isoimmunization, Shastri, Manhar, and Talwar (1981) carried out experiments with decapeptide LH-RH. LH-RH has an essentially conserved structure and is a "self" protein in mice as well as humans. Linkage of LH-RH to tetanus toxoid gave far better response than the conjugates with the conventionally used carrier, bovine serum albumin or keyhole limpet hemocyanin.

3.2. Adjuvant Conjugation

Another mode employed to increase antigenicity is the linkage of the hormone to the adjuvant muramyl dipeptide (MDP). MDP was identified by Lederer *et al.* as the minimal structure responsible for the adjuvant property on the mycobacterial cell wall (review Lederer, 1980). A conjugate has been prepared by linking LH-RH through the free carboxyl group at position 10 with lysine-MDP. This conjugate is reported to induce the formation of high antibody titers against LH-RH, which render male rodents infertile (Carelli *et al.*, 1982).

"*Structured*" vaccines have thus been created by essentially two approaches, one in which a carrier is attached to the desired antigen and the other in which the candidate antigen is linked to an adjuvant such as MDP. The former, if properly designed, can help elicit antibody response against both moieties; if the carrier has immunoprophylactic potential, the combination has the potential of dual benefit. Although this principle was utilized in developing a vaccine against the pregnancy hormone hCG, the concept may be broadly useful in

1. Eliciting antibody response to any "self" protein or cellular constituents, be it a hormone or otherwise.
2. Developing polyvalent vaccines against communicable diseases, since the linkage may improve the immunogenicity of each partner.

A novel feature of the presently developed structured vaccines is that they are directed against an endogenous process and not only against an exogenous pathogen.

4. EXPERIENCE WITH Pr-β-hCG-TT VACCINE

The first prototype vaccine consisted of 80 μg of β-hCG linked to 10LF of column-purified tetanus toxoid (Talwar *et al.*, 1976a). As shown by Figure 4, it elicited the formation of both anti-hCG and antitetanus antibodies not only in test animals but also in women. The response was reversible; the duration varied, but in subjects forming antibodies of fairly good titers, it lasted between 300 and 500 days, after which antibodies declined to nearly zero level. The aims of the phase I clinical trials conducted in six centers located in five countries were (1) to determine whether the structured conjugate is indeed immunogenic in women; (2) to investigate whether this mode of immunization against a "self" hormone leads to a permanent antibody response with an internal buildup; (3) to determine the side effects, if any, on metabolic endocrine and organ function; and (4) to identify immunological aberrations, if any, such as the formation of autoimmune antibodies, unacceptable hypersensitivity, and so on. The protocol envisaged study in women of reproductive age of proven fertility who had opted for tubal ligation after completion of their planned families. In some centers, the ethics committee permitted the postponement of tubal surgery on the understanding that condoms would be employed during the latent period for induction and building up of antibodies. The subjects were examined clinically and a battery of 56 tests was performed at periodic intervals to assess various parameters. The results from all centers have now been published (Kumar *et al.*, 1976; Hingorani and Kumar, 1979; Shahani *et al.*, 1979; 1982; Nash *et al.*, 1980). The results show that the conjugate was immunogenic and that 61 of 63 women formed both anti-hCG and antitetanus antibodies. It may be mentioned that the study was not large enough to permit the testing of different doses and immunization schedules. In each recipient, the antibodies eventually declined to near-zero levels. Administration of hCG did not cause a booster response, even though antibodies recognized the hormone and formed biologically inactive complexes. The women reported their libido to be normal, and menstrual cyclicity was maintained. The hormonal profiles were essentially normal. No significant disturbances in metabolic or organ functions were noticeable. There was no evidence of formation of autoantibodies or of immunological aberrations. Some nontubectomized women became pregnant, but pregnancy in each case occurred at a time when the antibody titers were very low. In most of such cases, the regime of immunization was not completed. The pregnancies were terminated, but the subjects volunteered to complete the course. In some cases the completion of the immunization schedule led to the formation of high antibody titers lasting for several months thereafter. These cases were unprotected and reported pregnancy only when the titers had declined again to low levels. The phase I clinical trials did not have the formal objective of investigating efficacy, but experience on a rather limited number of such cases has furnished valuable information on the levels of anti-

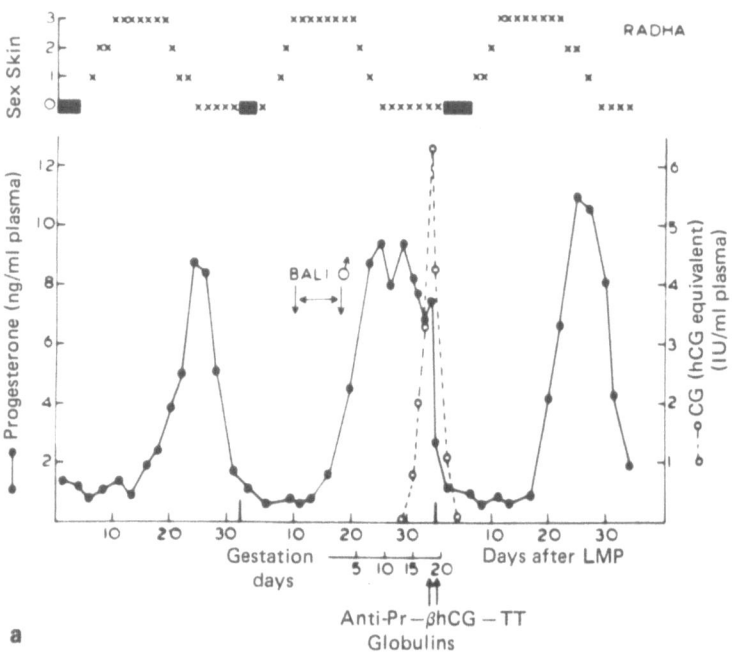

a

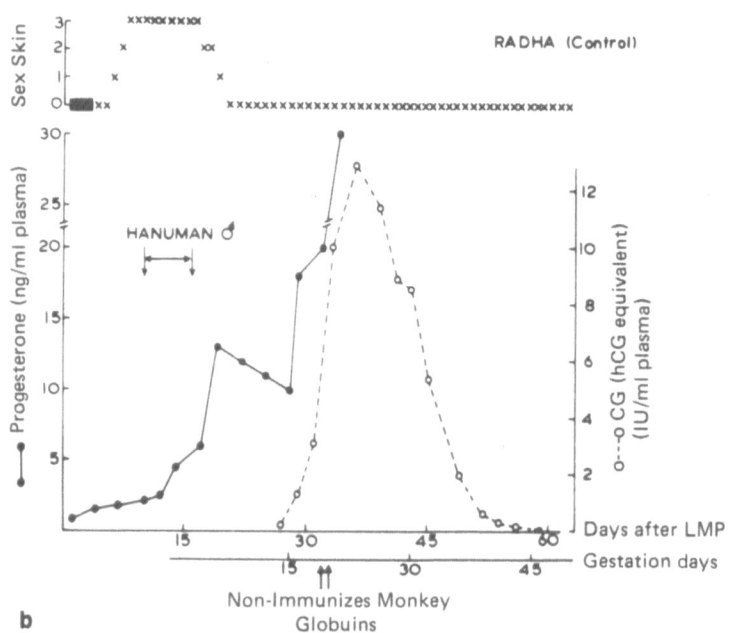

b

body titers insufficient for protection. It is also apparent that antibodies do decline to near zero levels and that, at this time, women can conceive and engender normal progeny.

4.1. Efficacy

A pertinent question relates to on the efficacy of the antibodies produced by the Pr-β-hCG-TT vaccine. Active immunization of marmosets and baboons with β-hCG has been shown by several investigators to protect these animals against pregnancy (references cited above). Lest the conjugation with tetanus toxoid should alter β-hCG in a detrimental manner, efficacy studies were carried out with the β-hCG-TT conjugate (Talwar *et al.*, 1980) and independently by Hulme, Fehilly, and Hearn (1980) with positive results. More stringent evidence for efficacy is provided by passive immunization experiments. Rhesus monkeys were immunized with Pr-β-hCG-TT and globulins fractionated from sera. Sera from control monkeys injected with only the vehicle and adjuvant were processed in a similar manner. Baboons were mated and, at a time when pregnancy was confirmed by appearance in circulation of chorionic gonadotropin, the animals were injected with globulins from either the Pr-β-hCG-TT immunized or control animals. Figure 5 gives typical results obtained. Administration of antibodies caused a drop in chorionic gonadotropin and progesterone, which was followed by termination of pregnancy. Figure 5b presents the results with control animal globulins. They did not exercise any noxious action on continuation of pregnancy. Data is given on the animal, in which pregnancy was terminated in a previous cycle by anti Pr-β-hCG-TT antibodies. Her ability to conceive in a subsequent cycle and carry pregnancy to full term points to the reversibility of the procedure and lack of residual side effects. The offspring from such animals have been normal and have shown normal developmental landmarks.

4.2. Limitations of Pr-β-hCG-TT

Figure 6 is a summary of data from 16 representative subjects studied in phase I clinical trials. What is obvious is the variability of titers; some elicit good

---

Figure 5.   (a) Termination of pregnancy in a baboon with anti-Pr-β-hCG-TT antibodies. Pregnancy was confirmed by the appearance in the circulation of chorionic gonadotropin when antibodies were administered (two injections at 24 hr intervals). The decline in chorionic gonadotropin and progesterone was followed by bleeding and termination of pregnancy. The animal returned to normal cyclicity. The figure shows the progesterone profiles; estrogenic activity is indicated by the sex skin swelling. (b) In a subsequent cycle, the baboon whose pregnancy was terminated by anti-hCG antibodies was mated again and became pregnant. Globulins from a normal non-hCG-immunized monkey were given on a schedule similar to that shown in Figure 5a. These failed to interrupt the pregnancy. (Data from Tandon *et al.*, 1981.)

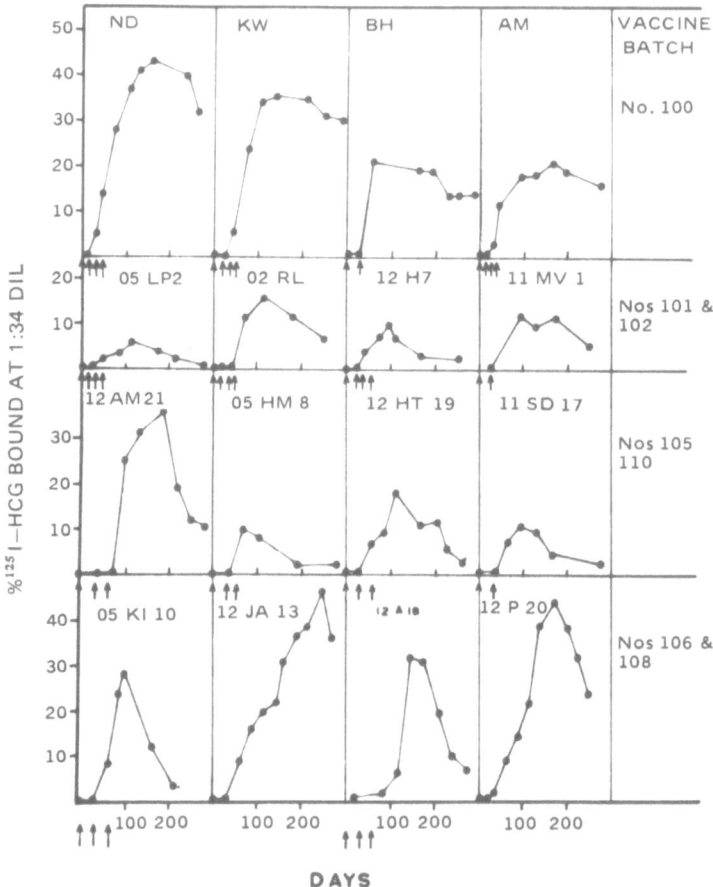

Figure 6.   Variability of antibody titers in women immunized with Pr-β-hCG-TT. The figure gives representative data on 16 women studied during phase I clinical trials.

antibody response; others, moderate; and still others, low antibody titers. As antibody is the intercepting agent, pregnancy will not be prevented unless it is present in adequate amounts. Variability may not be a feature limited to this vaccine. The response to other proteinic vaccines used for immunoprophylaxis is not observed to be equal in all human recipients. In community-based immunoprophylaxis, however, every individual may not get the infection; if a fair percentage are protected, the benefit of vaccination is perceptible. The antifertility vaccines, on the other hand, are likely to be primarily employed by those who have had the desired number of children and are thus of proven fertility. They will be exposed to pregnancy in the event that interception is not effective.

Monitoring of antibody titers can no doubt identify the subjects at risk, but again, this facility may not be readily available everywhere, especially in the remote areas of developing countries where the population problem is acute. It will therefore be necessary to improve the formulation to overcome these shortcomings. Adjuvants may have to be incorporated to raise the general threshold of antibody titers and ways and means found to minimize individual nonresponsiveness.

4.3. Immunopotentiation by Adjuvants

Freund's complete adjuvant (FCA) has been used traditionally to attain high antibody titers in experimental animals. It produces severe granulomas and one of its components, the mineral oil, was observed to be carcinogenic in Balb/c mice when administered intraperitoneally. FCA is therefore not appropriate for use in humans. Many research and industrial laboratories have been actively engaged in developing alternative immunopotentiating agents. The lipopolysaccharides (LPS) from gram-negative bacterial cell walls are potent adjuvants, but they have other toxic effects. The toxicity can be minimized by using derivatives of LPS, and sodium pthalyl and/or succinyl derivative of LPS have greatly reduced toxicity with retention of adjuvant properties. These derivatives, however, remain somewhat pyrogenic and would not be the first choice in a formulation. Ribi has recently prepared a detoxified preparation that is nonpyrogenic and also potent in its adjuvant action (Ribi *et al.*, 1982). Ayme *et al.* (1980) obtained a nontoxic lipid A from *Bordetella pertussis*. These have recently been evaluated and found to be good adjuvants for this task. Lederer (1980) obtained two fractions, the cord factor and a glycopeptide, the MDP from mycobacterial cell walls. Both have adjuvant properties. MDP itself is pyrogenic, but a large number of MDP derivatives have been prepared with the object of eliminating or suppressing to a great extent the pyrogenicity and toxicity while retaining the adjuvant property. The Institute Pasteur group led by Chedid are proceeding with a nontoxic derivative of MDP, murabutide, that is apparently on clinical trials with tetanus toxoid (personal communication). Among the compounds that we and the Population Council scientists have investigated, MDP-A$_1$ and MDP-A$_5$ (which is N-acetyl nor muramyl-L-alanine-D-isoglutamine) are the most suitable in the series. BCG is an excellent adjuvant, but it can probably be utilized only once.

For secondary immunization, a totally nontoxic lipidic emulsion of soya phosphatides, glycerine, and lecithin (manufactured by Leiras, a Finnish company) was found eminently suitable. Figure 7 is an example of the type of response that can be generated with these adjuvants in subhuman primates. The vaccine was LHRH-TT; LHRH is a "self" decapeptide in the species and so would not normally elicit an antigen response. Conjugation with tetanus toxoid

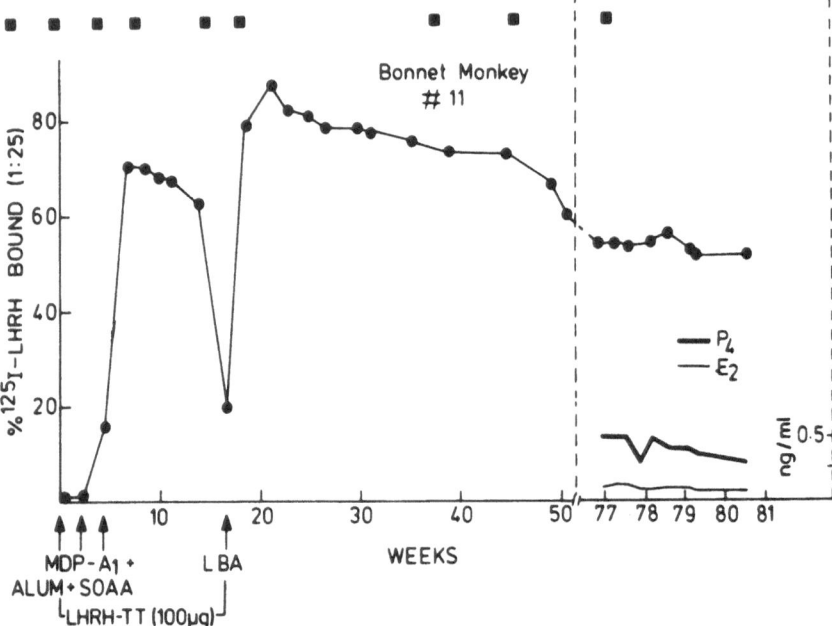

Figure 7. Induction of long-term biologically effective antibody response in a bonnet monkey immunized with LH-RH-TT. Primary immunization of three injections was carried out using alum, MDP-A emulsified with sesame oil, and Arlacel A. Booster immunization was done with a nontoxic metabolizable emulsion, the Leiras basic adjuvant (LBA), which gave rise to high antibody titers sustained to biologically efficacious levels for over 60 weeks. The solid squares along the upper abscissa are the menstrual cycles. P_4 (progesterone) and E_2 (estradiol) levels remained depressed with block of pituitary gonadotropins. (Data from Talwar *et al.*, 1983c.)

overcomes the tolerance. This mode of immunization without recourse to FCA produced a long-lasting high-antibody response with biological efficacy and control of fertility.

4.4. The Problem of Constitutional Variability

From studies in mice and guinea pigs, the role of genetics·in immune response is clearly apparent. One of the ways to overcome constitutional variability and ensure response in the overwhelming number of eventual users may be to offer a mixed or polyvalent vaccine instead of a vaccine directed against a single hormone or protein. The existence of several sites vulnerable to immunological control in the reproductive system has been pointed out above and elsewhere (Talwar, 1980).

5. IMMUNOCONTRACEPTION WITH PREFORMED ANTIBODIES

If antibodies are indeed effective agents in inactivating a critical hormone or masking an important site to prevent conception, it should be possible to use preformed antibodies for this purpose. The advantage would be the elimination of the uncertainty inherent in active immunization and the variable antibody response associated with it. The preformed antibody could be selected for its specificity (or desired cross-reactivity), affinity, subclass, and other traits. It could be utilized in amounts large enough to ensure efficacy in every case.

A major requirement for the passive immunization approach would be the production in unlimited amounts of antibody with the desired characteristics. The recent introduction and perfection of hybridoma technology has made this possible. A number of clones making antibodies against various reproductive tract antigens have been developed, and the ability of individual or mixed monoclonals to block fertility has been demonstrated (Talwar *et al.*, 1983b, 1984).

Passive use of antibodies has inherent advantages and disadvantages. The effect is short-lived, since it depends on the half-life of antibodies in circulation. This characteristic could be employed with advantage for finite events, for example, for the termination of pregnancy. The effect of conventional polyclonal antibodies against hCG has been described above. Clones making anti-hCG antibodies of high affinity and specificity have also been generated (Gupta and Talwar, 1980); see Figure 8. They have the capability of neutralization of hCG bioactivity. Highly sensitive and simple kits for the diagnosis of very early pregnancy and hCG synthesizing tumors have also been developed (Talwar *et al.*, 1983a). Pregnancy can be terminated in baboons and mice (Table I) by monoclonals reacting against LH-RH (Talwar *et al.*, 1983b, 1984). LH-RH is observed to be present in placenta, and it has been suggested that its stimulation leads to the secretion of hCG (Silver-Khodr and Khodr, 1978, 1979). Passive use of appropriate antibodies can in principle, provide a new surgical method for the termination of early pregnancy. Anti–LH-RH monoclonals can also be useful for the suppression of estrus in female dogs Figure 9 (Talwar *et al.*, 1983b, 1984).

It is interesting to note that some antibodies, such as those against the zona pellucida, become firmly attached to the target structure. Thus a single injection of anti-zona pellucida antibodies renders mice infertile for six to eight cycles. Studies in progress in monkeys also support long-term effects on fertility accruing from a single injection of the antibody. This is a situation where a passive approach, with all its advantages, attains also the advantages of an active immunization approach in terms of the duration of the effect. Dr. Isojima in Japan, our laboratory, and perhaps others have developed a number of stabilized clones against porcine zona pellucida that are cross-reactive with the human zona.

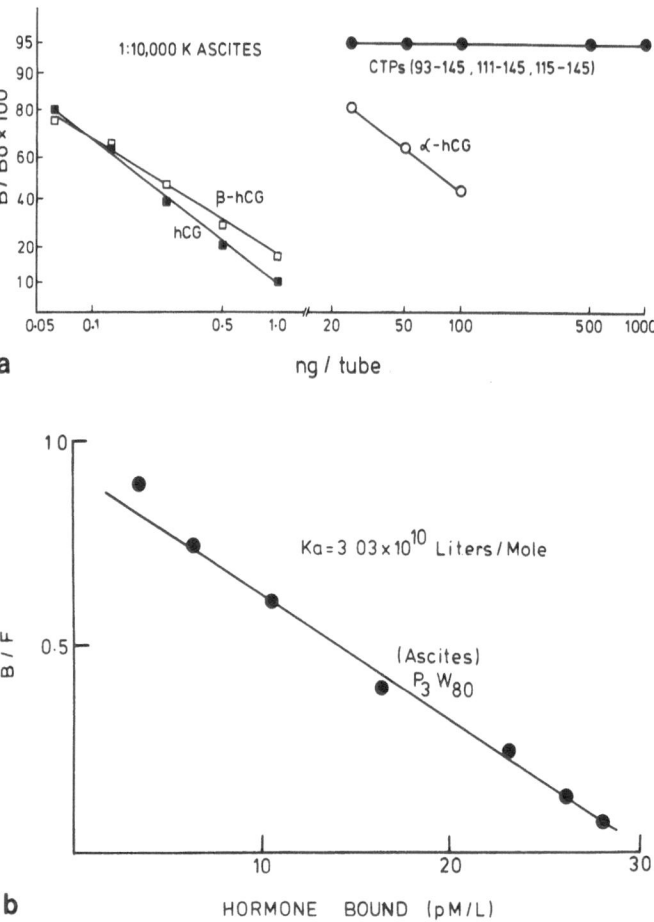

Figure 8. Recognition characteristics (8a) and affinity (8b) of the products of the clone P_3W_{80}. The antibody bound hCG and the β-subunit of hCG best; the binding to α-hCG was substantially lower. CTP, of β-hCG of 31, 35, and 53 amino acid units were not bound at all. The Ka of the antibody was 3.03×10^{10} M.$^{-1}$

Table I

Effect of Monoclonal Anti-LH-RH on Pregnancy in Mice

Group	Treatment	No. of animals	Implantation sites (mean ± S.E.)
I	Control	10	6.5 ± 0.2
II	Anti-LH-RH	15	0
			Partially resorbed 2 mice, mean = 6

[a]0.1 ml of ascites or saline was given I.P. on day 7 of pregnancy.

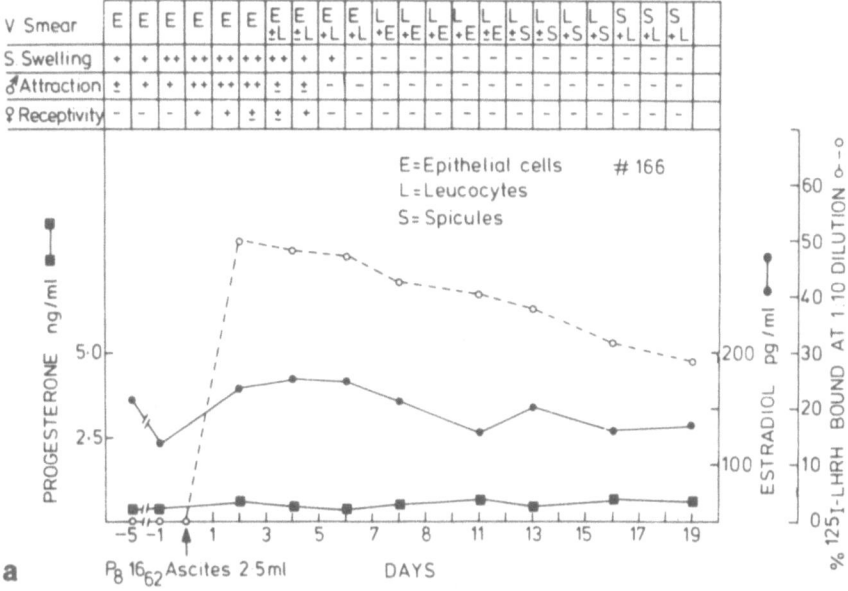

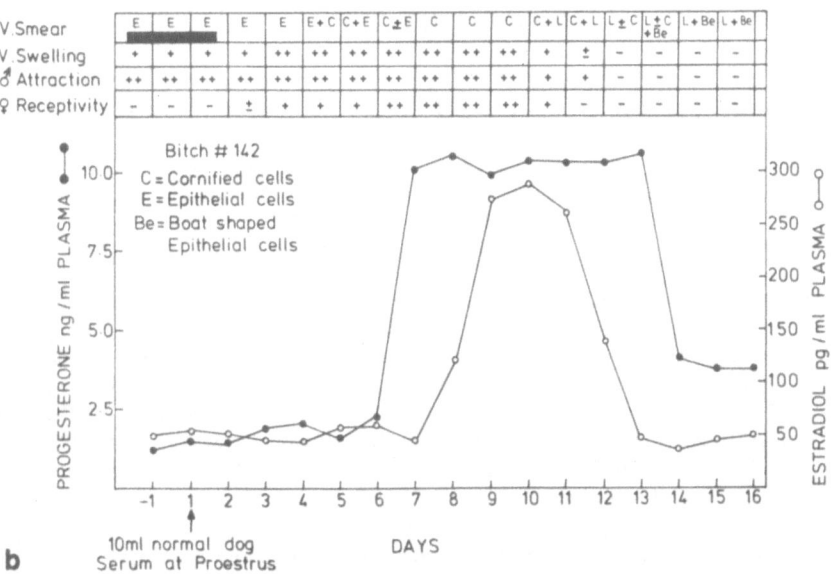

Figure 9. (a) Suppression of estrus in a female dog with monoclonal anti-LH-RH antibody. 2.5 ml of the ascites fluid of the clone $P_8 16_{82}$ was given as a single injection. The dotted line shows the antibody levels in blood on various days following injection. (b) A control that received 10 ml of normal dog serum instead of the anti-LH-RH antibody.

The monoclonals developed so far against the reproductive tract antigens are primarily derived from mouse cell lines. Their repeated use in other species may be contraindicated due to possible sensitization against mouse immunoglobulins. This may, however, be avoidable. Recent observations in cancer patients indicate that the mouse monoclonals, when given intravenously in an appropriate regimen, tolerize the immunological response against heterospecific globulins (Koprowski, 1983). Attempts are nonetheless being made in many laboratories to develop the human hybridomas. In both cases, the risk of forming anti-idiotype antibodies remains, and its consequences require careful study.

ACKNOWLEDGMENT. I would like to express my thanks to Dr. Harold Nash for going through the manuscript and making valuable suggestions.

REFERENCES

Ayme, G., Caroff, M., Chaby, R., Haeffner-Cavaillon, N., Le Duv, A., Moreau, M., Muset, M., Mynard, M. C., Roumiantzeff, M., Schulz, D., and Szabo, L., 1980, Biological activities of fragments derived from *Bordetella pertussis* endotoxin: Isolation of a nontoxic Shwartzman-negative lipid A possessing high adjuvant properties, *Infect. Immun.* 27:739.

Birken, S., Canfield, R. E., Laurer, R., Agosto, G., and Gabel, M., 1980, Immunochemical determinants unique to human chorionic gonadotropin: Importance of sialic acid for anti-sera generated to the human chorionic gonadotropin β-subunit COOH-terminal peptide, *Endocrinology* 106:1659.

Birken, S., Canfield, R., Agosto, G., and Lewis, J., 1982, Preparation and characterization of an improved β carboxyl terminal immunogen for generation of specific and sensitive antisera to human chorionic gonadotropin, *Endocrinology* 110:1555.

Carelli, C., Audibert, F., Gaillard, J., and Chedid, L., 1982, Immunological castration of male mice by a totally synthetic vaccine administered in saline, *Proc. Nat. Acad. Sci. U.S.A.* 79:5392.

Chang, C., Tsong, Y., Rone, J. D., Segal, S. J., Chang, D., Leban, J., and Folkers, K., 1981, A synthetic peptide capable of eliciting antibodies that neutralize human chorionic gonadotropin, *Fertil. Steril.* 36:659.

Chen, H.-C., Matsuura, S., and Ohashi, M., 1980, Limitations and problems of hCG-specific antisera, in: *Chorionic Gonadotropin* (S. J. Segal, ed.), Plenum Press, New York, p. 231.

Das, C., Salahuddin, M., and Talwar, G. P., 1976, Investigations on the ability of antisera produced by Pr-β-hCG-TT to neutralize the biological activity of hCG, *Contraception* 13:71.

Das, C., Talwar, G. P., Ramakrishnan, S., Salahuddin, M., Kumar, S., Hingorani, V., Coutinho, E., Croxatto, H., Hemmingson, E., Johansson, E., Luukainen, T., Shahani, S., Sundaram, K., Nash, H., and Segal, S. J., 1978, Discriminatory effect of anti Pr-βhCG-TT antibodies on the neutralization of the biological activity of placental and pituitary gonadotropins, *Contraception* 18:35.

Gupta, P. D., Nath, I., and Talwar, G. P., 1978, Immunofluorescence and electron microscopic studies on kidney, choroid plexus and pituitary in rhesus monkeys immunized with the Anti-hCG-TT, *Contraception* 18:91.

Gupta, S. K., and Talwar, G. P., 1980, Development of hybridomas secreting anti-human chorionic gonadotropin antibodies, *Ind. J. Exp. Biol.* 18:361.

Hearn, J. P., 1979, Long term suppression of fertility by immunization with hCG-β and its reversibility in female marmoset monkeys, in: *Recent Advances in Reproduction and Regulation of Fertility* (G. P. Talwar, ed.), Elsevier/North Holland, Amsterdam, p. 427.

Hingorani, V., and Kumar, S., 1979, Anti-hCG immunization—Phase I clinical trials, in: *Recent Advances in Reproduction and Regulation of Fertility* (G. P. Talwar, ed.), Elsevier/North Holland, Amsterdam, p. 467.

Hulme, M. J., Fehilly, C. B., and Hearn, J. P., 1980, The immune response to hCG-β subunit in rats and the effects of active immunization on their fertility, *J. Reprod. Immunol.* 1:329.

Koprowski, H., 1983, Monoclonal antibodies *in vivo*, *Proceedings of the A. Hammer Symposium* (R. Dulbecco, ed.) (in press).

Kumar, S., Sharma, N. C., Bajaj, J. S., Talwar, G. P., and Hingorani, V., 1976, Clinical profile and toxicology studies on four women immunized with Pr-β-hCG-TT, *Contraception* 13:253.

Landsteiner, K., 1899, *Cbl. Bakt.* 25:546.

Lederer, E., 1980, Synthetic immunostimulants derived from the bacterial cell wall, *J. Med. Chem.* 23:819.

Louvet, J. P., Ross, G. T., Birken, S., and Canfield, R. E., 1974, Absence of neutralizing effect of antisera to the unique structural region of human chorionic gonadotropin, *J. Clin. Endocrinol. Metab.* 39:1155.

Matsuura, S., Chen, H. C., and Hodgen, G. D., 1978, Antibodies to the carboxyl-terminal fragment of human chorionic gonadotropin β-subunits characterization of antibody recognition sites using synthetic peptide analogues, *Biochemistry* 17:575.

Metchnikoff, E., 1899, *Ann. Inst. Pasteur* 13:737.

Mohini, P., Chapekar, T. N., Raj, A. B., Shastri, N., Dubey, S. K., and Talwar, G. P., 1978, Differences between the discriminatory activity of antisera raised against the total gonadotropins and the Pr-β-hCG-TT for neutralization of hCG and LH action, *Contraception* 18:59.

Nash, H., Talwar, G. P., Segal, S., Luukainen, T., Johansson, E. D. B., Vasquez, J., Coutinho, E., and Sundaram, K., 1980, Observations on the antigenicity and clinical effects of a candidate antipregnancy vaccine: β-subunit of human chorionic gonadotropin linked to tetanus toxoid, *Fertil. Steril.* 34:328.

Nath, I., Gupta, P. D., Bhuyan, V. N., and Talwar, G. P., 1976, Autopsy report on rhesus monkeys immunized with Pr-β-hCG-TT vaccine, *Contraception* 13:213.

Ohashi, M., Matsuura, S., Chen, H. C., and Hodgen, G. D., 1980, Comparison of *in vivo* and *in vitro* neutralization of human chorionic gonadotropin activities by antisera to hCG and a carboxy-terminal fragment of the β-subunit, *Endocrinology* 107:2034.

Powell, J. E., Lee, A. C., Tregear, G. F., Niall, G. D., and Stevens, V. C., 1980, Characteristics of antibodies raised to carboxy-terminal peptides of hCG-β-subunit, *J. Reprod. Immunol.* 2:1.

Ramakrishnan, S., Das, C., and Talwar, G. P., 1978a, Recognition of the β-subunit of human chorionic gonadotropin and subdeterminants by target tissue receptors, *Biochem. J.* 176:599.

Ramakrishnan, S., Das, C., and Talwar, G. P. 1978b, Progesterone levels in monkeys immunized with Pr-β-hCG-TT after injection of hLH and hCG during luteal phase, *Contraception* 18:51.

Ramakrishnan, S., Das, C., Dubey, S. K., Salahuddin, M., and Talwar, G. P., 1979, Immunogenicity of three C-terminal synthetic peptide of the β-subunit of human chorionic gonadotropin and properties of the antibodies raised against 45 amino acid C-terminal peptide, *J. Reprod. Immunol.* 1:249.

Ramakrishnan, S., and Talwar, G. P., 1980, Immunobiological studies with β-subunit of human chorionic gonadotropin and its subfragments, in: *Chorionic Gonadotropin* (S. J. Segal, ed.), Plenum Press, New York, p. 213.

Ribi, E., Amano, K., Cantrell, J., Schwartzman, S., Parker, R., and Takayama, K., 1982, Preparation and antitumour activity of nontoxic lipid A, *Cancer Immunol. Immunother.* 12:91.

Sahal, D., Ramakrishnan, S., Iyer, K. S. N., Das, C., and Talwar, G. P., 1982, Immunobiological characteristics of carboxy-terminal-53-amino acid peptide of β-subunit of human chorionic gonadotropin, *J. Reprod. Immunol.* 4:145.

Salahuddin, M., Ramakrishnan, S., Dubey, S. K., and Talwar, G. P., 1976, Immunological reactivity of antibodies produced by Pr-β-hCG-TT with different hormones, *Contraception* 13:163.

Shahani, S. M., Kulkarni, P. P., and Patel, K. L., 1979, in: *Recent Advances in Reproduction and Regulation of Fertility* (G. P. Talwar, ed.), Elsevier/North Holland, Amsterdam, p. 473.

Shahani, S. M., Kulkarni, P. P., Patel, K. L., Salahuddin, M., Das, C., and Talwar, G. P., 1982, Clinical and immunological responses with Pr-β-hCG-TT vaccine, *Contraception* 25:421.

Shastri, N., Dubey, S. K., Vijaya Reghvan, S., Salahuddin, M. and Talwar, G. P., 1978, Differential affinity of anti-Pr-β-hCG-TT antibodies for hCG and hLH, *Contraception* 18:23.

Shastri, N., Manhar, S. K., and Talwar, G. P., 1981, Important role of the carrier in the induction of antibody response without Freund's complete adjuvant against a ''self'' peptide luteinizing hormone release hormone (LHRH), *Am. J. Reprod. Immunol.* 1:262.

Silver-Khodr, T. M., and Khodr, G. S., 1979, Extra hypothalamic luteinizing hormone-releasing factor (LRF): Release of immunoreactive LRF *in vitro*, *Fertil. Steril.* 32:294.

Silver-Khodr, T. M., and Khodr, G. S., 1981, Dose response analysis of GnRH stimulation of hCG release from human term placenta, *Biol. Reprod.* 25:353.

Stevens, V. C., 1976, Perspectives of development of a fertility control vaccine from hormonal antigens of the trophoblast, in: *Development of Vaccines for Fertility Regulation*, Scriptor, Copenhagen.

Stevens, V. C., Cinader, B., Powell, J. E., Lee, A. E., and Koh, S. W., 1981a, Preparation and formulation of a human chorionic gonadotropin antifertility vaccine: Selection of a peptide immunogen; selection of adjuvant and vehicle, *Am. J. Reprod. Immunol.* 1:307, 314.

Stevens, V. C., Powell, J. E., Lee, A. C., and Griffin, D., 1981b, Antifertility effects of immunization of female baboons with C-terminal peptides of the β-subunit of human chorionic gonadotropin, *Fertil. Steril.* 36:98.

Sundaram, K., Change, C. C., Laurence, K. A., Brinson, A. O., Atkinson, L. E., Segal, S. J., and Ward, D. N., 1976, The effectiveness of rhesus monkeys of an antifertility vaccine based on neutralization of chorionic gonadotropin, *Contraception* 14:639.

Talwar, G. P., 1980, *Immunology of Contraception*, Edward Arnold, London.

Talwar, G. P., Sharma, N. C., Dubey, S. K., Salahuddin, M., Das, C., Ramakrishnan, S., Kumar, S., and Hingorani, V., 1976a, Isoimmunization against human chorionic gonadotropin with conjugates of processed β-subunit of the hormone and tetanus toxoid, *Proc. Nat. Acad. Sci. U.S.A.* 73:218.

Talwar, G. P., Dubey, S. K., Salahuddin, M., and Shastri, N. 1976b, Kinetics of antibody response in animals injected with processed β-subunit conjugated to hCG, *Contraception* 13:153.

Talwar, G. P., Das, C., Tandon, A., Sharma, M. G., Salahuddin, M., and Dubey, S. K., 1980, in: *Non-Human Primate Models for Study of Human Reproduction* (T. C. Anand Kumar, ed.), S. Karger, Basel, Switzerland, p. 190.

Talwar, G. P., Gaur, A., Singh, A. K., and Gupta, S. K., 1983a, Two simple and sensitive methods for detection of pregnancy and hCG synthesizing tumours amenable to both qualitative and quantitative assays, *Ind. J. Med. Res.* 77:231.

Talwar, G. P., Gupta, S. K., Singh, O., Singh, V., and Das, C., 1983b, New approaches for contraceptive vaccine, in: *Advances in Immunopharmacology* (J. Hadden, P. Mullen, L. Chedid, and F. Spreafico, eds.), Pergamon Press, New York, pp. 415–420.

Talwar, G. P., Singh, V., Singh, O., Das, C., Gupta, S. K., and Singh, G., 1984, Pituitary and extrapituitary sites of action of LHRH-potential uses of active and passive immunization against LHRH, in: *Hormone Receptors in Growth and Reproduction* (B. B. Saxena, K. J. Catt, L. Birmhauma, and L. Martini, eds.), Raven Press, New York, pp. 351–359.

Tandon, A., Das, C., Jailkhani, B. L., and Talwar, G. P., 1981, Efficacy of antibodies generated by Pr-β-hCG-TT to terminate pregnancy in baboons: Its reversibility and rescue by medroxyprogesterone acetate, *Contraception* 24:83.

Thanavala, Y. M., Hay, F. C., and Stevens, V. C., 1978, Immunological control of fertility: Measurement of affinity of antibody to human chorionic gonadotropin, *Clin. Exp. Immunol.* 33:403.

Thanavala, Y. M., Hearn, J. P., Hay, F. C., and Hulme, M., 1979, Characterization of the immunological response in marmoset monkeys immunized against hCG β-subunit and its relationship with their subsequent fertility, *J. Reprod. Immunol.* 1:263.

Thanavala, Y. M., Hay, F. C., and Stevens, V. C., 1980, Affinity, cross-reactivity and biological effectiveness of rabbit antibodies against a 37 amino acid C-terminal of human chorionic gonadotropin, *Clin. Exp. Immunol.* 39:112.

Thau, R. B., and Sundaram, K., 1980, The mechanism of action of an antifertility vaccine in the rhesus monkey: Reversal of the effects of the antisera to the β subunit of ovine luteinizing hormone by medroxyprogesterone acetate, *Fertil. Steril.* 33:317.

Thau, R. B., Sundaram, K., Thornton, Y. S., and Seidman, L. S., 1979, Effects of immunization with the β subunit of ovine luteinizing hormone on corpus luteum function in the rhesus monkey, *Fertil. Steril.* 31:200.

Thau, R. B., Yamamoto, Y., Sundaram, K., and Spinola, P. G., 1983, Human chorionic gonadotropin stimulates luteal function in rhesus monkeys immunized against the β-subunit of ovine luteinizing hormone, *Endocrinology* 112:277.

Yamamoto, Y., Gunsalus, G. L., Sundaram, K., and Thau, R. B., 1982, Characterization of anti OLH-β antibodies acting as contraceptives in rhesus monkeys, *J. Reprod. Immunol.* 4:295.

Index